Craniometry and Biological Distance

Biocultural Continuity and Change at the Late-Woodland–Mississippian Interface

Center for American Archeology

DAVID L. ASCH, EDITOR

At Northwestern University
2000 Sheridan Road
Evanston, Illinois 60201

Research Series

Judith Droessler. Craniometry and Biological Distance: Biocultural Continuity and Change at the Late-Woodland–Mississippian Interface

Christopher Carr. Handbook on Soil Resistivity Surveying: Interpretation of Data from Earthen Archeological Sites

Kampsville Archeological Seminars

Robert Whallon and James A. Brown. (Editors). Essays on Archaeological Typology

Distributor of Research Volumes for Northwestern University Archeological Program

David L. Asch. The Middle Woodland Population of the Lower Illinois Valley: A Study in Paleodemographic Methods

Jane E. Buikstra. Hopewell in the Lower Illinois Valley: A Regional Approach to the Study of Human Biological Variability and Prehistoric Behavior

Jane E. Buikstra (Editor). Prehistoric Tuberculosis in the Americas

Thomas Genn Cook. Koster: An Artifact Analysis of Two Archaic Phases in Westcentral Illinois

Lynn Gail Goldstein. Mississippian Mortuary Practices: A Case Study of Two Cemeteries in the Lower Illinois Valley

John Winfield Rick. Heat-Altered Cherts of the Lower Illinois Valley: An Experimental Study in Prehistoric Technology

Bonnie Whatley Styles. Faunal Exploitation and Resource Selection: Early Late Woodland Subsistence in the Lower Illinois Valley

Craniometry and Biological Distance

Biocultural Continuity and Change at the Late-Woodland–Mississippian Interface

JUDITH DROESSLER
Texas A&M University

CENTER FOR AMERICAN ARCHEOLOGY
At Northwestern University
Evanston, Illinois

Center for American Archeology
Research Series, Volume 1

CENTER FOR AMERICAN ARCHEOLOGY
At Northwestern University
Evanston, Illinois 60201

Library of Congress Cataloging in Publication Data

Droessler, Judith B. (Date)

Craniometry and biological distance.

(Research series / Center for American Archeology at Northwestern University; 1)
Bibliography: p.
Includes index.
1. Indians of North America—Illinois—Anthropometry. 2. Woodland Indians—Anthropometry. 3. Mississippian culture. 4. Craniology—Illinois. I. Title. II. Series: Research series (Center for American Archeology at Northwestern University) (Evanston, Ill.); 1
[DNLM: 1. Anthropology, Physical—United States. 2. Craniometry. 3. Archaeology—United States. GN 75.A2 D783c]
E78.I3D76 977.3'00497 81-11009
AACR2

PRINTED IN THE UNITED STATES OF AMERICA

TO MY PARENTS

Contents

Center for American Archeology xi
Preface xv

1

The Problem

Introduction 1
Statement of the Problem 4

2

Archeological Background

Late Woodland 9
Mississippian 19
The Late-Woodland–Mississippian Interface 25

3

Material

The Study Series 33
Sex and Age Determination 44
Demography 47

4

Methods

Craniometrics as a Basis for Biological Distance Estimates 55
Measurement Techniques 67
Statistical Procedures 74
Variable and Case Selection 86

5

Artificial Cranial Deformation

Cranial Deformation in North America 89
Cranial Deformation in the Study Series 97
Cranial Deformation and Biological Distance 110

6

Adult Age and Cranial Morphology

Previous Research 117
Age Effects in the Study Series 122
Dental Loss and Age Changes in Morphology 131
Adult Age Changes and Biological Distance 135

7

Late Woodland Biological Distances

Univariate Results 140
Multivariate Distance Results Based on Face Measurements 149
Results from Alternative Data Sets 161
Summary and Discussion 164

8

Late Woodland and Mississippian Biological Distances

Univariate Results 167
Multivariate Distance Results Based on Face Measurements 171

Results from Alternative Data Sets 187
Summary and Discussion 192

9

Summary and Discussion

Summary 197
Discussion 202

APPENDIX

Master Data File 207

References Cited 231

Subject Index 247

Center for American Archeology
At Northwestern University

To realize its potential, archeology faces the formidable task of devising new approaches to research that will increase its capacity to interpret the remains of extinct cultures. Archeology today attempts to reconstruct, from excavated remains alone, important elements of three prehistoric systems—culture, environment, and human biology. It seeks to develop and to test hypotheses that explain observed relationships within and between aspects of the three systems. All have left traces in the soil.

But the most brilliant archeologists cannot possibly control the range of knowledge necessary to interpret the archeological remains of the three extinct systems. It will take an interdisciplinary effort among specialists who together possess the necessary expertise.

In recent years, there have been major advances in the physical and biological sciences. These have an enormous potential for increasing the archeologist's capacity for interpreting the prehistoric record of culture, environment, and human biology. The difficulty has been that many of the new methods in physics, chemistry, mathematics, mining engineering, and medicine, to mention a few, have not been regularly applied to archeological problem-solving because they require expertise that is unavailable and capital expenditures that are not feasible in conventional archeological research efforts.

Most of these interfaces between archeology and other sciences entail the development of new research methods by specialists using expensive instrumentation in a framework of long-term research. Application of these methods to archeological problem-solving can occur only when institutional frameworks within which archeology is conducted have themselves evolved to a level capable of sustaining the diverse specialities that today offer so much potential for the growth of the discipline.

In 1964, archeologists at Northwestern University began an attempt to create an institutional framework capable of sustaining the diverse research expertise and substantial facilities and budgetary levels required to conduct long-term, regional research of the kind archeology today increasingly defines for itself. From the beginning, this research effort carried the name "Northwestern Archeological Program" (NAP). In June, 1981, the *Center for American Archeology* (CAA) was founded as a nonprofit research institution affiliated with Northwestern University. Headquarters of the new institution is Northwestern's Evanston, Illinois, campus.

The geographic focus of the Center and the antecedent NAP has been a 64 × 112-km (40 × 70-mile) area of west–central Illinois situated immediately north of the confluence of the Illinois and Mississippi Rivers. The human record here, preserved in the more than 2000 known archeological sites, is at least 12,000 years long. Three major river valleys (Mississippi, Illinois, and Missouri) converge here, a factor partially responsible for the complex culture history that is beginning to emerge from recent archeological investigations. The Mississippi–Illinois–Missouri confluence area appears to have been a major center of prehistoric cultural development for thousands of years, a factor relating to the rich and stable resources of the river floodplains.

The intensity of focus that the CAA and NAP have given this area since 1964 is unusual in North American archeology. There are both practical and philosophical reasons for the lack of long-term regional research projects of this kind. It is believed, nonetheless, that such an intense focus can produce a data base that enhances observation of the relationships between cultural variables and environmental and human biological factors, enhancing the opportunity for archeologists to generate explanatory models.

By 1981, Center archeologists and their colleagues from various other universities, have excavated 16 prehistoric habitation and mortuary sites in the 7200-km^2 research universe surrounding the Kampsville Archeological Center. These projects have focused on delineating economic patterns, population changes, and various interdependent cultural and biological processes that characterize the Archaic, Woodland, and Mississippian periods of this region.

Only time will tell whether this geographically focused archeological research effort will produce a significantly higher level of interpretation. What is clear is that the Center for American Archeology is attempting to develop an organizational structure that can accommodate the specialized expertise backed by facilities and supported by an institutional budget adequate to capitalize and to sustain the research program. In this, it represents an unusual experiment in modern archeology.

The Lower Illinois Valley as a Field Laboratory

There are practical reasons why the lower Illinois River Valley is an ideal field laboratory for development of new methods and approaches in archeology: First, today this region is sparsely populated farmland, its southern limits separated from the St. Louis metropolitan area by the Mississippi River which has acted as an effective barrier to the northward spread of the city. Thus the lower Illinois Valley has escaped the widespread destruction that has greatly reduced the archeological research potential of many comparable river valleys throughout the United States. Second, the cost of performing research in the lower Illinois Valley is as low as can be expected anywhere in the world. Third, extensive information on climate, landforms, soils, water resources, plants, and animals is available for this region. These data provide an essential baseline for the cultural–ecological studies which are a major focus of CAA research.

The cost of doing archeological research has been too long overlooked as a significant factor affecting both the limitations archeologists impose on the goals of their research and the outcomes of that research.

As long as archeological dollars are scarce, cost and accessibility are key factors when selecting an area for long-term archeological research. The factors to be considered are (*a*) cost of transportation between the university and the field; (*b*) cost of maintaining and operating a field headquarters; (*c*) accessibility to cooperating natural scientists; (*d*) accessibility to supplies and equipment; (*e*) cost of transporting and maintaining students in the field; (*f*) ability to maintain continuity in the field program in terms of political and economic factors; (*g*) the prior availability of information on the natural environment (past and present); and (*h*) the ease of transporting artifacts to the home institution and technical specialists to the field. With respect to all these factors, the lower Illinois Valley is an ideal location for testing new archeological methods.

The Kampsville Archeological Center

To serve the research and teaching efforts of CAA, a permanent field center is under development at Kampsville. Kampsville is ideally suited for this purpose, since it is located in a region rich in archeological sites, yet one in which real estate values are modest enough to make feasible the purchase and construction of the facilities required to operate the Center for American Archeology's research and teaching programs.

During the late 1950s, I directed the excavation of Hopewell sites on the Illinois River near the small village of Kampsville. This area could be reached from Chicago in six hours and from St. Louis Airport in two. In steamboat days, Kampsville had been a major river port but had steadily declined since the 1920s. The facilities needed to create CAA's archeological field campus might be obtained most economically by purchasing a series of contiguous store buildings and houses in what had been the central business district of nineteenth-century Kampsville.

The purchase in 1968 of the building that formerly housed the Getz Hardware Store began the development of what has, by 1981, become a 39-building teaching and research center.

The Kampsville Archeological Center includes eight private residences that have been converted into student dorm houses. Several former store buildings are now laboratories for archeologists, zoologists, botanists, geologists, and other specialists. The 15,000-volume library at Kampsville represents an important resource, as does the PDP 11-34 computer. A small museum has been established to interpret the results of the Kampsville-based research.

Research Publications

During the 1960s, and early 1970s, the Northwestern Archeological Program published research monographs in cooperation with the Illinois State Museum. The growth of archeological programs in both institutions made this cooperative arrangement less practical over the years, and beginning in 1976 Northwestern began to publish under its own imprint the research of its in-house faculty and students, as well as that of cooperating scholars from other institutions.

The Center for American Archeology will carry this publication program forward. The present volume, by Judith Droessler, is the sixteenth in a continuing series of monographs and collected works that represent the research results of the Center and the Northwestern Archeological Program before it.

Stuart Struever
EVANSTON, ILLINOIS

Preface

This monograph is a revised version of my Ph.D. dissertation submitted to the Graduate School of Indiana University in 1979. I am grateful to Della Cook, chairperson of my doctoral committee, and to Robert Meier and Paul Jamison, who served on my committee, for their assistance with this research and for their support throughout my graduate program. I also wish to thank Patrick Munson and Don Bennett for their interest in this investigation and for serving on my doctoral committee.

I wish to express appreciation to Jane Buikstra and Northwestern University for permitting me to study the Ledders series. I would also like to thank Dr. Buikstra for her interest and support in this project.

Gregory Perino excavated the Schild, Yokem, Klunk, and Koster series. I am indebted to him for his appreciation of skeletal remains as a data base of value within the framework of archeological investigation. I am also grateful to the late Georg Neumann for the considerable effort he devoted to accumulating and curating the Indiana University skeletal collections, and for his tutelage in cranial measurement.

Many people assisted in processing the skeletal material. I wish especially to thank Sari Amick-Allen, Della Cook, Carol Cottom, Dave Jackson, Mary Pat Lynch, Emily Sherfey, Susan Sherfey, Paul Snyder, Tish White, Sue Winder, and Mike Wray.

I am grateful for friendship and idea exchange with Dona Thompson-Jacob, Sue Winder, Brian Fields, Julie McCarthy, Paul Snyder, and Lynne Goldstein. Valerie Wolfe, Joyce O'Rear, Wade Birch, and Rita Marsh provided much needed moral support.

The manuscript benefited significantly from the critical comments and editorial assistance of David Asch, and for this I am most grateful. I also wish to thank Betty Aulenbach for editorial assistance, Brenda Lott for keypunching the data, and Pat Picou for typing the manuscript.

Finally, I wish to thank my family. My parents contributed a great deal of moral as well as financial support, and I am sincerely appreciative of their help. I would also like to thank my husband Vern. His support and professional assistance throughout this project were vital to its completion.

I am grateful for financial assistance from Sigma Xi (The Scientific Research Society of North America), the Indiana Academy of Science, the Indiana University Office of Research and Development, and the Social Sciences and Humanities Research Council of Canada.

1

The Problem

Introduction

The description of skeletal material frequently appended to mortuary site reports testifies to the traditional contribution of the physical anthropologist to studies of American Indian prehistory. In the past, skeletal material was usually described in terms of vital statistics, unusual pathologies, and cranial measurements and indices. Analysis was most often limited to the identification of morphological types represented in particular skeletal series and the association of these physical types with particular archeological cultures. Well-preserved, undeformed male crania were most often selected for this purpose. Evidence for prehistoric migrations was sought in the correspondence of discontinuities in cultural and physical types.

The range of archeological questions which can be dealt with using skeletal data has been expanded in recent years through methodological advances and theoretical reorientations in both archeology and physical anthropology. In the field of archeology, the "process school," led by Lewis Binford, emphasizes an ecological approach to studies of extinct human cultures and embraces systems theory as an interpretive and investigatory framework (Watson, LeBlanc, and Redman 1971). Within this framework it is held that

> culture is made up of parts, structurally different from each other, but articulated within the total system. More broadly, culture and its environments represent a number of articulated systems in which change occurs through a series of minor, linked variations in one or more of these systems. A major objective of archaeology is to understand the linkages

> between parts in both the cultural and environmental systems as reflected in the archaeological data [Struever 1971:10].

Adoption of this theoretical approach leads logically to the use of a multidisciplinary research program in which archeologists draw upon the expertise of many specialists, including physical anthropologists, both to define and to pursue research goals.

At the same time, theoretical shifts and expanded methodologies in the field of physical anthropology enable the biological anthropologist to deal more effectively with questions of archeological importance. For example, there has been a reorientation in recent years in the approach to biological relationships among extinct populations, which is the major concern of the present study. Emphasis on a population approach (Mayr 1970) has led to a movement away from the traditional goals of identifying and relating physical types. The application of models of microevolutionary change to skeletal data yields more biologically meaningful estimates of population distance. With the assistance of the computer, multivariate procedures can be used to examine variation in morphological complexes. Since variation within and between a number of groups can be compared simultaneously, we are able to examine dynamic patterns of both biological distances and variability within and between groups along temporal, spatial, and cultural dimensions. If we assume that skeletal series represent breeding units defined by social factors operative during the time period represented by a particular mortuary site component, patterns of variation in inherited morphology among skeletal series can be interpreted as a reflection of patterns of social interaction among the groups they represent. In this respect, biological data can be used to derive hypotheses concerning prehistoric behavior.

Binford (1964) has discussed the advantages of a "regional approach"—the detailed and systematic study of the articulations among sociocultural, biological, and environmental systems on a regional level—in the context of archeological research design. West–central Illinois (Figure 1) has been the focus of a multidisciplinary research program to study the dynamics of prehistoric human ecology in the region (Brown and Struever 1973; Buikstra 1977; T. G. Cook 1976). Originally, this program centered on the lower Illinois Valley—the lower 113 km of the Illinois River, its floodplain, and adjacent uplands. It now includes the adjacent Mississippi Valley in Illinois. The area encompasses a number of rich natural resource zones. It is also rich in archeological remains, having been occupied for thousands of years beginning with Paleo-Indian hunter–gatherers and extending to Mississippian horticulturalists who lived in the region until about A.D. 1300.

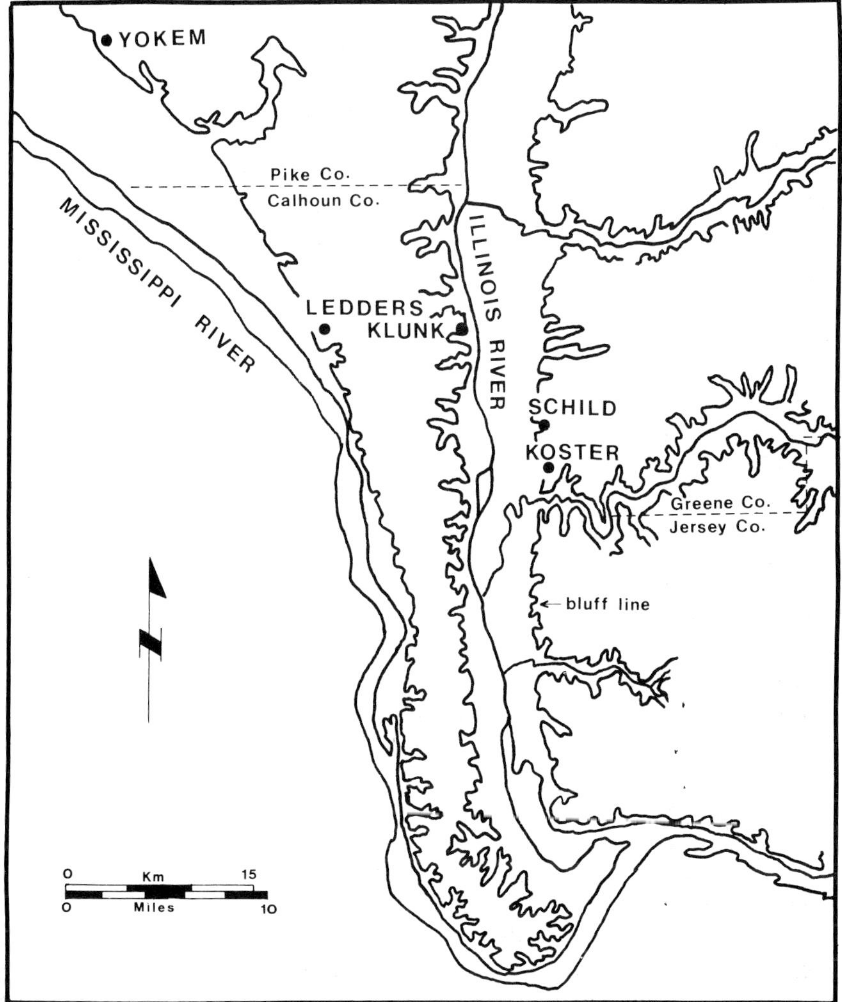

FIGURE 1. Location of the Yokem, Ledders, Klunk, Schild, and Koster mound groups in west–central Illinois.

The west–central Illinois region has been conceived of as a natural laboratory wherein the interaction of biological, cultural, and environmental systems can be traced through time (Buikstra 1975; T. G. Cook 1976).

Within the west–central Illinois research program, physical anthropologists have demonstrated that the study of the skeletal remains of the region's prehistoric inhabitants provides data which, when integrated with cultural and environmental information, can be applied to questions of archeological importance. For example, Buikstra (1974, 1976) has shown through analysis of skeletal variants and mortuary site structure that Middle Woodland populations probably had a social rank system at least partially dependent upon inherited status, and that adult behavior patterns were differentially distributed among these social subgroups. She has also identified subregional patterns of biosocial interaction during the Middle Woodland period which parallel the results of microstyle analysis of Middle Woodland ceramics (Houart 1975). D. C. Cook has also used biological data to deal with questions of an archeological nature. Cook (1975a, 1975b, 1981) has examined developmental disturbances and disease patterns in Middle and Late Woodland skeletal series in order to assess the biological effects of subsistence shifts during the Woodland period. Her results indicated greater environmental stress, or less effective ability to maintain health, in the Late Woodland period as compared to the Middle Woodland period. These results are consistent with those of O'Connell (1975, 1976), who examined the fluctuating asymmetry of nonmetric skeletal traits as a reflection of the biological adaptive efficiency of west–central Illinois Woodland populations.

The present study is also designed to address problems in the prehistory of the west–central Illinois region from a biological perspective. Following the population approach referred to above, craniometric data are used here to examine patterns of biological microvariability among Late Woodland and Middle Mississippian groups who inhabited the area from approximately A.D. 600 to A.D. 1300. This research is closely related to that of Buikstra (1975, 1977) who used nonmetric skeletal variants to determine patterns of biological relationships in the region from Middle Woodland through Mississippian times. The use in the present investigation of an alternative data base, craniometrics, provides a test of certain biobehavioral models generated by Buikstra's research. In addition, questions relating to change in patterns of within and between group variability—which can be most effectively dealt with using interval scale measures—are addressed.

Statement of the Problem

According to the systemic model referred to earlier, culture history is the product of complex, dynamic articulations through time among interdependent human biological, physical environmental, and sociocultural systems. Change in one of these subsystems is likely, either directly or indirectly, to stimulate change in other subsystems. The archeological record provides relatively direct evidence of some dimensions involved in this interactive model. For example, floral and faunal remains reflect local resource availability, and tool and weapon inventories reflect exploitive patterns. Similarly, site survey data can be used to reconstruct settlement patterns and population density, and distributions of artifact types can provide information regarding prehistoric trade networks.

Other, more intangible aspects of prehistoric societies—such as kinship systems, social status systems, and marriage patterns—are more difficult to deduce from archeological remains. This study represents an attempt to use biological distance data to examine one such dimension—biosocial interactions—among prehistoric Indian communities in the west–central Illinois region. Patterns of biological distance and variability among prehistoric skeletal series are used here as indirect measures of degree of social exchange between the groups they represent. It is assumed that the likelihood of gene flow—a result of the exchange of marriage partners between groups—was proportional to the degree of social intercourse between local communities. Skeletal series are regarded as approximately representative of local community breeding units, or demes, and similarities and differences in cranial morphology are assumed to reflect genetic similarities and differences among groups. Thus patterns of morphological variability among cranial series are interpreted as a reflection of patterning in an extinct network of social interactions.

Following this approach, two questions concerning the prehistory of the region are addressed in this study. The first question is as follows:

> *Was change in subsistence–settlement systems from Middle Woodland to Late Woodland times accompanied by change in the structure of biosocial interactions among west–central Illinois communities?*

There is archeological evidence (discussed in Chapter 2) that Middle Woodland sociocultural and economic systems were altered in the Late Woodland period, especially in the latter part. Trade apparently declined, ceramic styles and exploitive patterns became more localized, population numbers increased, and settlements extended over physiographic zones far removed from the major river valleys. It seems reasonable to expect, according to the systemic model, that these changes would have stimulated modifications in existing patterns of both cooperation and competition among local communities in the region. Modification of these patterns was, in turn, likely to have resulted in altered networks of intergroup social and biological exchange.

Buikstra (1976) has presented evidence of subregional epigenetic variability among local Middle Woodland communities in the lower Illinois Valley region. This intergroup variability appears to be associated with spatial factors, especially intersite distance by river. Patterns of biological distance among Late Woodland inhabitants of the region were studied here to see if the Middle Woodland pattern of subregional differentiation continued through Late Woodland times, or if biological distance relationships changed along with changes in subsistence–settlement systems. It was expected that alterations in the structure of biosocial relationships, which might have accompanied subsistence–settlement changes, would be reflected by altered patterns of intergroup craniometric variability.

The second question dealt with here concerns the relationship between Late Woodland and later, Mississippian occupations in west–central Illinois. This question can be stated as follows:

> *Were the cultural and ecological changes associated with the emergence of a Mississippian pattern in the west–central Illinois region associated with large-scale population movement into the region at the Late Woodland–Mississippian interface?*

The development of Mississippian has been associated archeologically with marked changes in subsistence–settlement systems and sociopolitical organization (J. A. Brown 1977; Dragoo 1976). One view of the emergence of the Mississippian complex in the area assumes a movement of substantial numbers of people up the Mississippi River from a center to the south, perhaps Cahokia (Maxwell 1947:29; Wray 1952:157). According to this view, local Late Woodland populations were either assimilated or displaced by Mississippian newcomers. Such a series of events would likely have had biological consequences. In particular, if large numbers of people moved into the region at this time, one would expect that the introduction of new genetic material would have resulted in alteration of the gene pool such that Mississippian skeletal series can be clearly distinguished morphologically from earlier Late Woodland series. Alternatively, if the Late-Woodland–Mississippian transition did not involve population movement into the region, this should be reflected by genetic continuity on a regional level.

Methodological Subproblems

Several methodological subproblems are also dealt with in this investigation. They are: (1) the effects of artificial cranial deformation on craniometric-based biological distance estimates, (2) the effects of age on adult cranial morphology, and (3) congruence of biological distance results based on different data sets.

In a study of biological distance based on craniometric data, it is assumed that differences in cranial morphology reflect inherited differences between groups. Artificial cranial deformation, which is present in several of the study series, is a potential source of noninherited variation in cranial morphology. To facilitate the interpretation of the biological distance results, that is, to assess the reliability of the distance estimates as a measure of biological relatedness among the groups in question, analyses were directed toward the following questions: What are the effects on craniometric-based biological distance estimates of including deformed crania in the samples? Is it possible to select a set of measurements which are relatively free of the effects of cranial deformation?

Since cranial morphology has been shown to change in adulthood in the living (Baer 1956; Goldstein 1936; Israel 1968, 1973a), age differences were examined as a second source of noninherited variation in the study series. The questions posed in this regard are as follows: Is there a discernible pattern of change in cranial morphology with age in the study series? If so, is this pattern of age change in prehistoric American Indians comparable to that found in living populations? Are age effects a significant source of variation between the study series?

Finally, congruence of biological distance estimates obtained from alternative data sets is examined. Separate analyses were carried out using four different sets of cranial measurements, selected so as to reflect broadly defined functional components of the skull.

In addition to investigating the stability of patterns of biological distance over different craniometric data sets, the results of the present study are compared with the results obtained by Buikstra from nonmetric cranial variants. Buikstra's (1975, 1977) study focused on the same general problems in lower Illinois Valley prehistory as does the present investigation. The two studies represent separate tests, using biological data, of models of prehistoric biocultural dynamics. The degree to which our results are congruent can be interpreted as an indication of the strength of our conclusions regarding Late-Woodland–Mississippian biosocial relationships in the region.

The examination of congruence of results based on alternative craniometric data sets, as well as congruence between distance patterns derived from craniometric and nonmetric cranial variants, provides a test of the "hypothesis of nonspecificity" of Sokal and Sneath (1963: 85). This hypothesis states that "there are no distinct classes of genes affecting exclusively one class of characters. . . . Although a given gene may have a main effect on one region or kind of character, it is likely to have side effects or chain reaction effects on other regions and characters." Since both craniometrics and nonmetric cranial variants have been shown by previous research to have a hereditary basis, this hypothesis predicts that the biodistance results obtained in both cases will be similar.

The degree to which the alternative data sets yield congruent results also provides some indication of the reliability of using any of these data sets alone in future biodistance studies. Since sources of error encountered in the alternative data sets are somewhat different (environmental effects and sampling vary, for example), variations in results may provide some indication of the potential for particular error effects to distort biological distance estimates.

2

Archeological Background

This investigation is concerned with interactions among Late Woodland and Mississippian populations in west–central Illinois, as reflected by intergroup biological relationships. This chapter is intended to provide an archeological context for this research by summarizing what is known of Late Woodland and Mississippian prehistory in the west–central Illinois area. For additional information on Late Woodland and Mississippian prehistory in the Midwest, the following sources should be consulted: J. A. Brown (1977), Buikstra (1977), Dragoo (1976), Ford (1974), L. G. Goldstein (1976, 1980), and Griffin (1964, 1967).

Late Woodland

The Late Woodland period in west–central Illinois extends from approximately A.D. 400 to A.D. 1000. By about A.D. 400, the Middle Woodland Illinois Hopewell complex, with its extensive trade networks and elaborate mortuary system, all but disappears from the region's archeological record. The Late Woodland period, which follows the dissolution of the "Hopewell interaction sphere" (Caldwell 1964; Struever 1964, 1965), has been described as a time of cultural decline, a "dark age" (Deuel 1958:34) of Illinois prehistory. Griffin's (1964:247) characterization of the Late Woodland period in Illinois is typical: "The culture products that identify Hopewellian gradually decline in quality and . . . the cultural intensity that produced excellent and distinctive art forms gradually fades into the production of drab and uninspired material." Perhaps because of the unspectacular nature of Late Woodland remains as compared to the material culture of Middle Woodland and Mississippian peoples, less research attention has been given to the Late Woodland period than to the periods of cultural florescence immediately preceding and following it.

A comprehensive analysis of Late Woodland ceramics in west–central Illinois has not been undertaken to date, although there seems to be general agreement that Late Woodland ceramics tend to show more local variability in form and craftsmanship than Middle Woodland ceramics. Griffin (1964:247) mentions the following general characteristics of Late Woodland pottery in Illinois: vessels noticeably thinner than Middle Woodland vessels; predominantly simple jar form with a conoidal to rounded base; grit, limestone, or clay temper; surfaces plain or cordmarked; decoration simple and usually limited to lip notching, crimping, or punching, with occasional incisions or punctates on outer rim.

Several attempts have been made to divide the Late Woodland period in west–central Illinois into phases according to ceramic characteristics. The early White Hall phase, dating from A.D. 400 to A.D. 700 (or slightly later) has been proposed by Struever (1964, 1968). White Hall ceramics are typically thin-walled vessels of extremely sandy paste and temper. Body decoration is usually limited to coarse cordmarking. Exterior rim decorations frequently consist of cord-wrapped stick impressions on the exterior lip, with a row of annular or hemiconoidal punctates beneath the lip (Houart 1971:9). Struever (1964) notes that some White Hall decorative and morphological attributes occur in earlier Middle Woodland ceramic series. Griffin *et al.* (1970:10) also remark on the carryover of some Hopewell decorative techniques and motifs in White Hall pottery, and note its similarity to pottery from the Pool and Irving sites (McGregor 1958) in the lower Illinois Valley and to Weaver wares (Wray and MacNeish 1961) in the central Illinois Valley.

Griffin *et al.* (1970) have proposed a Fox Creek phase for early Late Woodland occupations of the extreme lower Illinois Valley, the adjacent Mississippi Valley, and the Cahokia area. Evidence for the development of Fox Creek from the preceding Middle Woodland Pike phase was found at the Knight mound group, which overlooks the Mississippi River in Calhoun County, Illinois. A number of different types of Canteen wares from the Knight site are associated with the Fox Creek phase. General characteristics of Canteen wares include grit temper, simple conoidal vessel form, basal thickening, and cord-marked body decoration. Although the Canteen complex is simple in both form and decoration, vessels are generally as well made as earlier Havana wares (Griffin *et al.* 1970:23). Some Canteen vessels found in the Knight mounds were considerably smaller than similar pots from village contexts and showed no evidence of having been used for cooking. Griffin *et al.* (1970:23) interpret these vessels as evidence for the continuation into Late Woodland times of the manufacture of vessels specifically for burial purposes.

Munson (1971a), following a survey of the Wood River Terrace area of the American Bottoms near Cahokia, distinguished two Late Woodland phases, Early Bluff and Late Bluff. Radiocarbon dates from area sites which contain Early Bluff materials average to A.D. 755 ± 126. The average radiocarbon date for bottoms sites containing Late Bluff materials is A.D. 1070 ± 86 (Munson 1971a:14). Bowls and conoidal-based jars are typical Early Bluff pottery forms. Cordmarking typically decorates the body. Lips are rounded or tapered, and frequently decorated with exterior or interior plain dowl impressions. Impressions were occasionally made with a cordwrapped stick, and were sometimes applied to the lip crest. Vessels are predominantly grit-tempered, occasionally grog-tempered. Chert inclusions are common in the paste. "Stump ware" does not occur in Early Bluff contexts. Near the end of the Early Bluff phase, there appear cordmarked bowls with flattened lips. Jars with smoothed rims, flattened lips, and diagonally stamped interior rims are also found in terminal Early Bluff. Both of these vessel forms continue to be found in Late Bluff. Typical Late Bluff pottery forms are cordmarked, conoidal-based jars with smoothed rims. Vessel lips, which are sometimes notched, are either flattened and undecorated or thickened and flared. Grit, grog, and limestone were used as temper. Two new forms appear in Late Bluff: grog-tempered "stump ware," and Monks Mound Red, which is characterized by globular shape, limestone temper, and red film (Munson 1971a:10–11).

In regard to nonceramic artifacts, Griffin (1964:247) notes that the use of bone and stone gorgets continues from Middle Woodland to Late Woodland, while the platform pipe style gives way to the elbow pipe form. Projectile points become smaller in Late Woodland, probably indicating a shift to the bow and arrow during this period. Steuben points, characteristic of early Late Woodland White Hall and Weaver assemblages, are too large to be used as arrow points, suggesting that the bow and arrow was not commonly used until after the initial phases of the Late Woodland period (D. L. Asch, personal communication). Munson (1971a:10), in his American Bottoms survey, found both large points and arrow-sized points at Early Bluff sites. The corner-notched, flake Koster point occurred with the greatest frequency in Early Bluff assemblages. In addition to a variety of other flake projectile points, Munson also found Dickson Broad Bladed knives, ovate and triangular knives, stemmed knives, single-shouldered knives, drills, small end scrapers, side scrapers, hoes, and manos at sites with Early Bluff occupations.

According to Munson's survey, projectile points, and to a lesser extent knives and scrapers, decrease in frequency from Early to Late Bluff. Koster points are found less frequently in Late Bluff than in Early Bluff, while two new point types proposed by Munson, "Wanda" and "Roxana," are found in greater numbers. Wanda points are very poorly made, side-notched flake points. Roxana points are flaked, with wide side notches. Dickson Broad Bladed knives all but disappear in Late Bluff times. Polished hoe-sharpening flakes are found in greater quantities in Late Bluff than in Early Bluff contexts (Munson 1971a:11).

The absence of far-flung trade networks, such as existed during the Middle Woodland period, is a frequently cited characteristic of the Late Woodland period. Although trade did not cease, it apparently diminished, and the structure of trade relationships changed significantly. Munson (1971a:13) notes the presence of trade items in Bluff contexts. As in the Middle Woodland period, Late Woodland peoples appear to have traded cherts, although different chert sources were emphasized than in Middle Woodland times. According to Munson, there is evidence that hematite, copper, *Marginella* shells (from the Gulf and Atlantic Coasts), and *Anculosa* snail shells (perhaps from the Wabash and lower Ohio Valleys) were also traded in the Late Woodland period. Porter (1973:156) discusses the importance of Late Woodland redistributive systems in the development of the extensive Mississippian trade systems.

West–central Illinois encompasses a number of ecological zones which provided a great wealth and diversity of natural food resources for the region's prehistoric inhabitants. Several descriptions of the prehistoric ecology of the region are available (Zawacki and Hausfater 1969; Asch and Asch 1978; Whatley and Asch 1975). As in the preceding Middle Woodland period, subsistence in early Late Woodland times appears to be characterized by intensive hunting and gathering of a few rich natural food resources, supplemented by the cultivation of several native North American plant species. Struever (1968:299) reports that food remains associated with White Hall occupations at the Apple Creek site indicate that a wide range of fauna was exploited, although there was an emphasis on deer, turkey, ducks and geese, and fish. In addition to hickory nuts and acorns, *Chenopodium* and *Polygonum* seeds were utilized.

Munson (1971b) describes a similar intensive hunting and gathering economy at Scovill, a Weaver village site (ca. A.D. 450) near the Spoon

River in the central Illinois Valley drainage. As at Apple Creek, environmental potential was rich and there appears to have been a good deal of specialization. White-tailed deer, turkey, and fish comprised meat staples. Nuts were gathered according to seasonal availability, with little evidence of selective bias. There is evidence at Scovill for the cultivation of squash and gourds. Wild plant foods, however, appear to have been at least of equal importance in the diet. The occupants of Scovill appear to have led a semisedentary way of life, relocating seasonally according to resource availability (Munson 1971b).

Asch and Asch (1978, 1980) and Asch, Farnsworth, and Asch (1979), in their study of botanical remains from Woodland sites in west–central Illinois, find that there was little change in patterns of plant utilization from Middle Woodland to early Late Woodland. Although the importance of premaize cultivation as a supplement to hunting and wild plant food collecting is uncertain at the present time, Asch and Asch present evidence that Middle and early Late Woodland groups cultivated five species of native eastern North American seed annuals. Three of these species—*Chenopodium bushianum* (goosefoot), *Polygonum erectum* (knotweed), and *Phalaris caroliniana* (maygrass)—produce starchy seeds, and two species—*Iva annua* (sumpweed) and *Helianthus annuus* (sunflower)—yield oily seeds. As in the Middle Woodland period, there appears to have been an emphasis on starchy seeds. Squash and gourd remains also continue into early Late Woodland times as a common variety of plant remains. Nuts, on the other hand, are found less frequently at early Late Woodland sites than they are at Middle Woodland sites. Asch *et al.* (1979) suggest that the decline in nut remains may indicate that the need for fall nut harvests was lessened by the cultivation of seed plants in quantities sufficient to provide a secure food source in years of poor nut production.

Asch and Asch's research also indicates that a distinct subsistence shift took place in late Late Woodland times. Maize remains, which are either absent or extremely scarce at Middle Woodland and early Late Woodland sites, are common in late Late Woodland sites in the area. Although the cultivation of both starchy and oily seed crops continued, seed cultivation begins to receive less emphasis with the increase in maize production in the late Late Woodland period. There is also a decline in nut collection and the use of squash and gourds. Archeobotanical evidence from the Koster East site, which has both Early and Late components, indicates that maize was adopted as a staple cultigen in Late Bluff times (D. Asch, personal communication).

Survey data also support a Late Bluff date for the adoption of maize as a food staple and decreased emphasis on hunting. Munson (1971a:12), in his American Bottoms survey, notes that polished hoe-sharpening flakes are more common in Late Bluff contexts, whereas lithic artifacts associated with hunting are found in lower frequencies. Harn (1971a:33), in another American Bottoms survey, also found that hoes and sharpening flakes are more common in Late Bluff contexts, whereas the frequency of arrowpoints and butchering tools is lower than in Early Bluff sites.

Middle Woodland village sites in the lower Illinois Valley region are characteristically located in major valleys near large, nonstagnant channels (Asch *et al.* 1979). There is considerable evidence that these settlements were characterized by a high level of residential stability (Struever 1968:308). Survey data indicate only minor changes in settlement pattern from Middle Woodland to early Late Woodland (Asch *et al.* 1979).

A major shift in settlement pattern appears to have taken place in late Late Woodland (Jersey Bluff) times at approximately the same time that maize cultivation becomes important. Settlements still are abundant on the floors of major river valleys, but they also are found in large numbers on the bluff crests far above the valley floodplains and along minor streams and tributaries. Harn (1971b:69) has observed that nearly every tributary of the Illinois River is dotted with Late Woodland sites. Munson (1971a), in his American Bottoms survey, also found Late Bluff sites to be more widely distributed and to occupy a greater diversity of physiographic zones than Early Bluff sites. Farnsworth, in an archeological survey of the Macoupin Valley, found a great number of Jersey Bluff sites, while evidence of earlier Late Woodland White Hall occupations was absent. He suggests (1973:27) that the

> Jersey Bluff tradition may have developed in major secondary valleys like Macoupin where it was, in effect, an adaptive response to a stressful situation created when the harvestable backwater-lake fish populations and migratory waterfowl characteristic of the Lower Illinois Valley were deleted from the subsistence repertoire of groups moving into large secondary valleys adjacent to the Illinois. It is likely that the migratory shift would have involved major changes in the pattern of subsistence, perhaps including increased reliance upon agricultural food sources to round out nutritional needs.

House forms in early Late Woodland (Bluff) sites tend to be circular or oval and only occasionally rectangular (Griffin 1964:247). Later in the Late Woodland period, house forms were more often rectangular in form. At Cahokia, where Late Woodland occupations were quite extensive, houses were of small, individual post construction, usually set in basins 30–90 cm (1 to 3 ft) deep, with no central fireplace (Griffin

1964:250). At the late Late Woodland Kane Village site in the American Bottoms in Madison County, five house floors were excavated. All houses were placed in rectangular or square basins ranging in depth from 36 to 76 cm. As at Cahokia, they were of small post construction and lacked interior fireplaces. They appear to have been bent pole, arbor-shaped structures, which were covered with mats (Munson and Anderson 1973:35).

The changes in subsistence and settlement systems evidenced in the Late Woodland period may have been the result, at least in part, of increased population pressure in Late Woodland times. Estimates of population density calculated by DeRousseau (1973) indicate an increase in population numbers from Middle Woodland to Late Woodland and continuing throughout the Late Woodland period. DeRousseau and Braverman's intensive survey of burial mounds in two transects of the lower Illinois Valley indicate that this population increase was more marked on the east side of the Illinois River, where the rich, arable floodplain is considerably broader than it is on the west side of the river (DeRousseau 1973).

Compared to the Middle Woodland period, a relatively high frequency of violent deaths is indicated in the Late Woodland period by numerous instances of projectile points lodged in bones or situated in the body cavity (Perino 1973c:135). Intergroup conflict apparently increased in Late Woodland times, perhaps in response to factors such as increasing population pressure, competition for resources (such as arable land), and breakdown of Middle Woodland patterns of structured interaction (Struever and Houart 1972) and resource redistribution among groups in the region.

There is considerable evidence that Late Woodland populations of west–central Illinois were generally less healthy than people in the preceding Middle Woodland period. Results of a study of the epidemiologic pattern shown by circular caries and related dental lesions suggest that the environment was substantially more stressful for children in the Late Woodland period than it was in the Middle Woodland period (Cook and Buikstra 1973).

Similar indications were found in subsequent studies by D. C. Cook (1974, 1975a, 1975b, 1981). Her comparison of Middle Woodland and Late Woodland mortality data suggests that Late Woodland populations underwent a more rigorous mortality experience than Middle Woodland populations, and had a lower life expectancy (D. C. Cook 1974:7,9). Cook's (1975a, 1975b) epidemiological study of skeletal markers indicative of environmental stress—such as Harris lines, dental hypoplasia, cortical thickening, growth retardation, and nutritionally related diseases—has yielded further evidence that populations in the Late Woodland period, especially in the terminal phase, were less able to maintain health than Middle Woodland populations. She suggests that the lower health status of Late Woodland populations may be related to the ecological changes noted for Late Woodland (D. C. Cook 1975a:13).

The findings related to the health of Woodland populations are supported by the fluctuating asymmetry research of O'Connell (1976). Her model was as follows: Assuming that both sides of symmetrical organisms are controlled by the same genes, nondirectional differences in bilateral structures can be presumed to be environmental effects. If it is further assumed that development will be least stable and fluctuating asymmetry greatest during periods of environmental change, when an organism has not adapted fully to a new environment, then the degree of asymmetry of bilateral structures can be interpreted as a measure of a population's ability to buffer environmental stress. This model was tested through examination of asymmetry of cranial nonmetric traits in Middle and Late Woodland skeletal series from west–central Illinois. O'Connell (1976:9) found that asymmetry measures tended to be highest in terminal Middle Woodland and terminal Late Woodland skeletal series, which represent populations living during periods of environmental change.

Since burial mounds containing early Late Woodland White Hall ceramics have not yet been excavated (or not recognized), virtually nothing is known of White Hall mortuary practices (Asch 1976:54). The following discussion of Late Woodland burial customs is therefore limited to data from *late* Late Woodland (Bluff) phases.[1]

The practice of interring the dead in mounded, bluff–crest cemeteries continued from Middle Woodland to Late Woodland. Late Woodland mounds, however, tend to be smaller and elliptical in shape, whereas Middle Woodland mounds tend to be larger and of circular or oval shape (DeRousseau 1973:11). Density of burials within mounds also varies through time. Early Late Woodland (Early Bluff) mounds contain a considerably lower average number of burials per mound than Middle Woodland mounds. However, burial density appears to have increased markedly by late Late Woodland; late Late Woodland mounds contain a slightly greater mean number of burials than Middle Woodland mounds (DeRousseau 1973:15).

Cremation was practiced more frequently in the Late Woodland period than in the preceding Middle Woodland period. There is evidence

[1] Data pertaining to Late Woodland mortuary practices are primarily from Perino (n.d., 1973a, 1973b, 1973c).

in Late Woodland of cremations associated both with blufftop burial mounds and in the valley unassociated with a cemetery. Cremations associated with mound groups have been reported at the Joe Gay site (D. C. Cook 1974), the Helton site (Tainter 1975), and possibly[2] the Klunk, Yokem, and Schild sites (Perino n.d., 1973b, 1973c). The Perrins Ledge crematory (Buikstra and Goldstein 1973) represents a Late Woodland valley crematory.

Between Mounds 6 and 7 at the Klunk site, Perino (1973b) excavated a circular limestone basin which may represent a mound-associated Late Woodland crematory. Limestone slabs, some of them set on edge, defined a circular area approximately 3.35 m (11 ft) in diameter. The floor of this area, which was partly covered with limestone slabs, contained scattered charred and unburned bone fragments. Some of the bones were in articulation. A child had been buried in flexed position in the crematory floor; charred bone in the grave fill indicated that this individual had been buried after the crematory had been used. A Late Woodland pottery vessel, clay pipe, and discoidal were found in the crematory basin (Perino 1973b).

The valley crematory at Perrins Ledge in Calhoun County has been analyzed by Buikstra and Goldstein (1973). This crematory site contains an 2.44 × 2.44 m (8 × 8 ft) central crematory base circled by a ring of limestone slabs. There is evidence for at least two burning episodes. Cremation fires were apparently built on top of flesh-covered corpses. Although at least 13 individuals were represented by the skeletal remains, only 2 individuals were represented by approximately complete skeletons. These two people had been placed in flexed position on their right side. There is no strong evidence to indicate that differential access to the crematory was accorded to any particular age or sex category. A pottery elbow pipe, the base of a pot, a flake knife, and possibly a brachiopod were associated with the Perrins Ledge crematory (Buikstra and Goldstein 1973).

Middle Woodland mounds in west–central Illinois typically contain burials arranged around a central log tomb, in which selected individuals were placed temporarily, to be later reburied in bundle form outside the central charnel structure. It appears that Late Woodland people also processed deceased individuals through charnel structures. These features were generally less elaborately constructed than Middle Woodland central tombs, while showing considerable structural variability. Perino (n.d., 1973a, 1973b, 1973c) describes the remains of Late Woodland charnel structures at the Klunk, Schild, Koster, and Yokem sites. The

[2] Perino's interpretation of these "crematories" is dealt with later in this section.

structures, situated both on and below the original ground surface, were almost always rectangular to square in shape, with rounded corners. Limestone slabs were frequently used to line floors and walls, although walls were occasionally of log construction. The roof was most commonly constructed of logs weighted down with limestone slabs and/or soil. Doorways to the tombs were identified in several structures at the Yokem site. Most of the structures at the Schild and Klunk sites contained only one or two individuals or a few bone fragments. Tomb A in Schild Mound 9, however, contained eight individuals which had been placed there in varying states of decomposition and articulation. Tombs at the Yokem site usually contained more individuals than structures at the Schild and Klunk sites did. Individuals recovered from the charnel structures were buried in bundle, flexed, and extended positions. A high incidence of missing bones, the frequent presence of disarticulated bone in and near the charnel structure, and the presence of bundle burials in surrounding areas of the mound indicate that the charnel structure was used as a processing facility. In most cases, the structure was covered with an earth mound when use as a charnel house was terminated (Perino n.d., 1973a, 1973b, 1973c).

In a number of instances, the charnel structures contained evidence that both bones and structural elements had been burned. Perino (1973b) initially interpreted areas of charred bone and soil at the Klunk site as crematories. Later, after he had excavated the remains of several structures at the Yokem site, he reinterpreted these charred areas as probable charnel structures which had been accidentally or intentionally burned. Tainter (1975) prefers Perino's original interpretation of the Klunk features as crematories.

At the Koster site, Perino (1973a:195) found evidence suggesting that the dead were sometimes exhumed from single graves for reburial elsewhere without being processed through a charnel structure. The skeleton was not completely removed in most cases, indicating that this practice was carried out after the flesh had decayed. Usually the individual was originally buried in extended position and later reburied in bundle form.

Group burials occur with greater frequency in Late Woodland mounds than in Middle Woodland mounds. In Mound 1 at the Koster site, 11 individuals were apparently placed on a level ridge and covered with earth. Some of these skeletons were articulated, suggesting that the deaths of these individuals occurred at approximately the same time. Others, possibly individuals who died earlier, were in bundle form. Similar group burials, ranging from 6 to 12 individuals, were found in Mound 3 and Knoll 8 at the Koster site and in the Late Woodland portion of Mound 3 at the Yokem site. Perino notes that in some instances individuals who died at the same time appear to have met violent deaths, and speculates that they were perhaps victims of the same violent event. Another type of group burial, in which all individuals represent secondary burials, was found at the Yokem site. The disarticulated remains of 12 individuals found in Mound 4 appear to represent individuals who had been temporarily interred in a charnel pit or structure (Perino n.d., 1973a).

D. C. Cook (1974) mentions that many individuals were interred in large, multiple graves at the Late Woodland Homer Adams site. The age/sex structure of the multiple burials appeared to reflect the age/sex structure of the rest of the cemetery (D. C. Cook 1974:4), indicating that burial in group contexts was probably independent of age and sex classes.

The majority of Late Woodland individuals were interred singly in grave pits, on the original ground surface, or in the mound fill. Grave pits were usually round to oval in shape. Limestone slabs were frequently used to line or cover the grave; log roofs were used occasionally. Burials on the original ground surface were individually covered with small earthen mounds, which were later incorporated into the larger mound. Individuals were buried in the mound fill both during and following mound construction (Perino 1973a, 1973b, 1973c).

Skeletons in Late Woodland mounds are most frequently found in flexed position, somewhat less frequently bundled or in semiflexed position, and only rarely in extended position (Perino 1973c). At the Koster site, burial in extended position appears to have been reserved for principal burials, usually found in a central position in the mound and often in a log-covered grave (Perino 1973a:156).

Grave goods associated with Late Woodland burials are largely utilitarian. They occur in lower frequencies and are considerably less elaborate in style than grave furniture associated with Middle Woodland and Mississippian interments. Typical grave items include small, flake, side-notched projectile points, dart points, discoidals, Canteen and Bluff pottery, Late Woodland style pipes, ornaments of shell and animal bone, and *Anculosa* shell beads (Perino 1973b, 1973c).

Mississippian

The term "Mississippian" is used here to refer to the very complex and extensive cultural system which dominated the Mississippi drainage system in the eastern United States beginning about A.D. 900. Mississippian culture is distinguished by a level of technological and social complexity unparalleled among prehistoric aboriginal populations north of Mexico. The following are generally recognized characteristics of Mississippian cultures: shell-tempered ceramics which vary greatly in form and decoration; ceramic workmanship reflective of specialized potters; earthen temple mounds shaped like truncated pyramids and arranged around a plaza; large towns, frequently palisaded; a well-developed agricultural system based on cultivation of corn, beans, and squash; and a priest class and ruling elite, reflected in mass human sacrifice and retainer burial (O'Brien 1972:1).

There exists a large body of archeological data pertaining to the Mississippian cultural tradition and its many regional variants. The following description of Mississippian archeology is very brief and general, since more detailed, analytic treatments of Mississippian cultural systems are readily available. Dragoo (1976), Griffin (1967), Jennings (1968), and Willey (1966) are among sources containing general descriptions of Mississippian cultures in the eastern United States. Regional manifestations of Mississippian have been described and analyzed by J. A. Brown (1971), Cole *et al.* (1951), Fowler (1973, 1974), L. G. Goldstein (1976, 1980), Harn (1971b, 1975), Larson (1971), Lewis and Kneberg (1946), O'Brien (1972), Peebles (1971), and Perino (1971a, 1971b), among others. Goldstein, Fowler, and Perino deal primarily with Mississippian cultures in or near the west–central Illinois region. For this reason, these sources, together with Griffin's general summary, were the most heavily relied upon references for the present discussion.

The reasons for the development and spread of the Mississippian complex are not clearly understood at the present time. Explanation almost certainly lies in understanding complex interactions among a number of variables. Griffin (1967:189) views the cultivation of domesticated food crops as an important causal factor in Mississippian development. He suggests that the shift to an agricultural food base led to a sedentary way of life, territoriality, marked increase in population numbers, specialization of labor, a market exchange system, and elaborate religious ceremonies associated with crop production. Porter (1973:158) sees the establishment and growth of a far-flung market exchange system, with influences from Mexico (probably via traders) as a major factor in the development of Middle Mississippian culture.[3]

[3] Mississippian manifestations in the northern, central, and southern portions of the Mississippi Valley area are sometimes described as "Upper," "Middle," and "Lower" Mississippian, respectively.

Others (e.g., Peebles 1971) emphasize the role of ecological factors in Mississippian development, stressing the importance in the organization of Mississippian society of a redistributive and political network for the purpose of exploitation and control of various resource zones. Finally, Chmurny (1973) suggests that the organization of Mississippian society is at least partially attributable to the adoption of a divided risk strategy for crop production. According to this model, expansion into a number of areas encompassing a variety of local weather and soil conditions reduced the risk of crippling crop failures.

There appears to be general agreement that the Mississippian cultural complex developed in the lower and central portions of the Mississippi Valley, in the fertile bottomlands which extend south from the St. Louis, Missouri area to the mouth of the Arkansas River (Dragoo 1976:20; Griffin 1967:189). From here, the Mississippian pattern apparently spread along the major river valleys from the Gulf Coast to as far north as Wisconsin, and from the Atlantic Coast to as far west as Texas and Oklahoma. In some areas, the Mississippian way of life persisted up to contact times. Early accounts of Natchez Indian culture, for example, indicate that this group was practicing an essentially Mississippian way of life when first contacted by Europeans. In other areas, Mississippian culture disappears from the archeological record prior to contact times. The west–central Illinois region and adjacent areas were evidently abandoned by Mississippian peoples some time before the Europeans passed through this area in the latter half of the seventeenth century.

Although hunting, fishing, and the gathering of wild plant foods continued to provide important elements of the diet, agriculture played a major role in the Mississippian subsistence system. Impetus for this shift may have come from increased productivity of maize varieties adapted to northern latitudes, and the development of hoe cultivation techniques (Fowler 1974:33). In addition to maize, crops such as beans, squash, pumpkins, gourds, and sunflowers were cultivated (Griffin 1967:189). Storage areas and domesticated plant remains at Mississippian sites indicate that food was stored for use after the growing season had ended. Mississippian sites are concentrated near the major river and stream valleys, where broad, rich bottomlands were easily worked with digging sticks and hoes of flint, shell, and bone. Nearby oxbow lakes provided an abundance of fish and bird life (Griffin 1967:189).

A wide trade network was evidently in existence in Mississippian times. Both raw materials and finished products were traded over long distances. Trade materials included marine gastropods from the Gulf Coast, copper from Michigan and Isle Royale, bauxite from Oklahoma or Arkansas, flint, salt, kaolin, and mica (Griffin 1967:190; Perino 1971b:138). O'Brien (1973:103) has also presented evidence of trade in ceramics between Cahokia and the Caddoan and lower Mississippi Valley regions.

The Mississippian period is characterized by a highly organized system of graded settlements ranging from very large, populous, urban centers to single farmsteads. Large towns or cities, such as Cahokia (Illinois), Moundville (Alabama), Angel (southern Indiana), and Etowah (Georgia) apparently functioned as political, ceremonial, and redistributive centers. These major centers, which Fowler (1974) terms "first line communities," share certain characteristics such as large size, organizational complexity, temple mounds arranged around a plaza, and central location within an area of smaller communities strategically located to control resources, communication, and transportation over a wide area. Cahokia, situated approximately 65 km south of the lower Illinois Valley near the present site of St. Louis, is of particular interest here since Mississippian occupants of the study region were undoubtedly within Cahokia's sphere of influence. Strategically located on extremely fertile bottomland just below the confluence of the Illinois, Missouri, and Mississippi rivers, Cahokia is a very large, complex site. It was the most populous of the major Mississippian centers in North America. Population estimates vary from 10,000 to 38,000 people, with a density of from 780 to 3125 people per square kilometer (2000 to 8000 per square mile, Fowler 1974:25). The Cahokia site extends over an area of approximately 30 km^2 (6 mi^2) and includes well over 100 mounds of various types—truncated square or rectangular platform mounds, conical mounds, and ridgetop or lineal mounds. The distribution of habitation debris over the Cahokia site suggests that certain areas of the site were used for specialized activities, such as the manufacture of particular items (Fowler 1974:8; Perino 1971a:109). The site is dominated by Monks Mound, a four-terraced, earthen, flat-topped mound which is larger than any other structure built by prehistoric man north of Mexico. Adjacent to Monks Mound, and associated with several additional platform mounds, is a large, rectangular plaza. Large buildings, possibly temples, public buildings, and residences of important people, were built on top of the flat-topped mounds. Occasionally, platform mounds are closely associated with conical burial mounds. Fowler (1974:25) cites ethnographic data from the southeast (Swanton 1946:726) which indicate that the remains of the dead were placed temporarily in charnel structures supported by platform mounds, and later buried in associated conical burial mounds. As was the case in some other major Mississippian towns, a portion of Cahokia, including the major platform mounds and plaza, was fortified with a stockade. Important people—social, political, and religious leaders—are thought to have resided and been buried within the central, palisaded area (Fowler 1974:25; Griffin 1967:190).

The major urban centers were surrounded by smaller towns which usually had several temple mounds, a smaller plaza, and sizable residence areas. In the case of Cahokia, four of these "second line communities" are represented nearby at the Mitchell, East St. Louis, St. Louis, and Pulcher sites. According to Fowler's (1974:31) community stratification model,[4] these communities likely monitored trade and communication along the rivers for the Cahokia area. A series of yet smaller "third line communities," characterized by a single mound and surrounding habitation debris, appear to have been occupied with exploitation of specific local resources which were tied to the Cahokia redistributive system. Finally, a series of small, moundless sites represents individual farmsteads, hamlets, or villages. Fowler (1974:32) terms this level of settlement "fourth line communities." Mississippian sites in the west–central Illinois region generally represent this small village–farmstead level of Mississippian society. Goldstein, using surface survey data from the region, notes that Mississippian sites in the region tend to be small, located in areas of rich agricultural soils, and approximately evenly spaced along creek and river bottoms. These settlements were likely part of the resource procurement and redistributive systems centered at Cahokia (L. G. Goldstein 1980:22–23).

The complexity of Mississippian society is reflected in the great formal and functional diversity of Mississippian artifacts. The more complex and heavily populated Mississippian sites tend to have more diverse and elaborate artifact forms, a reflection of the fact that large centers could support more varied and specialized activities than smaller villages and hamlets (L. G. Goldstein 1980:14–15).

While the Mississippian ceramic complex is remarkably varied in form and decoration, regularity in basic vessel shapes, clay sources, and firing techniques suggests that pottery was made by specialized potters (O'Brien 1972:36). Basic vessel shapes include jars, deep and shallow bowls, plates, pans for evaporating salt water, beakers, and bottles. These basic shapes were varied with such additions as spouts, handles, and bases of various styles. Animal and human effigy forms were

[4] An alternate model for the Cahokia settlement system has been proposed by Harn. He has suggested that the third and fourth line communities were occupied earlier than the first and second line communities, representing a stage in the development of the Cahokia system which preceded nucleation of population to the first and second line communities (Fowler 1974:32).

produced in addition to the basic shapes. A wide variety of decorative techniques were used, such as polishing, engraving, incising, fabric impressing, stamping, painting (bichrome, polychrome, and negative), and red filming. Pottery appears to have been manufactured for ceremonial use as well as for general use. Utilitarian wares were usually undecorated, or decorated with incising and cordmarking. Ceremonial pots were considerably more elaborate in form and decoration. While the presence of shell temper has often been used to identify Mississippian ceramics, grit, grog, and clay temper were also commonly used (Vogel 1975; L. G. Goldstein 1980:15; Griffin 1967:190; O'Brien 1972).

As in the Late Woodland period, the bow and arrow was used for hunting. Arrowpoints were typically small, triangular, notched, and finely chipped. Fish hooks were usually made of bone, occasionally of copper. A variety of tools, including digging sticks; hoes of stone, shell, or animal bone; manos; and metates reflect agricultural activities. Other utilitarian tools included bone or antler shaft straighteners; sandstone abraders; chipped stone knives, scrapers, drills, and microdrills; ground stone celts, adzes, and axes; bone and antler awls, pins, and needles. Items of personal adornment included beads, hair and ear ornaments, wing bone fans, and gorgets and breast plates. The latter were often made of exotic materials and elaborately engraved; they were perhaps worn by important people as badges of office. Discoidals, or chunky stones, are also characteristic of Mississippian; they were probably used to play a game (Griffin 1967:190).

Diversity also characterizes the Mississippian mortuary complex. The multiplicity of burial treatments reflects the ranked character of Mississippian society. While some individuals were buried with few or no grave goods, others, evidently persons of great importance, were interred with great quantities of exotic raw materials, hundreds of artifacts, and a number of retainers. Individuals were buried in mounds, in cemeteries, in the sides of or under temple mounds, in middens, in house floors, and in burial urns. The extended burial position is most common, although other positions were used as well. Graves consist of oval, round, or rectangular pits, or stone- or log-lined tombs. People were buried both singly and in groups (L. G. Goldstein 1980:15–16).

As with Mississippian material culture, the complexity of the burial program is less in areas removed from the major urban centers. The elaborate social hierarchy evident at major centers is apparently not characteristic of smaller Mississippian communities. Goldstein has examined rural Mississippian social structure in the lower Illinois Valley region. She found that outlying Mississippian mortuary sites reflect a generally egalitarian form of social organization, with a communal rather than an individualized emphasis (L. G. Goldstein 1980:135).

The Late-Woodland–Mississippian Interface

This section is intended to review very briefly existing theories regarding the emergence of the Mississippian complex and its relationship to indigenous Late Woodland cultures in the eastern United States. These theories are presented within the framework of four basic questions of increasing specificity:

1. Where did Mississippian come from?
2. How did the Mississippian culture complex spread throughout the eastern United States?
3. How and why did Cahokia emerge as a major Mississippian center?
4. What was the vehicle of the expansion of Middle Mississippian elements out of the American Bottoms into areas such as the lower Illinois Valley?

Origin of the Mississippian Tradition

The source of the Mississippian tradition in the eastern United States has been debated for many years. Mississippian cultural features are apparent by about A.D. 900 in the lower Mississippi Valley, in the American Bottoms area of the central Mississippi Valley, and in the Caddoan area of Oklahoma, East Texas, Louisiana, and Arkansas. Each of these areas has at one time or another been considered as a candidate for the "origin" area from which the Mississippian pattern spread to other areas of the eastern United States. At this time, most authorities agree that the precise geographical area of initial Mississippian development cannot be pinpointed from available evidence. There appears, however, to be general agreement that the major development of Mississippian culture probably took place in the lower and central Mississippi Valley, where Mississippian sites are earliest and most numerous (Caldwell 1959:33; Griffin 1967:189; Jennings 1968:216; Sears 1964:277).

The question of the relationship between Mississippian peoples and indigenous Woodland groups has also been argued extensively. A wide range of hypotheses has been put forward to explain this relationship. At one extreme, it has been proposed that the Mississippian tradition was introduced by a large group of Mesoamerican invaders who moved throughout the eastern United States, conquering or displacing local Woodland tribes. Thus Mississippian was regarded as approximately representative of a single ethnic or linguistic group. While Mesoamerican influence is clearly present in the Mississippian religious–ceremonial complex and in certain artifact styles and motifs (Caldwell 1959:33; Griffin 1964:248, 1967:190; Willey 1966:297), it appears unlikely that Mississippian culture arrived in the Mississippi Valley via large-scale migrations from Mexico. Willey's (1966:293) view that Mesoamerican elements in Mississippian culture probabaly derived from "diffusion, intermittent contact, and occasional immigration rather than by mass movements of Mesoamerican tribes into the Mississippi Valley" appears to approximate the majority opinion at the present time.

It has also been argued that the Mississippian period represents an *in situ* evolutionary development stimulated by the shift to an agricultural economy by indigenous Late Woodland groups. Cultural ties between Mississippian cultures and local Woodland cultures have been recognized in several areas of major Mississippian development (Dragoo 1976:20; Fowler 1974:33; Hall 1975:18). For example, local Late Woodland elements appear in Mississippian assemblages in the American Bottoms (O'Brien 1972:47) and in the central Illinois Valley region (Harn 1971b:69). However, indigenous Late Woodland elements are perhaps most clearly seen in situations peripheral to the major centers of early Mississippian development. For example, Upper Mississippian cultures such as Fort Ancient and Oneota have been described as a blend of indigenous Late Woodland and Mississippian elements (Caldwell 1959:37; Dragoo 1976:21; Willey 1966:309). Sears (1964:281) describes similar situations in the Southeast, where the cultures of local peoples appear to have been modified by Mississippian influence.

The general question of Woodland–Mississippian relationships in the context of Mississippian origins remains moot at the present time. Many investigators tend now, however, to emphasize interaction processes both within and between regions, recognizing variation from area to area in the processes of Mississippian development.

Spread of the Mississippian Tradition

It is generally acknowledged that Mississippian cultures were present in the central and lower Mississippi Valley by about A.D. 900. A short time later, Mississippian manifestations are recognizable in other areas of the eastern United States. A variety of migration and diffusion hypotheses have been offered concerning the spread of Mississippian culture out of the Mississippi Valley "core" area. To the north, early

Mississippian remains have been found at Aztalan in southern Wisconsin. The Aztalan pottery series shows ties with the Cahokia ceramic complex. In the Southeast, early Mississippian sites are located in eastern Tennessee (Hiwasee Island), central Georgia (Macon Plateau), and on the Florida Gulf Coast (Weeden Island). Sears (1964:277) believes that the Macon site represents a clear case of population movement out of the Mississippian core area. Willey (1966:298) suggests that migrations out of the American Bottoms were responsible for the colonization of the Aztalan and Macon, Georgia areas. Griffin (1967:189) also believes that this expansion was at least in part attributable to migration. He suggests that Cahokia was probably the source of northward migrants, while the lower Tennessee–Cumberland–Ohio area was the source of population movements into the Southeast as far as central Georgia.

The proposition that Mississippian culture spread via migration from the American Bottoms area of the central Mississippi Valley to other regions of the eastern United States has recently been tested from a biological standpoint by David Wolf (1976). Wolf compared craniometric and discrete trait data among six Mississippian skeletal series from sites in coastal Georgia, the lower central Mississippi Valley, the American Bottoms, and the central Illinois Valley region. The results of his analyses suggested that the various regional skeletal samples were probably drawn from several biologically distinct populations. Thus support was not obtained for the proposition that Mississippian manifestations in the Southeast and in the central Illinois Valley are attributable to a single biological population which migrated outward from the American Bottoms (Wolf 1976:182). It seems likely that migration, diffusion, and *in situ* development may all have been involved to different degrees in various local situations.

Mississippian at Cahokia

The period of Late Woodland occupations at the Cahokia site and environs prior to A.D. 800 has been termed the Patrick phase.[5] The Patrick phase is a "pure" Late Woodland, pre-Mississippian phase. The Patrick ceramic complex has much in common with the Raymond pottery series south of Cahokia, and with Early Bluff wares found on the

[5] The Mississippian period at Cahokia was orginally divided into two phases: Old Village (A.D. 800–1250) and Trappist (A.D. 1250–1500). In 1971, the Collinsville conference of archeologists defined eight ceramic phases to replace the old two-phase scheme. These eight phases are: Patrick (pre-A.D. 800), Unnamed I (A.D. 800–900), Fairmount (A.D. 900–1050), Stirling (A.D. 1050–1150), Moorehead (A.D. 1150–1250), Sand Prairie (A.D. 1250–1500), Unnamed II (A.D. 1500–1700), Historic (A.D. 1700+) (Fowler and Hall 1972).

bluffs bordering the American Bottoms. Patrick wares are typically grit-tempered, globular in form, and decorated with cordmarking, smoothed-over cordmarking, lip notching, or wrapped-stick impressions. In regard to house forms, rectangular structures built by individually placing posts in subterranean pits are characteristic of the Patrick phase; wall trench construction is typical of later, Mississippian structures (Fowler and Hall 1972:2).

An "Unnamed" phase (A.D. 800–900) has been tentatively included in the Cahokia sequence to represent the period of interaction between peoples of the Late Woodland Patrick phase and the succeeding Fairmount phase (A.D. 900–1050), which is the first definitely Mississippian phase at Cahokia. This Unnamed phase is tentative because the Late-Woodland–Mississippian interface period is not clearly understood at the present time. It is possible that new data will indicate that the Unnamed phase should be included in either the Patrick or the Fairmount phase, rather than be distinguished as a separate phase (Fowler and Hall 1972:4).

The impetus for the development of a complex Mississippian center at Cahokia has been widely debated. Porter (1973:158) has suggested that the emergence of Cahokia was associated with the evolution, out of a redistributive system already well-established in the area in Late Woodland times, of a mesoamerican-type market exchange system, together with an influx of ideas from the south via traders. Sears (1964:278) has also suggested that the development of Middle Mississippian was significantly influenced by cultures south of the American Bottoms. He has hypothesized that the basic economic, social, and religious elements of Mississippian spread northward from the Caddoan area to the American Bottoms, where they were integrated with indigenous cultural systems.

Fowler (1974:33), on the other hand, does not regard diffusion from the south as an adequate explanation for the development of Cahokia, pointing out that the diffusionist model explains neither the reasons for the development of Cahokia in this particular locality nor the actual processes of integration and development. Fowler emphasizes local development in the emergence of a complex Mississippian society at Cahokia. He has proposed that

> The basis of Cahokia formation was in the development of intensive agriculture as a major subsistence base. This probably came about as a result of adaptation of the maize plant and the technique of hoe cultivation. Village farming communities and a demographic growth resulted. . . . the combination of rich soils, confluences of major river systems and the closeness of a variety of physiographic zones made this a fortuitous area for such development.

Following this model, Fowler (1974:19) believes that the Patrick phase occupants of Cahokia were fully agricultural, and that the Patrick phase represents the beginning of the population growth and *in situ* development that resulted in the Mississippian cultural tradition at Cahokia.

There is evidence of continuity between Woodland and Mississippian settlements adjacent to the Cahokia area. Bareis' (1976) work at the Knoebel site, 24 km southeast of Cahokia, has provided evidence, on a local village level, of *in situ* culture change from Late Woodland to Mississippian. Bareis found indications of an evolutionary sequence of house structures through four construction periods, extending from Late Bluff through Early Mississippian. He interprets this continuity in settlement pattern as a reflection of culture change over a relatively short period of time, perhaps no more than three generations, in response to contact and interaction with larger Mississippian centers in the area, such as Cahokia (Bareis 1976:14).

Many questions remain as to the precise nature of the interaction between Woodland and Mississippian peoples in the American Bottoms. Current and planned research in the Cahokia area will undoubtedly amplify our understanding of this complex transitional period.

Spread of Cahokia Mississippian

There is firm evidence that by the Stirling phase (A.D. 1050–1150) Mississippian culture was being felt outside the American Bottoms area (Fowler and Hall 1972:7). A Mississippian community, with close ties to Cahokia, was beginning to develop in the central Illinois Valley region by about A.D. 1000, according to the analysis of remains from the Dickson site in Fulton County, Illinois (Harn 1971b:74). Mississippian sites in west–central Illinois date primarily to the Stirling and Moorehead phases (A.D. 1050–1250). Radiocarbon dates from the Mississippian component at the Schild site in Greene County, Illinois, center at about A.D. 1065 (Perino 1971a:136). At the Yokem site in Pike County, two radiocarbon dates of A.D. 1190 and A.D. 1430 were obtained for the Mississippian component. Perino (1971b:183) believes that the earlier date is more nearly correct, and suggests that Mississippian use of the Yokem site extended from about A.D. 1200 to 1300. L. G. Goldstein (1980:38) believes that Moss, a third Mississippian mortuary site in the region, probably dates between A.D. 1050 and A.D. 1250, according to pottery found at this site.

Prior to the development and refinement of carbon-14 dating techniques, there was little doubt that Mississippian culture spread northward by mass migrations of people out of the Cahokia area. Wray (1952:157), for example, states that "Old Village was . . . spread up the Illinois Valley [from the Cahokia region] by actual settlement, at least as far as the central area and possibly farther north." Maxwell (1947:29) states a similar view:

> For some reason, as Old Village was developing into Trappist at Cahokia, a group broke away from the parent city and started northward along the Mississippi. . . . They settled for a short time along the Apple River, then pushed on, presumably fighting their way through hostile Woodland groups, to the Rock River in Wisconsin where they founded the fortified village of Aztalan.

This migration theory was consistent with the chronology adhered to at this time. According to the dendrochronological scheme developed at the University of Chicago for the lower Ohio and middle Mississippi Valley, the entire Mississippian tradition spanned barely 100 years, from ca. A.D. 1513 to A.D. 1613 (Maxwell 1947:32). Clearly, *in situ* evolution of a Mississippian pattern from a Late Woodland base was a less reasonable hypothesis than migration, given only 100 years for the entire process of Mississippian development and spread to take place in the central Mississippi Valley.

The application of radiocarbon dating techniques has since greatly expanded the time range of the Mississippian cultural complex. There is still no general agreement, however, as to the relative importance of migration and diffusion processes in the spread of Mississippian culture northward out of the American Bottoms. Griffin (1967:189) has suggested that Mississippian peoples migrated northward up the Illinois and Mississippi Rivers from Cahokia. Similarly, Caldwell (1959:37) has stated that Mississippian communities in Wisconsin and central Illinois may represent a radiation of people from the Cahokia area. Caldwell (1967:139) has since reevaluated his position, however, in the light of more recent evidence from the central Illinois Valley region. He states that the "hypothesis of Cahokian invaders does not fit the newly discovered facts nearly as well as an hypothesis that a resident Late Woodland population somehow became 'acculturated' under the influence of Cahokian ideas and customs."

Similarly, Harn (1975:427) views Mississippian in the central Illinois Valley as a Cahokia-influenced but predominantly local development: "There is nothing in the Spoon River area which would suggest more than a short period of Cahokia immigration, suggesting that the Spoon River variant was largely composed of a Woodland population whose development became integrated with the Cahokia-Mississippian movement."

Blakely has completed a biological distance study of Late Woodland

and Mississippian skeletal series from the Dickson site. Blakely sees evidence from his biodistance results that Mississippian culture was introduced into the central Illinois Valley from outside the region. He suggests that the Dickson Mound Mississippians were probably not evolutionary descendants of the local Sepo Late Woodland people (Blakely 1973:155).

With reference to the lower Illinois Valley region, Perino (1971a) has put forward an acculturation hypothesis similar to those of Caldwell (1967) and Harn (1975) for the development of Mississippian in the central Illinois Valley. Although he finds much evidence for close ties between Cahokia and the Mississippian people represented at the Schild site, Perino (1971a:141, 1971b:184) believes that Mississippian sites in the lower Illinois Valley region do not represent major population movement into the region from Cahokia. Rather, he suggests that Mississippian manifestations in the region resulted from the acculturation of local Late Woodland Jersey Bluff peoples and that this acculturation process could have been initiated by a relatively small group of Mississippian newcomers to the region. According to Perino's view, the great majority of people buried in Mississippian cemeteries at the Schild and Yokem sites are most likely the descendants of indigenous Late Woodland populations which adopted a Mississippian way of life, rather than Mississippian invaders and their descendants.

To summarize, there is archeological evidence that the Mississippian pattern had spread to the lower and central Illinois Valley regions by about A.D. 1000–1100. The precise nature of this spread, however, is debated. Prior to the use of carbon-14 dating techniques, it was generally agreed that the Mississippian culture spread northward by means of mass migrations of people out of the Cahokia area. With the expansion of the Mississippian time range as a result of radiocarbon dating, the *in situ* evolution of a Mississippian pattern became a reasonable alternative hypothesis. At the present time, there is no general agreement as to the relative importance of migration and diffusion processes in the spread of Mississippian culture northward out of the American Bottoms.

3

Material

The Study Series

The cranial series examined were from five bluff-edge mortuary sites along the Mississippi and Illinois Rivers in west–central Illinois (Figure 1, page 3). The Yokem site in Pike County and the Ledders site in Calhoun County overlook the eastern floodplain of the Mississippi River. The Klunk site, also in Calhoun County, is located on the western bluffs of the Illinois River. Across the river to the south of the Klunk site, the Schild and Koster sites overlook the eastern floodplain of the Illinois River in Greene County.

The seven study series and the approximate date for each series are listed in Table 1. Late Woodland series from all five of the sites were studied. In addition, Mississippian series were examined from two sites—Schild and Yokem. These series together represent a time span of about 630 years, according to available radiocarbon dates (Tainter 1975). The number of crania measured are also indicated in Table 1. Generally, these numbers are smaller than the total number of excavated individuals. Of a total of 507 crania measured, 331 individuals provided sufficiently complete data to be included in the biological distance analyses. The burial numbers, ages, and sexes of these individuals are listed in the appendix.

Koster Mounds

The Koster mound group (Figure 2) was excavated in the summers of 1961 and 1962 by Perino (1973a), under the sponsorship of the Gilcrease Institute of Tulsa, Oklahoma. The site is located on bluffs and a high

TABLE 1
The Skeletal Series

Site	Component	Approximate date[a] (A.D.)	Total sample[b]		Biodistance sample[c]	
			Male	Female	Male	Female
Koster	Late Woodland	660	48	49	31	35
Klunk	Late Woodland	700	11	12	8	12
Schild	Late Woodland	800	44	51	11	19
Yokem	Late Woodland	870	30	40	14	25
Ledders	Late Woodland	1020	21	20	14	12
Schild	Mississippian	1070	60	72	53	58
Yokem	Mississippian	1290	19	30	15	24

[a] Based on radiocarbon dates reported by Tainter (1975).
[b] Total number of crania measured.
[c] Number of crania included in biological distance analyses.

terrace approximately 9.7 km south of the town of Eldred and 2.4 km north of the point where Macoupin Creek intersects the Illinois floodplain. Seven mounds and eight natural knolls, which contained burials, were excavated.

On the basis of artifacts associated with the burials and burial style, Perino concluded that the mounds were constructed and used by people of the Late Woodland period. This Late Woodland cultural association is supported by three radiocarbon dates. Charred bone from Mound 2 yielded a date of around A.D. 673 ± 130, and bone collagen dates from two burials in Mound 5 averaged to A.D. 648 ± 51 (Tainter 1975:134). Perino (1973a:203) suggests that this mortuary site was in intermittent use throughout the Late Woodland period. He feels that Mounds 1 through 3 and most of the knoll burials are earlier than Mounds 4 through 7. He also notes elements reminiscent of Middle Woodland associated with Burials 8, 9, and 13 from Knoll A, and the presence of a Mississippian-type pottery sherd in Knoll G.

The Koster Late Woodland mound site overlooks an extensive habitation site located at the bluff base and on the high terrace. Late Woodland ceramics are represented chiefly by Early Bluff and Late Bluff pottery; there is also a very minor White Hall component (Houart 1971:9; D. Asch personal communication). It is the deeply stratified Archaic deposits in the north field area that have been the object of extensive excavations in recent years and that have come to be called "the Koster site." Unless otherwise specified, references to Koster in the present study refer to the mortuary site rather than to the habitation areas.

Following the excavation of the Koster mound group, the skeletal

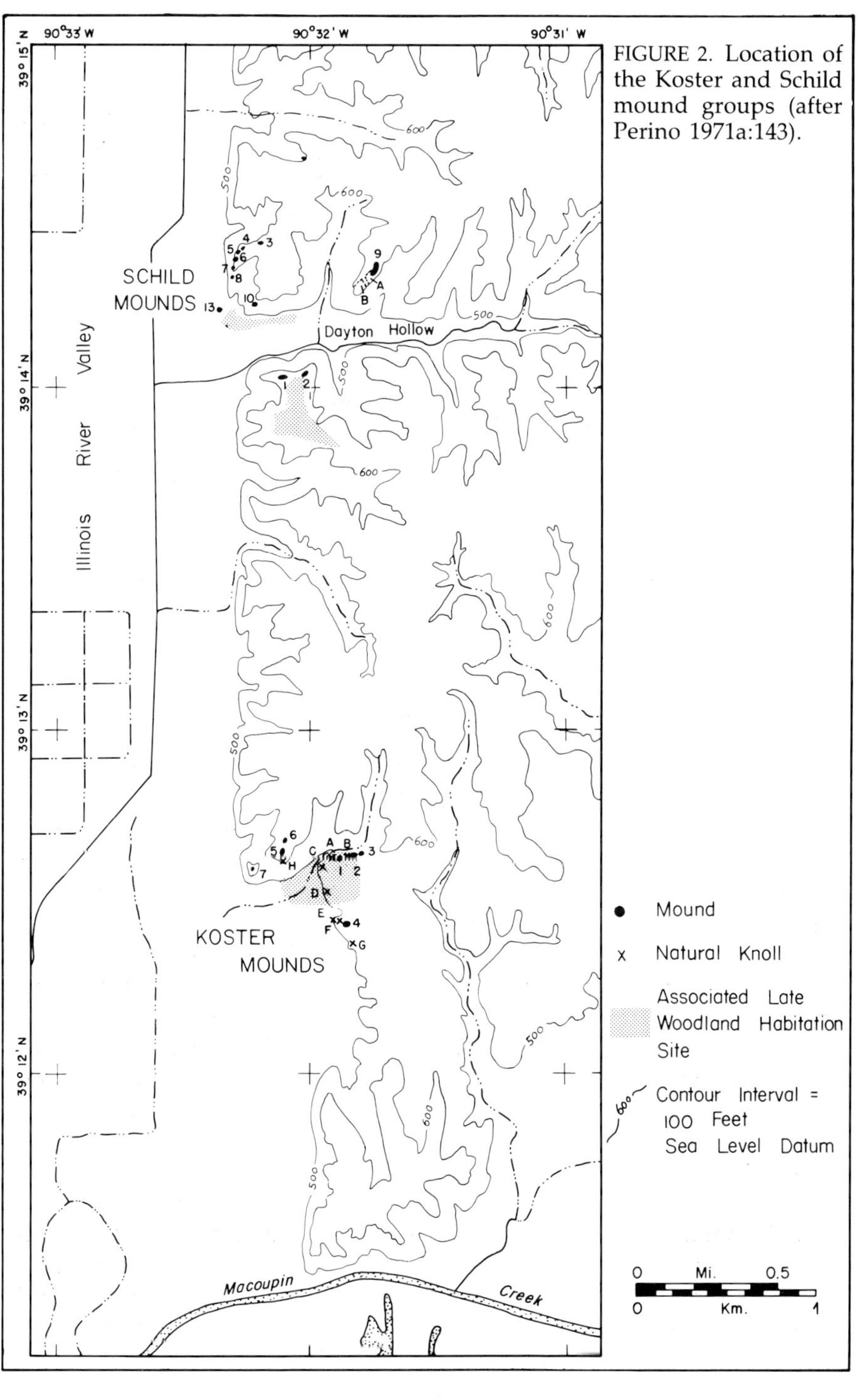

FIGURE 2. Location of the Koster and Schild mound groups (after Perino 1971a:143).

material was removed to Indiana University where it is now housed. The Indiana University inventory of the material, which was completed following processing of the material during the summer of 1974, indicates that a total of 318 individuals are represented in the Koster series. Of this total, 97 adult crania were measured; 31 male and 35 female crania provided sufficient craniometric data to be included in the biological distance analysis. In both male and female study samples, the early and later portions of the site are approximately equally represented.

Perino has raised the possibility that Knoll G may have been used by Mississippian people rather than by Late Woodland people, because a Mississippian pottery sherd was recovered from mound fill about 51 cm above the burial. Results of the biological distance analysis (reported in Chapters 7 and 8) did not support a Mississippian affiliation for this knoll. For the purposes of this study, it was assumed that Knoll G is comparable in time to the remaining knoll burials.

Perino has also suggested that Burials 8, 9, and 13 from Knoll A may be of Late Hopewell origin. These individuals were not included in the study series.

Klunk Late Woodland

The Klunk skeletal series was excavated from mounds located on land owned by Peter Klunk on the Illinois Valley bluff crest northwest of the present village of Kampsville (Figure 3). This mound group—named the Pete Klunk mound group by Perino—is oriented in a north–south direction along the bluff crest. The excavation, sponsored by the Gilcrease Institute, was carried out by Perino (1968, 1973b) during the summers of 1960 and 1961. A nearby mound group was named the Ben Klunk group by Perino. In this study, references to the Klunk mound group pertain only to the Pete Klunk mounds.

The Klunk site included Archaic, Middle Woodland, and Late Woodland components. The three components were distingushed by Perino on the basis of burial position and associated artifacts. Skeletal material examined in the present study is from the Late Woodland component, which includes Mounds 8, 9, 10, and 14. Perino (1973b) has suggested that Mounds 8, 9, and 10 were early Late Woodland, while Mound 14, which contained certain Mississippian elements along with Late Woodland traits, was used at a later date. Two radiocarbon dates are available from the Late Woodland Klunk mounds. A charred log from Mound 8 has been dated at A.D. 622 ± 112, and charcoal from Mound 10 has been dated at A.D. 800 ± 130 (Tainter 1975:134). Thus the Klunk series appears to be slightly more recent than the Koster series.

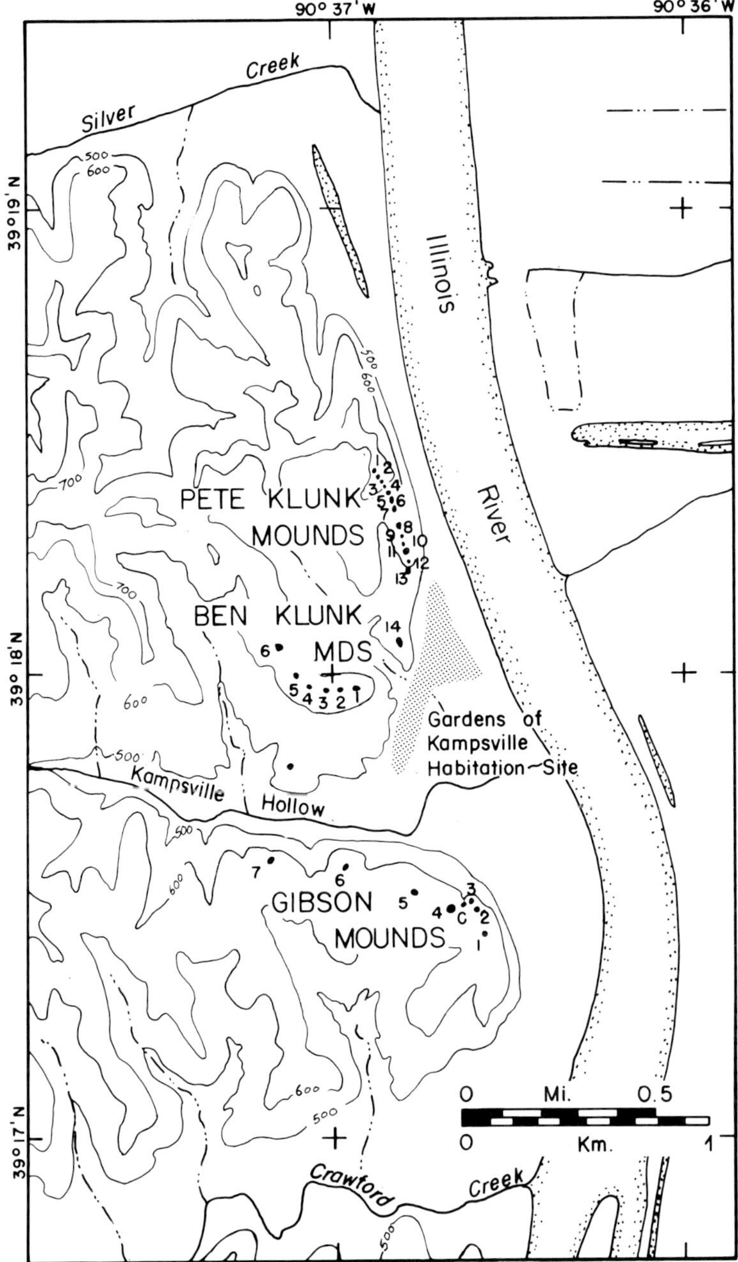

FIGURE 3. Location of the Ben and Pete Klunk mound groups. Contour interval = 100 feet; sea level datum. (After Asch 1976:14.)

According to Perino's (1973b) site report, approximately 55 individuals were excavated from the Late Woodland mounds. Of the total series, 23 adult crania were measured; 8 males and 12 females were sufficiently complete to provide data for the biological distance analysis. The male biodistance sample was made up of 3 individuals from Mound 8, 1 individual from Mound 10, and 4 individuals from Mound 14. All 12 of the female crania were from Mound 8.

The Klunk Late Woodland series is housed at Indiana University, along with the Middle Woodland and Archaic series from the Klunk site.

Ledders

The Ledders site is situated near Mozier, in Calhoun County (Figure 4). Two bluff-crest mounds were excavated by Buikstra (1971) in the fall of 1970 and the summer of 1971. Artifacts associated with the burials were typical of the Jersey Bluff phase of the Late Woodland period. Available bone collagen dates support this Late Woodland association; three bone samples from Mound 1 yielded an average date of A.D. 1018 ± 30 (Tainter 1975:138). Thus the Ledders series is the most recent of the five Late Woodland series considered here.

A total of 259 individuals were recovered from the Ledders mounds, according to the inventory on file at Northwestern University where the series is currently housed. Forty-one adult crania were measured for the present study. Of this total, 14 male and 12 female crania provided sufficiently complete data to be included in the biodistance analysis.

Schild

The Schild site is approximately 6.4 km south of the town of Eldred. This bluff-crest site overlooks the Illinois Valley floodplain to the west, and Dayton Hollow, a tributary valley, to the south (Figure 2). It is approximately 3.2 km north of the Koster mound group. At least 13 mounds, a Mississippian cemetery, scattered individual burials, and Late Woodland habitation areas were located. During the 1962 field season, Perino (1971a, 1973c) excavated nine Late Woodland mounds and a Mississippian cemetery located in natural knolls, designated Knolls A and B. Mounds 1 and 2 and a Late Woodland habitation area were located on the southern bluffs overlooking Dayton Hollow and the Illinois River valley. Mound 9 and the Mississippian cemetery were located across the hollow on the northern bluff crest. Mounds 3 through

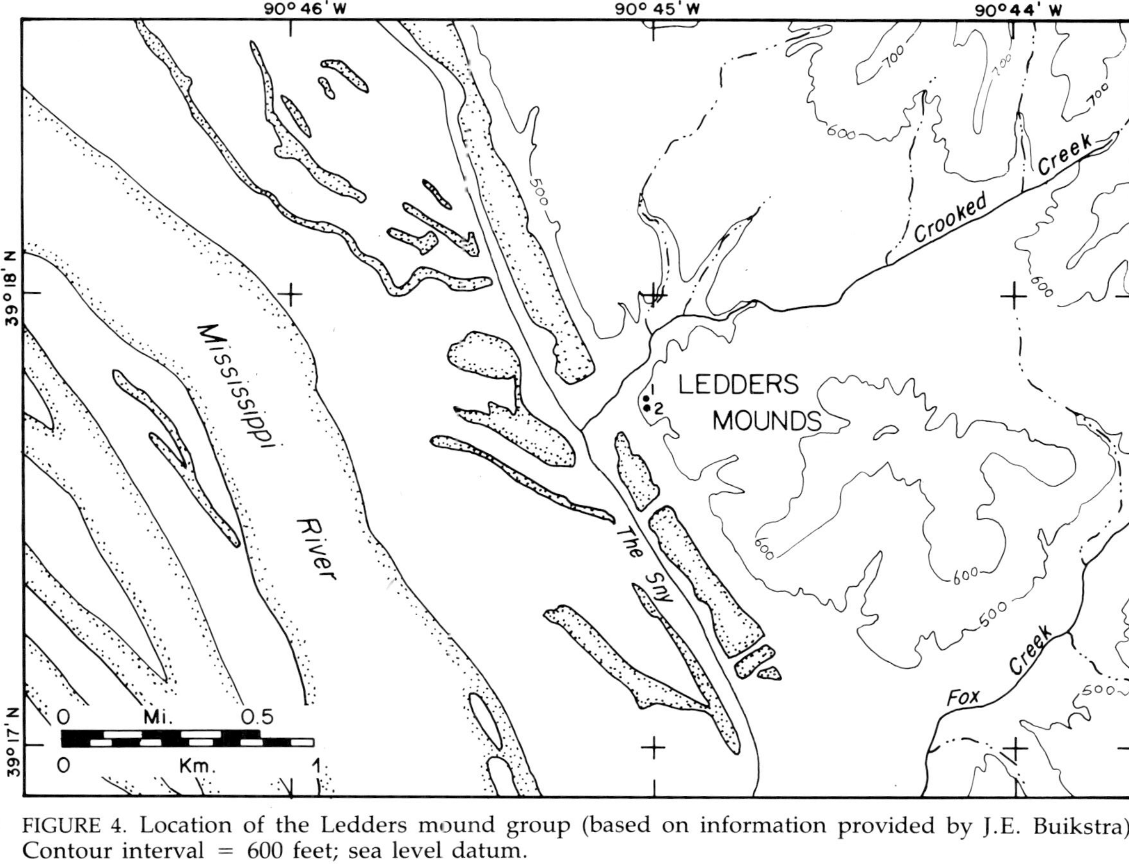

FIGURE 4. Location of the Ledders mound group (based on information provided by J.E. Buikstra). Contour interval = 600 feet; sea level datum.

8 overlooked the Illinois Valley to the northwest of Mound 9 and the Mississippian cemetery. A second Late Woodland habitation area was located on a ridge below the bluffs on the north side of Dayton Hollow (Perino 1971a).

The Schild Mississippian cemetery was large. If it was used by a single Mississippian community, this community would have been proportionately large. There is a small temple mound in the valley at the mouth of Dayton Hollow. However, there is very little evidence of Mississippian habitation in the area. Perino (1971a:8) suggests, therefore, that the habitation site(s) of the Schild Mississippians who used the cemetery may have been obliterated by natural erosional and depositional processes. He also raises the possibility that many of the individuals buried in the Schild Mississippian cemetery may have been transported there from other areas for burial. Mississippian mortuary practices at Schild were investigated in detail by L. G. Goldstein (1980).

Late Woodland and Mississippian components at the Schild site were distinguished by Perino (1971a, 1973c) on the basis of artifact typology and burial style. In regard to the Late Woodland component, Perino (1973c) suggests that Mounds 1, 2, and 9 may date to later in the Late Woodland period than Mounds 3 through 8. Radiocarbon dates (Tainter 1975:135) from the Late Woodland Schild mounds are consistent with the Late Woodland typological association, but they do not support the suggestion that Mounds 1, 2, and 9 are later than Mounds 3 through 8. Two collagen samples from Mound 9 yielded an average date of A.D. 759 ± 47. A date of A.D. 839 ± 71 was obtained from bone from Mound 3. Thus the Late Woodland component probably dates to around A.D. 800, aproximately 150 years later than the Koster mounds and about 100 years later than the Klunk Late Woodland remains.

Radiocarbon dates are also available for the Mississippian component of the Schild site. Charred wood, bone, and corn from Knoll B were dated at A.D. 943 ± 114, while charred wood, bone, and hickory nuts from Knoll A were dated at A.D. 1194 ± 114 (Tainter 1975). On typological grounds, Perino (1971a) suggests a reverse temporal relationship between the two knolls; artifacts found in Knoll A appear to be earlier in style than those found in Knoll B. However, Perino does accept an approximate date of A.D. 1069, the average of the two radiocarbon dates, for the Mississippian component as a whole. Thus the Mississippian component appears to postdate the Late Woodland component by approximately 250 years. Perino (1971a:136) describes the Schild Mississippian component as Mississippian "with Late Woodland affiliations." He suggests that the Schild people were basically Mississippian in terms of socioeconomic and religious organization, although Late

Woodland elements continue in certain ceramic and mortuary characteristics.

The skeletal material from the Schild site was processed and inventoried during the summers of 1973 and 1974, and is currently curated by Indiana University. The Indiana University inventory of the material indicates that 349 individuals were recovered from the Late Woodland mounds, and 449 individuals were excavated from the Mississippian cemetery. Although the total number of individuals represented in the Late Woodland series is large, the series is markedly less well-preserved than the Mississippian series. As a consequence, data from the Late Woodland series were considerably less complete than data from the Mississippian crania. A total of 95 adult Schild Late Woodland crania were measured; data from 11 male and 19 female skulls were used for the biological distance analysis. The major portion of the Late Woodland crania used in the biological distance analysis comes from Mounds 1, 3, and 9. The Schild Mississippian series, in contrast to the Late Woodland series, is remarkably well-preserved, and contains a large number of virtually complete crania. For the biological distance analysis, the male sample included 53 crania (21 from Knoll A and 32 from Knoll B), and the female sample contained 58 crania (32 from Knoll A and 26 from Knoll B).

Yokem

The Yokem site is located a short distance south of the intersection of Two Mile Creek with the Mississippi River floodplain (Figure 5), about 3.2 km south of the town of Atlas in Pike County. Yokem is a bluff-crest site which contained at least 18 mounds, a Late Woodland village area, and earlier Late Woodland refuse pits. Nine mounds were excavated by Perino (1971b, n.d.) during the 1967 and 1968 field seasons.

Perino (1971b) distinguished Late Woodland and Mississippian components at the Yokem site on the basis of associated artifacts and mortuary practices. The lower part of Mound 3, and Mounds 4 and 5 were attributed to Late Woodland Jersey Bluff peoples. Mounds 6, 7, 8, and 9, which contained stone tombs, were also Late Woodland, possibly predating the Jersey Bluff phase. The Mississippian component was represented by Mounds 1, 2, and the upper part of Mound 3. Available radiocarbon dates (Tainter 1975:135) support Perino's chronology. Charcoal from the crematory between Mounds 6 and 7 yielded a date of A.D. 924 ± 124, and charcoal samples from Mounds 7 and 8 were both dated at A.D. 886 ± 130. A bone collagen date of A.D. 790 ± 130 was obtained from Mound 9. These dates average to ca. A.D. 870. Thus the

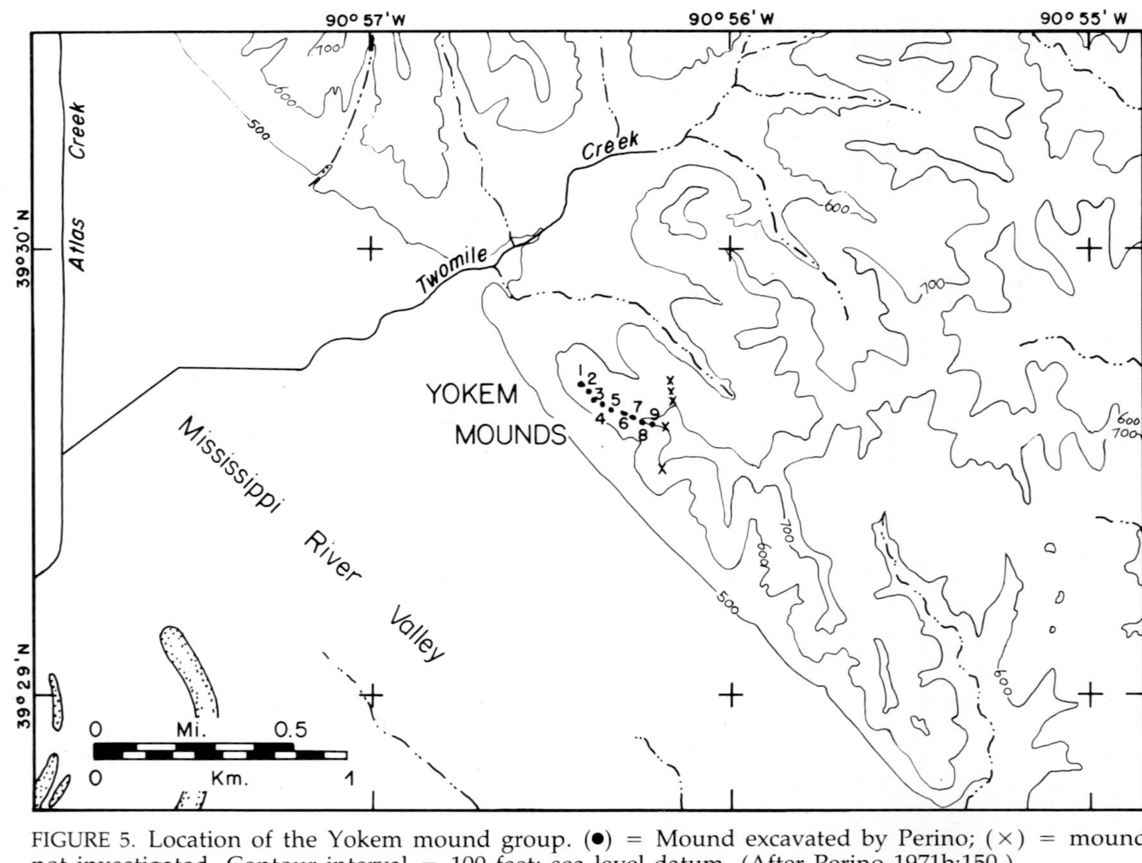

FIGURE 5. Location of the Yokem mound group. (●) = Mound excavated by Perino; (×) = mound not investigated. Contour interval = 100 feet; sea level datum. (After Perino 1971b:150.)

Yokem series appears to be somewhat more recent than the Schild, Klunk, and Koster Late Woodland series, and 100 to 150 years earlier than the Late Woodland Ledders series.

Two radiocarbon dates (Tainter 1975:136) were obtained from Mississippian materials at the Yokem site. Charred wood and bone from the wooden structure in Mound 3 were dated to A.D. 1185 ± 114, and charcoal from the wooden structure in Mound 2 yielded a date of A.D. 1399 ± 114. Perino believes that the date from Mound 3 is probably more accurate, and suggests a probable date of A.D. 1200–1300 for the Yokem Mississippian component (Perino 1971b:182). Thus, the Yokem Mississippian series appears to be 150 to 250 years younger than the Mississippian series from the Schild site. Like the Schild Mississippians, Perino (1971b:153) regards the people represented by the Yokem Mississippian component as an "acculturated Mississippian–Late Woodland group." In other words, he views the Mississippian skeletons as representing a Late Woodland people, or their descendants, who had adopted, or were in the process of adopting, a Mississippian way of life in response to influences from Cahokia to the south.

The skeletal remains of over 350 individuals were excavated from the Yokem mounds according to Perino's (1971b, n.d.) reports. Preservation at the Yokem site ranged widely, from excellent to very poor. Approximately 100 burials were associated with the Mississippian component, while the remainder were assocated with the Late Woodland component. A final inventory of the material, which is housed at Indiana University, is in progress at the present time.

The Yokem Late Woodland series measured for this study consisted of 70 adult crania. Of this total, 14 male and 25 female skulls were sufficiently complete to be included in the biodistance analysis. A total of 49 Mississippian crania were measured. The Mississippian series for the biological distance analysis was made up of 15 males and 24 females.

Perino's (1971b:153, n.d.:4) separation of components was followed in separating Late Woodland from Mississippian burials. That is, burials from Mounds 1 and 2—together with Burials 78, 91, 92, 97, 103, 104, 111, 112, 113, 115, 116, and 117 from Mound 3—were included in the Mississippian series. These Mound 3 burials were associated with a Mississippian charnel structure constructed along the eastern edge of the earlier Late Woodland mound. The remainder of the burials from Mound 3 and burials from Mounds 4 through 9 were included in the Late Woodland series. Due to factors of preservation, all but one male and one female in the Late Woodland series were from Mounds 3, 4, and 5, which Perino regarded as late Late Woodland Jersey Bluff.

Sex and Age Determination

Sex Determination

Metric data from male and female crania were treated separately in the biological distance analysis so as to exclude within-group variability contributed by sexual dimorphism. Sex assessments for the Schild, Koster, Klunk, and Yokem series were made by the writer following at least two observations separated by an interval of one month or more. Independent determinations were made by at least one additional observer. Whenever possible, discrepancies were resolved with the assistance of a third observer. Only one observation was made by the writer for the Ledders series; assessments were consistent with sex determinations made previously by Buikstra and her students at Northwestern University.

Sex was determined primarily on the basis of sexually dimorphic features of innominate, skull, and long bone morphology (Bass 1971; Brothwell 1965; Genovés 1959; Hrdlička 1939; Krogman 1962; Phenice 1969). All available parts of the skeleton were used in making final judgments. No attempt was made to assess the sex of subadults since sex indicators in juveniles are generally unreliable.

Innominate morphology, which reflects differences in reproductive functions between the sexes, is generally regarded as the most reliable morphological sex indicator (Bass 1971; Hrdlička 1939; Krogman 1962; Washburn 1948). Features of the bony pelvis were therefore weighted most heavily in determining the sex of individuals in the study series. Particular attention was paid to the shape of the pubis, size of the subpubic angle, shape of the obturator foramen, size and position of the acetabulum, breadth of the sciatic notch, incidence and size of the preauricular sulcus, and the presence or absence of scarring on the dorsal surface of the pubic bone.

In cases where the innominates were fragmentary or absent, cranial and femur morphology were used as a basis for sex determination. Features of the skull used as sex indicators included size and rugosity of the mastoid processes, nuchal lines, and other sites of muscle attachment; size of the supraorbital ridges, frontal and parietal bossing; chin form; and gonial angle. Size and shape of the head of the femur and size of the angle between the neck and shaft axes were observed in the femur. Finally, areas of muscle attachment on the long bones and general skeletal robusticity were considered.

The ischio–pubic index (Schultz 1930; Washburn 1948, 1949) was used to assign sex when morphological criteria did not provide a clear indication of sex. The distribution of this index in 100 essentially complete Schild Mississippian skeletons (Figure 6) was used as a standard of sexual dimorphism in the index.

Limited sexual dimorphism in the crania of prehistoric midwestern skeletal series has been noted previously (Buikstra 1976:8; Hrdlička 1910:103). Although sexual dimorphism in the skull was not marked in the study series, particularly in the Schild Mississippian series, sexual differences in the innominate were such that disagreements between observers were few. In virtually all cases where assessments differed between observers, the skeleton was incomplete, and insufficient craniometric data were obtained to include the individual in question in the samples for this investigation.

Age Determination

The majority of subadolescent individuals in the Schild, Koster, and Yokem series were aged by, or under the close supervision of, Della Cook. Estimates of age for the Schild and Koster adults are my own, following at least two observations separated by a minimum time period of one month. These adult series were also aged independently by at least one other observer. For the Yokem series, pubic symphysis age estimates were made by the author, Della Cook, Sue Winder, and Carol

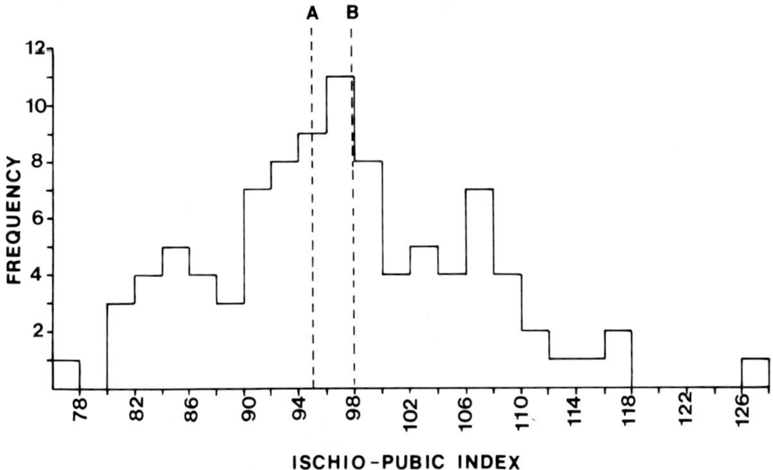

FIGURE 6. Distribution of the ischio-pubic index in the Schild Mississippian series. Sectioning points *A* and *B* represent, respectively, the lower limit of the female range and the upper limit of the male range. The index ranges from 77.4 to 97.8 in males and from 95.5 to 127.8 in females.

Cottom. Differences of opinion were resolved at the time of observation. Final age assessments for the Yokem series were made by the writer based on these pubic symphysis observations and subsequent examination of cranial age indicators. Age estimates for the Klunk Late Woodland series are those agreed upon by myself, Sue Winder, and Brian Fields, following independent observations. The Ledders series was aged by Jane Buikstra and her students. I reexamined a sample of adult Ledders individuals to assure that aging criteria were comparable to those applied to the other series.

Criteria used to determine skeletal age varied with the maturity and completeness of the skeleton. For infants and prepubescent children, standards of dental development (Schour and Massler 1941; Thoma and Goldman 1960), including crown formation, eruption, and root development, were used wherever possible. Other criteria included fusion of the mandibular symphysis, closure of the metopic suture, fusion of vertebral elements, development of the occipital bone (Redfield 1970), and long bone diaphysis length (D. C. Cook 1972; Johnson 1962). Adolescent individuals were aged primarily according to standards of epiphysial union in long bones (Johnson 1961; MacKay 1961). Dental development and, in particular, root development was also useful in aging adolescents.

The reliability of age estimates decreases significantly as age increases in adulthood. Incompleteness of skeletal material compounds the difficulties encountered in aging mature individuals. Furthermore, available aging standards have been developed largely on the basis of data from modern, white cadaver series. To the extent that aging processes are population specific, application of these standards to prehistoric American Indians involves an unknown degree of error. Due to limitations in the reliability of adult aging standards, precise age determinations were not attempted for adult individuals in the study series. Adults were assigned to 15-year age intervals: young (20–34.9), middle-aged (35–49.9), and old (50+). Individuals under 20 years of age were not included in the cranial samples used for the biological distance analyses.

Multiple criteria were considered in assigning ages to adult skeletons. In young adults, eruption of the third molar, closure of the spheno–occipital synchondrosis (basilar suture), fusion of the medial clavicular epiphysis, and fusion of the first and second sacral elements were useful indicators of age. In older adults, age changes in the pubic symphysis (Gilbert and McKern 1973; McKern and Stewart 1957; Todd 1920, 1921), generally regarded as the most reliable criterion for estimating age in adult skeletons (Bass 1971; Brooks 1955; Brothwell 1965;

Krogman 1962), was the most heavily weighted indicator in assigning age. In cases where the pubic symphysis was missing or anomalous, endocranial suture closure (Todd and Lyon 1924) provided a basis for age estimates. Other factors such as dental attrition (Brothwell 1965; Miles 1963), peridontosis, cementum apposition (Gustafson 1950), and arthritic changes were observed. These indicators were used only to corroborate assessments based on more reliable age criteria. Since analytic procedures in this study required that crania be relatively complete, pubic indicators were present in most individuals included in the samples, and suture closure standards could be applied in virtually all cases where observable pubes were lacking.

Demography

One of the basic assumptions of the population approach to problems of biological relationships is that the samples being compared represent breeding populations, or "demes."[1] Following this approach, it must be assumed that the seven skeletal series from the Schild, Koster, Yokem, Klunk, and Ledders sites are approximately representative of local populations, and that these local communities buried their dead exclusively at these sites. The validity of this assumption is assessed in this section through examination of age and sex structure in the study series.

If the mortuary sites in question were used by groups of people which approximated local populations or demes, the demographic structure of the skeletal series from these sites should conform to that of natural mortuary populations; that is, they should reflect the general pattern of human mortality experience. Human populations typically have a U-shaped mortality profile. The rate of mortality is normally very high at birth. It declines from birth onward, but remains very high throughout the first year of life. The probability of death declines steadily throughout childhood, reaching its lowest point during or just prior to adolescence. From adolescence through young and middle adulthood, mortality slowly increases, for both males and females. After middle age, the mortality rate accelerates more rapidly (Acsádi and Nemeskéri 1970:26; DeJong 1972:51; Howell 1973:257). According to this model, we would expect the greatest proportion of individuals in the

[1] Mayr (1969:401) defines "deme" as "a local population of a species; the community of potentially interbreeding individuals at a given locality."

study series to occur in the 0–5-year age category; within this category, we would expect a disproportionately large number of individuals to be under 1 year of age. The number of individuals in succeeding juvenile age categories should decrease, with the lowest number of individuals in the 10–20-year age categories. Relatively higher frequencies of individuals would be expected in the adult age classes.

The demographic structure of the study series was examined to see if age and sex distributions were typical of a natural mortuary population. Conformation to the general pattern of human mortality experience was interpreted as support for the assumption that the skeletal series can be regarded as approximately representative of local populations whose dead were buried primarily at these sites.

Before examining the demographic structure of the study series, several sources of error must be recognized. Discussions of sources of bias can be found in a number of recent paleodemographic studies, including those by Acsádi and Nemeskéri (1970), Buikstra (1976), D. C. Cook (1974), Moore, Swedlund, and Armelagos (1975), and Weiss (1973, 1975). These error sources can be grouped into three general categories: bias resulting from mortuary practices of the people who used the burial site, bias resulting from archeological excavation procedures, and bias introduced by osteological analytic techniques.

D. C. Cook (1974:1) notes two kinds of bias which can be introduced by mortuary practices of the populations under study. First, the remains of individuals of certain ages and classes may have been more likely than others to be disposed of in a manner which would make archeological recovery unlikely (such as tree and scaffold burials), thereby resulting in underrepresentation of these categories in the recoverable portion of the mortuary population. Second, certain segments of the population may have been buried in locations other than the principal disposal site. Burial of juveniles in village sites, for example, would introduce this kind of bias in that juveniles would be underrepresented at the primary disposal site. There is no archeological evidence for the practice of burial customs which would have biased the representation of particular age and sex classes in the study series. However, the existence of such burial practices is difficult to infer from archeological remains. If irregularities in the age and/or sex distributions are found in the study series, mortuary practice must be considered in attempting to explain these irregularities.

Another sort of bias can be introduced as a result of limitations in archeological field methodology. Certain segments of the burial population may have a lower probability of recovery than other segments. For example, the small size of both the graves and bones of infants can make them less likely to be recovered than adults. This situation arises most frequently when the excavator does not aim to recover the total mortuary population or when bone preservation is poor. The likelihood of serious recovery bias of this sort is relatively low in the case of the series under study, as preservation was generally good to excellent and the excavators set out to recover the total mortuary sample. Mounds were completely excavated, and mound floors and areas adjacent to the mounds were probed to locate subfloor and extra-mound burials. Exceptions to this occur at the Schild site, where 3 of 13 Late Woodland mounds were not excavated, and at the Yokem site, where approximately half of the total number of mounds were not excavated and preservation of some of the Late Woodland skeletal material was poor. Historic disturbance of burial sites can also result in recovery bias. The majority of the sites studied here had been disturbed to a certain extent by historical activities such as farming, road construction, previous excavations, and pot hunting (D. C. Cook 1974:4; Perino 1971a, 1971b, 1973a, 1973b, 1973c, n.d.). While it is impossible to determine precisely the effects of such disturbances on the age and sex structure of the skeletal series, it appears that in most instances relatively few individuals were lost. Perino (1973c:92) estimates that approximately 15 individuals were removed from the Schild Late Woodland mounds through the combined activities of treasure seekers and road construction. The excavations of pot collectors into the Mississippian remains at the Schild and Yokem sites (Perino 1971a:1, 1971b:149) likely resulted in the destruction of some burials as well. At the Koster site, Perino (1973a:142) notes that "a few" burials were destroyed in the process of land clearing operations.

The data presented here for the Koster Late Woodland, Schild Late Woodland, Ledders, and Schild Mississippian series come from inventory listings of all individuals recovered from these sites. Only individuals which could be assigned specific age and sex designations were included; adult individuals of questionable sex and individuals that could not be aged beyond "adult" or "infant" categories were not counted. Thus the number of individuals included in the age and sex tabulations is fewer than the total of individuals inventoried. The tabulations include approximately 72% of the total number of individuals identified in the Koster Late Woodland series, 74% of the total Schild Late Woodland series, 73% of the Ledders series, and 77% of the Schild Mississippian series. It is possible that these percentages are somewhat low, however. Most of the individuals excluded from the age and sex count were very fragmentary; all of the remains designated as burial units in the inventory may not actually represent separate individuals.

The three series from the Klunk and Yokem sites were excluded from most of the demographic tabulations because complete inventory listings of these series were not available at the time of writing. Available age and sex data from these sites are limited to adult individuals. The Klunk Late Woodland data presented here were obtained from an approximately complete inventory listing of adults compiled by Winder, Fields, and Droessler. The Yokem Late Woodland and Yokem Mississippian individuals included in the tabulations are those adult crania from which metric data were collected for the present study. Based on the ratio of measurable to unmeasurable crania in the completely inventoried series, it is estimated that the Yokem data presented here represent slightly under half of the total number of adults contained in the Yokem series.

Table 2 indicates the frequency of deaths in age categories under 20 years of age, and Table 3 shows the frequency of deaths in adult age and sex categories. Percentage of total series is also indicated for each age category. The data tabulated in Tables 2 and 3 are presented graphically in Figure 7.

Patterns of juvenile mortality in the study series (Figure 7) will be examined first. Juvenile data are available for the Koster, Schild Late Woodland, Ledders, and Schild Mississippian series. In all four series, the probability of death was greatest during the first year of life. Mortality remained high during early childhood, declining rapidly after about 5 years of age, and remaining low in the teen-age years. This pattern is consistent with the general pattern of human mortality experience discussed earlier. In the Koster series, approximately 45% of the total series is under 20 years of age, whereas 54% of the Schild Late Woodland series, 61% of the Ledders series, and 58% of the Schild Mississippian series are younger than 20. D. C. Cook (1976) is researching the effects of ecological factors (such as change in exploitative patterns, nutritional intake, and population density) on growth and

TABLE 2
Subadult Age Distributions

Series	0–.9		1–4		5–9		10–14		15–19	
	N	%	*N*	%	*N*	%	*N*	%	*N*	%
Koster Late Woodland	25	10.9	38	16.6	12	5.2	15	6.6	13	5.7
Schild Late Woodland	29	11.3	46	17.9	22	8.6	21	8.2	21	8.2
Ledders Late Woodland	36	19.1	34	18.1	23	12.2	10	5.3	12	6.4
Schild Mississippian	73	21.1	59	17.1	32	9.2	22	6.4	14	4.0

Note: Percentages calculated with respect to total number of individuals (adult and subadult) in skeletal series.

TABLE 3
Adult Age Distributions

	20–34		35–49		50+	
	N	%	N	%	N	%
Koster Late Woodland						
Males	32	14.0	25	10.9	9	3.9
Females	29	12.6	18	7.9	13	5.7
Total	61	26.6	43	18.8	22	9.6
Klunk Late Woodland						
Males	1	—	7	—	4	—
Females	6	—	6	—	3	—
Total	7	—	13	—	7	—
Schild Late Woodland						
Males	21	8.2	26	10.1	13	5.0
Females	26	10.1	20	7.8	12	4.7
Total	47	18.3	46	17.9	25	9.7
Yokem Late Woodland						
Males	7	—	14	—	9	—
Females	13	—	17	—	10	—
Total	20	—	31	—	19	—
Ledders Late Woodland						
Males	12	6.4	13	6.9	13	6.9
Females	20	10.6	9	4.8	6	3.2
Total	32	17.0	22	11.7	19	10.1
Schild Mississippian						
Males	33	9.5	18	5.2	17	4.9
Females	35	10.1	18	5.2	25	7.2
Total	68	19.6	36	10.4	42	12.1
Yokem Mississippian						
Males	11	—	5	—	3	—
Females	9	—	12	—	9	—
Total	20	—	17	—	12	—

Note: Percentages calculated with respect to total number of individuals (adult and subadult) in skeletal series.

mortality patterns of juvenile Late Woodland and Mississippian skeletal series from the lower Illinois Valley region.

The pattern of adult mortality (Figure 7) is also quite consistent among the seven study series. In all series except Klunk Late Woodland and Yokem Late Woodland, the highest frequency of adult deaths occurs in the 20–39-year age range. The lowest frequency occurs in the old adult (50+) category, except in the Schild Mississippian series where there are slightly fewer individuals in the 35–49 category, and the Klunk Late Woodland series, where there is an equal number of individuals in the 20–34 and 50+ categories. On the whole, males and females show similar patterns of mortality. There is only a very slight tendency for the number of females to exceed the number of males in the 20–34 age category. Trauma related to childbirth was likely a frequent cause

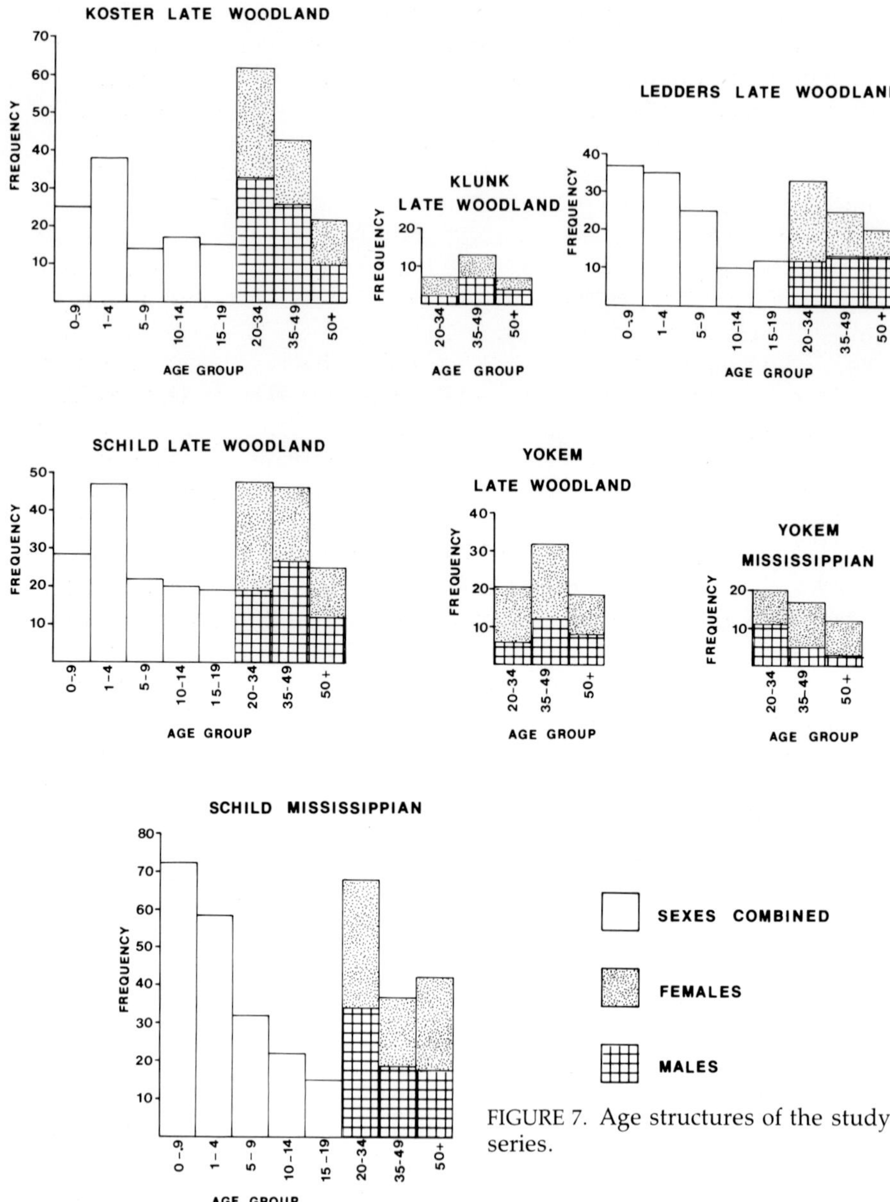

FIGURE 7. Age structures of the study series.

of death among young females. We can only speculate as to the causes of death among young males. Hazardous activity patterns and warfare may have contributed to the high young adult male mortality. Epidemic diseases, many of which do not affect bones, may have been a significant factor in both male and female mortality in early adulthood.

The adult mortality patterns observed in the study series reflect the findings of several other workers who have studied age structure in prehistoric American Indian mortuary populations. D. C. Cook (1974:6), in a demographic study of Late Woodland series from the Joe Gay and Homer Adams sites in the west–central Illinois region, found that the highest frequency of adult deaths occurred in the 20–34-year age category, and the lowest frequency occurred in the 50+ category. A high incidence of young adult deaths has also been noted by Blakely (1977:53) in the Etowah Mississippian series. Bennett's (1973:8) data from Point of Pines also indicate a relatively high frequency of deaths among young adults (20–35) as compared to adults over 40 years of age. Buikstra (1976:23) notes an underrepresentation of old adults in the Middle Woodland Gibson series when Gibson mortality data are compared to United Nations model life tables. A similar underrepresentation of old adults is evident in the age structure of both Late Woodland and Mississippian series from the Dickson site (Blakely 1973:71).

In general, adult males and females are approximately equally represented in human populations (Shryock, Siegel, *et al.* 1973:191). Therefore, the ratio of adult males to adult females can also be examined for evidence of systematic bias, according to sex, in access to prehistoric mortuary sites. Under normal circumstances— that is, in the absence of interactive behavioral practices or differential mortality factors—approximately equal representation of males and females is expected in the study series.

Adult sex ratios (Table 4) were calculated for the study series on the basis of the data used to examine age structure. Chi-square statistics (Thomas 1976:270) were calculated for each sex ratio. In each case, the null hypothesis was that males and females were equally represented in the series. None of the chi-square statistics was statistically significant at the .10 level. The Yokem Late Woodland and Mississippian series, which have more females than males, are most divergent from a one-to-one sex ratio. Although the Yokem sex ratios may be a reflection of sampling error rather than an indication of bias in access to the burial sites, the representativeness of the Yokem Late Woodland and Mississippian series should be reevaluated when inventories of these series are completed.

In summary, the study series appear to generally approximate natural

TABLE 4
Sex Ratios of Skeletal Series

Series	Male	Female	Sex ratio[a]	Chi-square[b]
Koster Late Woodland	66	60	110.0	0.286
Klunk Late Woodland	12	15	80.0	0.333
Schild Late Woodland	60	58	103.4	0.034
Yokem Late Woodland	30	40	75.0	1.429
Ledders Late Woodland	38	35	108.6	0.123
Schild Mississippian	68	78	87.2	0.685
Yokem Mississippian	19	30	63.3	2.469

[a] Sex ratio = (N males/N females) × 100.
[b] *Null hypothesis:* Males and females are equal in number. None of these values is statistically significant at the .10 level (critical value = 2.705, 1 df).

mortuary populations. Age structure in the study series generally reflects the normal pattern of human mortality experience. Although there were relatively more young adult deaths than predicted, mortality patterns in the adult series are not atypical of American Indian mortuary series. With the possible exception of the two Yokem series, males and females are represented in roughly equal proportions in the study series. These findings generally support the assumption that the skeletal series are approximately representative of local populations which buried their dead at these sites.

4

Methods

Craniometrics as a Basis for Biological Distance Estimates

Cranial measurements have long been used to describe biological differences between human groups. Most of the early racial typologies, for example, included head dimensions in the lists of traits associated with various races (Deniker 1900; Dixon 1923; Hooton 1946; Morton 1839; von Eickstedt 1934).

In more recent times, physical anthropology has shifted theoretically from "typological thinking" toward "population thinking" (Bennett 1969; Mayr 1963). The essence of this theoretical reorientation has been succinctly described by Mayr (1959:2): "For the typologist, the type (*eidos*) is real and the variation an illusion, while for the populationist the type (average) is an abstraction and only the variation is real."

Within this population framework, cranial measurements continue to provide a useful data base for studies of human variation. However, the current emphasis on variability and process has led both to an expansion of the range of questions applied to craniometric data and to the use of more complex analytic techniques to deal with these questions. Whereas craniometric data were used by typologists primarily to characterize races in terms of head form, morphological data are used by populationists to address a wide variety of problems ranging from the nature of plasticity responses to new environmental situations to the reconstruction of patterns of biocultural interaction among extinct human populations. With the assistance of electronic computers, a variety of multivariate statistical models are being used to deal with such questions. As Howells (1969a:456) has repeatedly pointed out, this multivariate approach represents a more "natural means of arithmetically handling whole organisms and structures, and of treating them in populations" than the traditional trait-by-trait comparisons of population averages.

Biological Distance Studies among the Living

Biological distance research in living populations has several advantages over similar studies of skeletal populations. First, it is possible to collect data from living people on traits for which the mode of inheritance is understood. Monogenic blood polymorphisms are examples of such traits. Since the mode of inheritance is known, it is possible to calculate gene frequencies within populations and to compare gene frequencies between populations. Furthermore, traits such as blood polymorphisms are not affected by environmental factors during the lifetime of the individual. Thus monogenic traits can be used to determine genetic differences, unconfounded by environmental effects, between populations.

In contrast to living populations, skeletal populations do not provide reliable serological data. For the most part, we must rely upon polygenic traits, such as osteometrics, as a basis for comparing microvariability in extinct human populations. The mode of inheritance of osteometric traits is complex, and not well understood at the present time. It is likely that similar phenotypes may result from a number of different combinations of genes (Hiernaux 1966:290). Gene frequencies, therefore, cannot be determined. In addition, osteometric traits are a product of both heredity and environment. Thus comparisons of skeletal populations on a purely genetic level are not possible.

Population studies of the living have a second advantage, in that data on population structure, marriage patterns, historical interactions between groups, intergroup migration rates, and linguistic relationships between groups are frequently available. From these types of information it is possible to define demes with more precision than is usually the case with skeletal populations. Such data are also useful to derive hypotheses of biological relationships between groups and to build models of microevolutionary change.

Several studies of biological distance in living human populations are briefly described below. These investigations demonstrate that polygenic anthropometric traits vary between populations in such a way as to reflect between-group variation in traits of known inheritance, as well as patterns of known historical and/or linguistic relationships between groups. Demonstration of these associations in living populations supports the use of craniometric data to approximate the genetic substrate in skeletal studies where data on traits of known inheritance are unobtainable and linguistic relationships, marriage patterns, and historical affiliations between groups are unknown.

THE SANGHVI STUDY

One of the earliest comparisons of population distance estimates based on gene frequencies and cephalometric variables was carried out by Sanghvi (1953). Serological and morphological data were collected from samples of 100 males from each of five endogamous groups living in or near Bombay. The serological data consisted of ABO, MN, and Rh blood types, PTC taste reactions, and red–green color blindness. The morphological data included 11 cephalic measurements—head length, head breadth, minimum frontal breadth, bizygomatic breadth, bigonial breadth, total facial height, upper facial height, nasal length, nasal breadth, biorbital breadth, and interorbital breadth. Measures of intergroup distance based on the five serological traits were computed by Sanghvi from chi-square values for the individual traits. Morphological intergroup distances were represented by a multivariate T^2-statistic. Similar relationships among the five groups were indicated by morphological and serological data sets.

THE SPIELMAN STUDY

Spielman (1973) has investigated the degree of correspondence between patterns of allele frequencies, anthropometrics, and geographical locations among 19 Yanomama Indian villages. Genetic distances (Ward 1972) were calculated on the basis of blood group data, erythrocyte enzymes, and serum protein types. The anthropometric data consisted of nine cranial measurements (forehead height, face height, nose height, nose breadth, head length, head breadth, bizygomatic breadth, bigonial breadth, head circumference) and three postcranial measurements (stature, sitting height, calf circumference). Mahalanobis generalized biological distance estimates (D^2) based on metric data from 19 villages were reported earlier by Spielman, da Rocha, Weitkamp, Ward, Neel, and Chagnon (1972). Geographic distances were represented by straight line distances between villages on a map. Spielman (1973:465) notes that proximity of villages to one another is in part determined by the degree of contact desired between the villages in question. Thus geographical distance can be regarded as a rough indicator of the extent of intervillage social and biological interaction.

Spielman (1973) determined the degree of correspondence of the three Yanomama data sets—allele frequencies, anthropometrics, and geo graphical separation—using two different methods. The first method tested the similarity of networks of intergroup relationships derived from the three data sets, while the second tested the degree of geometric congruence between the locations of populations in multidimensional space. The test for network correspondence indicated a high degree of correspondence among patterns of intergroup relationships based on anthropometrics, genetic data, and geographical distance. The test for geometric congruence, or superimposability, yielded somewhat different results. A rather poor fit was indicated between the patterns of geographical location and genetic distance based on allele frequencies. The degree of congruence between the anthropometric and geographical patterns, however, was high. In general, Spielman's analyses support the contention that intergroup variability in anthropometric traits generally reflects intergroup variability in blood traits of known inheritance, and that patterns of intergroup relationship based on anthropometrics correspond generally to predictions made from interaction patterns between groups as reflected by village locations.

THE FRIEDLAENDER STUDY

Friedlaender (1975) has presented the results of an extensive study of biological relationships among 18 villages, representing several diverse language groups, on Bougainville Island in the Southwest Pacific. Blood polymorphism frequencies were used to calculate genetic distances among the villages. Intervillage biological distances were also estimated on the basis of polygenetically determined traits—anthropometrics, dermatoglyphics, and odontometrics—and the results were compared to the genetic distance results. The genetic and biological distance patterns were then compared to patterns of intervillage relationship predicted from spatial relationships among the villages, linguistic affiliations, and patterns of intervillage migration.

Multiple discriminant analysis was used to test for intergroup differences in morphology, dental measurements, and dermatoglyphics. A total of 13 anthropometric variables were included in the analysis; 8 of them were cranial (head length, head breadth, minimum frontal breadth, bigonial breadth, total facial height, nose breadth, nose height, bizygomatic breadth); 5 were postcranial (sitting height, upper extremity length, chest breadth, stature, weight). A univariate analysis indicated that, on the whole, cranial measurements were more important than postcranial measurements in distinguishing between groups. Measurements related to bone growth were of higher discriminatory value than those related to soft tissue morphology. In addition, measurements with high discriminatory value also tended to have relatively high estimates of heritability according to the heritability studies of Hiernaux (1963) and Osborne and DeGeorge (1959). Anthropometrics proved to be better discriminators among villages than either odontometrics or dermatoglyphics. While finger and hand prints showed much intra-group variability, intergroup variability was limited.

Gower's (1971) R^2 statistic was used to compare patterns of intergroup relationships derived from blood polymorphisms, hand prints, dental measurements, anthropometrics, geographical distance, linguistic affiliations, and migration rates. Data from 14 villages were used for this comparison. The closest correspondence among the patterns produced by the various data sets was found to be between anthropometric and language patterns. The three next most congruent patterns were those produced by anthropometrics and blood polymorphisms, blood polymorphisms and geography, and geography and language. Dermatoglyphics patterns were the most different from the other patterns. A second congruence test, in which Kendall's τ was used as the test statistic, yielded similar results.

ADDITIONAL STUDIES

A number of additional studies support the proposition that morphological data can be used to approximate patterns of genetic distance between human populations. Basu, Namboodiri, Weitkamp, Brown, Pollitzer, and Spivey (1976), in a study of the relationship of several Haitian village populations to possible ancestral populations, found that biological distances based on anthropometrics approximated genetic distances computed from blood polymorphism data. Both data sets supported the hypothesis, generated from demographic and social history data, that Haitians are most similar biologically to African black populations, with lesser affinities to white and American Indian populations. Similarly, Pollitzer (1958) found correspondence between biological distances based on anthropometrics and genetic distances based on blood polymorphisms in a study of biological relationships among four samples—blacks from the vicinity of Charleston, South Carolina; West African blacks; American blacks; and whites. Chai (1972), in an investigation of biological variation in eight linguistically and culturally distinguishable Taiwanese tribes, found that the pattern of intertribe morphological differences corresponded to patterns of geographical and social isolation existing among the tribes. A study of population distance among Seminole Indian populations reported by Pollitzer, Rucknagel, Tashian, Shreffler, Leyshon, Namboodiri, and Elston (1970) also demonstrates congruity among serological data, anthropometric data, and known historical relationships.

To summarize, there is considerable research evidence that anthropometrics are characterized by much between-group variability, and can therefore be used effectively for the purpose of discriminating between human groups. In addition, it has been demonstrated that patterns of variation in polygenetically determined anthropometric traits frequently correspond closely to patterns of genetic variability derived from serological data. Finally, human variation studies in the living have demonstrated that anthropometric data, like blood polymorphisms, yield distance patterns that are generally consistent with those predicted from the intergroup interaction patterns suggested by language relationships, migration patterns, geographical separation, and other such factors.

Biological Distance Studies of Skeletal Series

Although certain data classes accessible in the living are unobtainable from skeletal series, skeletal studies permit the investigation of certain types of problems which cannot be dealt with in living populations. Biological distance studies of temporally sequential skeletal series permit the consideration of microevolutionary problems within a far broader time perspective than is possible in studies of the living. It is possible in extinct human populations to study the operation through time of slow microevolutionary processes. This section briefly outlines several studies which support the use of multivariate analysis of craniometric data from skeletal series to investigate microevolutionary change through time in extinct human populations.

THE LAUGHLIN AND JØRGENSEN STUDY

Laughlin and Jørgensen (1956) used both craniometric and cranial nonmetric discrete traits to test an hypothesis of biological relationships among Greenlandic Eskimo groups. This hypothesis was derived from archeological, linguistic, and ethnological data. All of the Eskimo populations appear to have entered Greenland in the Cape York area; from this area they migrated in opposite directions around the island. Since contact across the land was prevented by the presence of large ice sheets, gene flow was limited to contacts between neighboring groups along the island's coast. Four skeletal series, representing isolates on the northwest, southwest, southeast, and northeast peripheries of the island, were studied. Laughlin and Jørgensen (1956:6) hypothesized that crania from the northeast and southeast locations, which represented opposite terminal points of the two lines of migration around the island, would be most dissimilar morphologically due to their long temporal separation. Coefficients of divergence (Laughlin and Jørgensen, 1956:8) were calculated separately for two data sets. The first data set was composed of seven cranial discrete traits, whereas the second included seven cranial measurements and indices. Both cranial measurements and discrete trait data yielded coefficients of divergence which supported the hypothesis that the greatest intergroup biological distance among the four skeletal series would be found between the northeast and southeast terminal isolates.

THE HOWELLS STUDIES

One of the earliest biological distance studies in which multivariate discriminant analysis was applied to craniometric data was carried out by Howells (1966a). Howells' data consisted of 28 cranial measurements from Ainu and modern Japanese cranial series. The multivariate discriminant analysis clearly distinguished the Ainu cranial series from the modern Japanese series. Howells' conclusions regarding the origins of the present day Japanese were consistent with earlier archeological reconstructions.

Howells (1973) has more recently published the results of a much larger study in which cranial measurements from series representing all major geographical areas of the inhabited world were submitted to multivariate discriminant analysis. A clear pattern of population affinities emerged:

> Siberian Buriats, Africans, and Southwest Pacific peoples are a primary triangle of differentiation. Europeans and American Indians have a similarity couched in a lack of cranial differentiation and are broadly related in a northern hemisphere complex which also includes Greenland Eskimos and Hawaiians. The patterning is confirmed by the very detailed correspondence in results for the two sexes obtained separately, and by the ability of the functions to classify individuals to their proper populations [Howells 1973:155].

THE RIGHTMIRE STUDIES

Rightmire (1970a, 1970b) has used miltivariate discriminant analysis to clarify biological relationships among prehistoric and historic groups in southern Africa. His data consisted of 35 cranial measurements (analyzed in subsets ranging from 6 to 27 variables) from prehistoric Iron Age skeletal material from Zambia, Rhodesia, Botswana, and South Africa, and from modern South African Bushman, Hottentot, and Bantu series of both sexes. His results indicated that Iron Age remains from Rhodesia, classified previously as "large Khoisan" or "Bush–Boskopoid," share considerably greater morphological affinity with modern Bantu crania than with modern Bushman or Hottentot crania. Virtually all of the prehistoric crania examined fell within the range of variation found in modern Bantu, Hottentot, and Bushman crania, leading Rightmire to suggest that attempts to define strains or racial types from these prehistoric skeletons should be abandoned. Comparison of the modern Bushman, Hottentot, and South African Bantu series resulted in a small, nonsignificant Bushman–Hottentot biological distance, and greater, statistically significant ($p < .05$) Bushman–Bantu and Hottentot–Bantu distances. These results are consistent with blood group and serum protein data from these groups.

In another study, Rightmire (1972) compared biological distance estimates based on metric and nonmetric traits among several eastern and southern African groups. Several workers (e.g., A. C. Berry and R. J. Berry 1967; R. J. Berry 1968) have suggested that nonmetric or discrete traits are preferable to metrics for biological distance studies because they are more easily scored and analyzed, relatively uncorrelated with one another, show less sex variation, and, at least in some cases, appear to be under simple genetic control. Rightmire selected for comparison six well-documented series of male Bantu crania, two representing East African Bantu tribes and four representing South African Bantu tribes. Thirty-seven mesurements were taken and 18 nonmetric cranial traits were scored. Mahalanobis D^2 values were computed from the metric variables and C. A. B. Smith's measure of divergence statistics were computed from the nonmetric data. Biological relationships among the six series were predicted from linguistic evidence, archeological data, oral tradition, and the early accounts of explorers and traders.

The two sets of biological distances did not correspond well. The results of the D^2 analysis based on the cranial measurements reflected the pattern of tribal relationships predicted from linguistic, archeological, and historical data. The coefficient of divergence results, based on the nonmetric traits, did not reflect this pattern. Rightmire (1972:274) concluded that although patterns of biological variation cannot be expected to consistently reflect linguistic and cultural patterns, failure of the nonmetric data to reflect patterns of intergroup relationships based on nonbiological data "does nothing to support claims that . . . determinations [of biological distance based on nonmetric data] are somehow to be preferred as more accurate, or whatever, than conclusions stemming from the study of continuous measurements," and that "cranial measurements, properly treated in multivariate statistical fashion, provide at least as much information useful to the study of population movement and past history."

THE CORRUCCINI STUDY

Rightmire's conclusion regarding the utility of metric traits in population studies is supported by a later study by Corruccini (1974). Corruccini compared the ability of cranial measurements and cranial nonmetrics to discriminate between black and white series in the Terry skeletal collection. It was found that metrics and discrete traits discriminated approximately equally well between racial groups. While nonmetric traits appeared less subject to sex variation than metric traits, nonmetrics showed considerably more age-related variation than metrics. Corruccini concludes that nonmetrics are no more reliable than metrics for estimating inherited differences between groups, and advocates use of nonmetrics as a control against other data sets in assessing intergroup relationships (1974:440).

THE JANTZ STUDY

A number of studies dealing with prehistoric North American skeletal material have also used craniometric data to deal with problems of microevolutionary change. Jantz (1973) carried out a discriminant analysis of 15 cranial measurements from five male and female skeletal series representing a temporal sequence of prehistoric and historic Arikara populations. For both sexes, the resulting discriminant functions reflected the known temporal relationships among the series. This result was interpreted by Jantz (1973:15) as a reflection of "systematic microevolutionary change" through time in Arikara cranial morphology. In view of the nonrandom, directional nature of the morphological change and the relatively short time period (200–250 years) represented by the cranial series, Jantz hypothesized that gene flow was the most likely evolutionary process responsible for the differentiation of the five series. He tested this gene flow hypothesis through discriminant analysis of the Arikara data together with craniometric data from the two populations representing the most likely sources of gene flow—Mandan and historic white. The discriminant analysis indicated little overlap between the Arikara and White series, suggesting that the degree of white admixture was slight. The discrimination between the Arikara and Mandan samples was considerably less marked, supporting the hypothesis that microevolutionary change through time in Arikara cranial morphology was brought about by gene flow between Mandan and Arikara populations. Jantz's research illustrates the usefulness of craniometric data and the multivariate approach, both to reflect microevolutionary change in temporally sequential series and to test hypotheses regarding the specific evolutionary process(es) responsible for microdifferentiation.

THE ORTNER AND CORRUCCINI STUDY

Ortner and Corruccini (1976) also investigated processes of microevolutionary differentiation among prehistoric American Indian populations through multivariate analysis of craniometrics. Odontometric and cranial nonmetric data were collected and analyzed. Three skeletal series, representing geographically separated Virginia Indian populations, were examined. The 16 cranial measurements were analyzed using univariate t and F values, and multivariate Penrose coefficients, D^2, and canonical analysis. The three classes of skeletal data yielded consistent results. Biological distance among groups was found to reflect geographical distance. Greater between-group differences in cranial measurements among the male groups, as compared to female intergroup separation, suggested a pattern of gene flow involving exchange of females. Again, craniometrics proved useful for examining processes of microevolutionary change in extinct human populations.

ADDITIONAL STUDIES

Discriminant analysis of craniometric data has been used in a number of additional studies to test hypotheses of microevolutionary change in prehistoric American Indian populations. Mackey (1977) found that the pattern of microdifferentiation among 14 extinct Towa populations from the American southwest corresponds closely to the archeologically defined culture sequence for the area. Similarly, Blakely (1973, 1977), Wilkinson (1971), and Wolf (1976) have used multivariate analysis of cranial dimensions to test hypotheses derived from archeological data.

In summary, a considerable volume of research attests to the usefulness of multivariate analytic techniques and cranial morphological data for dealing with problems of microevolutionary differentiation in extinct human populations. Morphological data have proved useful both for estimating biological relationships among skeletal series and for investigating the specific evolutionary processes involved in microdifferentiation of the populations they represent. The demonstrated tendency for patterns of morphological variability to reflect known patterns of intergroup relationships based on nonbiological data (such as language and cultural affiliations) supports the use of morphological data to approximate hereditary similarities and differences. The use of cranial measurements to measure biological relationships is also supported by the correspondence, noted in several studies, of biological distances based on craniometrics with distance estimates derived from skeletal data thought to have a higher hereditary component of variation.

Heritability of Cranial Morphology

It is generally recognized that phenotypic cranial morphology is determined by the interaction of genetic and environmental factors. In order to accurately interpret the results of biological distance analyses based on craniometric data, it is necessary to estimate what proportion of the phenotypic variation in cranial measurements is genetically determined, and what proportion is environmentally determined. Twins have been used to compute estimates of "heritability"—the proportion of the variation in a trait which is genetically determined (Clark 1956:53). The twin method involves determining the variance within pairs of dizygotic (DZ) twins, and comparing it to the variance within pairs of monozygotic (MZ) twins. All of the variance within MZ twin pairs is necessarily due to environment because MZ twins, which develop from a single zygote, are genetically identical. On the other hand, the variance within pairs of DZ twins, which develop from two separate zygotes and share approximately 50% of their genomes, includes both environmental and genetic components. The difference between within-pair variances in MZ and DZ twins, divided by the within-pair DZ variance, is thus an estimate of heritability (h^2). F ratios are used to test heritability estimates for statistical significance. The twin model, its assumptions, and its limitations are discussed further in numerous sources including Bodmer and Cavalli-Sforza (1976), Clark (1956), and Vandenberg and Strandskov (1964).

A number of twin studies have been aimed at estimating the heritability of anthropometric traits (Clark 1956; Dahlberg 1926; Horowitz, Osborne, and DeGeorge 1960; Newman, Freeman, and Holzinger 1937; Osborne and DeGeorge 1959; Vandenberg and Strandskov 1964). Parent-offspring and sibling correlations (W. A. B. Brown 1973; Howells 1953, 1966b; Nakata, Yu, and Nance 1974; Susanne 1977; Wolánski and Charzewska 1967) have also been used to estimate the degree to which morphological traits are under genetic control. Although there are discrepancies in the results of the different heritability studies, certain generalizations can be made. The great majority of the measurements considered in these studies yielded statistically significant heritability estimates, suggesting that in most anthropometric traits a significantly large portion of the variance is genetically determined. Vandenberg (1962:333) compared the results of six twin studies and found that "In general the F ratios associated with the heritability estimates in the different studies are in loose agreement; in fact, occasionally, the agreement is remarkable." Vandenberg (1962:334) also noted that "F-ratios run higher for measures of length . . . than for measures of width or girth." This tendency has also been pointed out by Osborne and DeGeorge (1959) and Howells (1966b).

The heritability research referenced above was conducted using samples drawn from modern populations of European descent. As has been repeatedly pointed out (Clark 1956:53; Vandenberg and Strandskov 1964:48), heritability estimates are population specific—that is, they can be generalized only to the population from which the sample used to derive the heritability estimates was drawn. One cannot assume, therefore, that cranial measurements which have a high genetic component in modern European populations have a similarly high inherited component in other populations. Nevertheless, there is some evidence that available twin study heritability estimates may be useful for studying heredity–environment interactions in non-European populations. This evidence comes from the research of Hiernaux (1963) in Africa and of McHenry and Giles (1971) in New Guinea.

Hiernaux (1963), in a study of two Hutu subgroups from Rwanda, found that measurements of high heritability according to Osborne and DeGeorge's (1959) research tended to be less ecosensitive than measures of low heritability. The two genetically similar subgroups, which share a common culture and history, underwent a very recent ecological separation when one of the subgroups moved to an environment more favorable in terms of nutrition and malarial infestation. Hiernaux found that physical measurements among the Hutu group in the more favorable environment were larger than physical measurements among the Hutu groups in the less favorable environment, and that the increase in physical dimensions was inversely proportional ($r = -.65$ for cranial measurements) to estimates of heritability for these measurements. These results suggest that Osborne and DeGeorge's heritability estimates, although derived from a modern American sample, provide a reasonable estimate of the genetic component of variation in anthropometrics in a nonwhite, non-American population.

McHenry and Giles (1971), in a study of biological distance among these adjacent Waffa villages in New Guinea, found that anthropometric variables of relatively high heritability according to Osborne and DeGeorge's study were more effective in discriminating among the three villages than anthropometric variables of relatively low heritability. In order to assess the stability of heritability estimates in populations in different environmental situations, McHenry and Giles also derived heritability estimates from their Waffa data, using analysis of variance within and among Waffa sibships. McHenry and Giles (1971:250) found that in general the heritability estimates derived from the Waffa data corresponded reasonably well to Osborne and DeGeorge's estimates of heritability.

The available heritability research is useful for purposes of the present study in two ways. First, these studies support the use of cranial measurements as a basis for biological distance estimates. Although they are subject to envirnomental influence, cranial measurements appear to have a significantly high genetic component of variation. Second, the available heritability estimates can be used as an objective criterion for measurement selection. Since the genetic component of intergroup variation in cranial morphology is of primary interest here, it is reasonable to select measurements which have a relatively high measure of genetic control.

Measurement Techniques

The original variable list was composed of 57 cranial measurements and four angles. Table 5 lists the measurements, abbreviations, measuring points, and sources in which the measurements are defined. The purpose of this original variable list was to provide a data pool from which smaller subsets of variables could be drawn for the purpose of biological distance analysis (the criteria for selection of these variable subsets are discussed later in this chapter). The measurements in the original variable list were selected so as to provide a broad representation of cranial and facial morphology. In order to minimize missing data, an attempt was also made to include short measurements which are more likely than most longer measurements to be obtainable from incomplete crania. Martin's (1928) definitions were followed for the majority of the measurements. Several other measurements were taken according to Howells' (1973) and Neumann's (n.d.) definitions. Morant's (1936) definitions were followed for most of the mandibular measurements. The measuring points used to take these measurements are defined in Table 6.

In addition to the standard cranial measurements, five measurements were taken for which definitions were not found in the literature. Definitions of these previously undefined measurements are provided in Table 7.

All measurements were taken by the writer using standard anthropometric instruments and techniques. Instruments included calipers (sliding, spreading, and coordinate), goniometer, craniophor and auricular head spanner, and mandibulometer. All measurements were

TABLE 5
List of Cranial Measurements

Measurement[a]	Abbreviation	Measuring Points	Source of Definition[b]
Vault			
Glabello-occipital length	L	g–op	Martin (1)
Maximum cranial breadth	B	eu–eu	Martin (8)
Minimum frontal breadth	MF	ft–ft	Martin (9)
Maximum frontal breadth	XFB	co–co	Martin (10)
Basion-bregma height	H	ba–b	Martin (17)
Porion-apex height	PAH	a⊥po–po	Martin (21)
Length of cranial base	LB	n–ba	Martin (5)
Biasterionic breadth	ASB	ast–ast	Martin (12)
Frontal chord	FC	n–b	Martin (29)
Frontal subtense	FRS	max. subt.⊥FC	Howells (FRS)
Frontal subtense fraction	FRF	n–point of FRS	Howells (FRF)
Parietal chord	PAC	b–l	Martin (30)
Parietal subtense	PAS	max. subt.⊥PAC	Howells (PAS)
Parietal subtense fraction	PAF	b–point of PAS	Howells (PAF)
Occipital chord	OCC	l–o	Martin (31)
Occipital subtense	OCS	max. subt.⊥OCC	Howells (OCS)
Occipital subtense fraction	OCF	l–point of OCS	Howells (OCF)
Mastoid length 1 (left)	MDL	length⊥po–inf. margin artic. tub.	(Table 7)
Mastoid length 2 (left)	MLN	length from par. notch	(Table 7)
Mastoid breadth (left)	MDB	po-sup. digas. groove	(Table 7)
Face			
Total facial breadth	TFB	zy–zy	Martin (45)
Midfacial breadth	MFB	zmi–zmi	Martin (46)
Total facial height	TFH	n–gn	Martin (47)
Upper facial height	UFH	n–alv. pt.	Martin (48)
Internal biorbital breadth	IOB	fmo–fmo	Neumann (IOB)
Subtense to IOB	SIOB	n⊥fmo–fmo	Neumann (SIOB)
Biorbital breadth	BOB	ec–ec	Martin (44)
Anterior interorbital breadth	AIB	mf–mf	Martin (50)
Orbital breadth, mf (left)	LOBM	mf–ec	Martin (51)
Orbital breadth, d (left)	LOBD	d–ec	Martin(51a)
Orbital height (left)	LOH	⊥mf–ec	Martin (52)
Nasal height	NH	n–ns	Martin (55)
Nasal breadth	NB	max. aperture	Martin (54)
Dacryal chord	DC	d–d	Martin (49a)
Minimum breadth of nasals	MN	min. breadth nasalia	Martin (57)
Breadth of nasal bridge	BNB	zms–zms	Neumann (BNB)
Height of nasal bridge	HNB	max. ant. projection nasals⊥zms–zms	Neumann (HNB)
Malar length, inferior (left)	IML	zmi–inf. zygo-temporal suture	Howells (IML)
Malar length, maximum (left)	XML	zms–inf. zygo-temporal suture	Howells (XML)
Malar subtense (left)	MLS	max. subt.⊥XML	Howells (MLS)
Cheek height (left)	WMH	min. chord, inf. orb. border-inf. border max.	Howells (WMH)

TABLE 5 *(Cont.)*

Measurement[a]	Abbre-viation	Measuring Points	Source of Definition[b]
Maxillo-alveolar length	ML	pr–alv.	Martin (60)
Maxillo-alveolar breadth	MB	ecm–ecm	Martin (61)
Facial length, pr	FL	ba–pr	Martin (40)
Facial length, alv. pt.	FLA	ba–alv. pt.	Neumann (FLA)
Angle total facial prognathism	FP∠	∠ n–pr	Martin (72)
Angle midfacial prognathism	MP∠	∠ n–ns	Martin (73)
Angle alveolar prognathism	AP∠	∠ ns–pr	Martin (74)
Base			
Basion-porion height	BPH	ba⊥po–po	Neumann (BPH)
Foramen magnum length	FML	ba–o	Martin (7)
Length occipital condyle (left)	LCD	maximum length	(Table 7)
Breadth occ. condyle (left)	BCD	maximum breadth	(Table 7)
Mandible			
Height of mandibular symphysis	SH	it–gn	Morant (Hl)
Biangular breadth	BA	go–go	Martin (66)
Breadth of ascending ramus (left)	RL	minimum breadth	Martin (71a)
Bicondylar breadth	BCB	cdl–cdl	Morant (Wl)
Coronial breadth	CrCr	cr–cr	Morant (CrCr)
Maximum condylar length (left)	CyL	maximum length	Morant (CyL)
Breadth at mental foramen	ZZ	minimum chord	Morant (ZZ)
Length of mandible	LM	length of corpus	Morant (CpL)
Gonial angle	G ∠	∠ between horizontal and rameal planes	Morant (M)

[a] Defined in Tables 6 and 7.

[b] Figures in parentheses indicate the corresponding measurements defined by Howells (1973), Martin (1928), Morant (1936), and Neumann (n.d.). See Table 7 for previously undefined measurements.

TABLE 6
Definitions of Cranial Measuring Points[a]

Alveolar point (alv pt) The lowest point of the intermaxillary suture on the alveolar margin between the two medial incisors.

Alveolon (alv) A point on the bony palate where a line drawn through the termini of the alveolar ridges crosses the median line. It is projected into space, not on the bone.

Apex (a) A point in the median sagittal plane where it intersects the porionic plane (a plane passing through the two poria, perpendicular to the ear-eye plane).

Asterion (ast) The common meeting points of the temporal, parietal, and occipital bones on either side of the skull. If the meeting point is occupied by a wormian bone, extend the lambdoid suture onto its surface and then extend the other two sutures to the first line, finding asterion as the point midway between the intersections if they do not coincide. If the lambdoid suture is very complex, use the main axis of the suture (Howells 1973:166).

Basion (ba) The lowest point in the median sagittal plane on the anterior margin of the foramen magnum.

(continued)

TABLE 6 *(Cont.)*

Bregma (b) The point of intersection of the coronal and sagittal sutures. When a bregmatic bone is present, the sutures are projected across it.

Condylion laterale (cdl) The most lateral point on the surface of the condyle of the mandible.

Coronale (co) The two points on the lateral margins of the frontal bone, on the coronal suture, which mark the termini of maximum breadth of the frontal bone. These points must be symmetrically placed with reference to the median line.

Coronion (cr) The most superior points of the coronoid processes. The coronia can be located by inverting the mandible on a sheet of carbon paper, so that the carbon paper contacts both coronoid processes and at least one condyle. The carbon impressions left on the tips of the coronoid processes mark the coronia (Morant 1936:5).

Dacryon (d) A point on the inner side of the orbit, where the lacrimo-maxillary suture meets the frontal bone.

Ectoconchion (ec) The point where the orbital length line from maxillofrontale, roughly parallel to the upper orbital margin, meets the outer rim. The most anterior edge of this rounded outer rim can be found by drawing the side of the point of a pencil along it.

Ectomolare (ecm) The most lateral point on the outer surface of the upper alveolar process, usually opposite the middle of the second molar.

Euryon (eu) The two points opposite each other on the sides of the braincase which form the termini of the line of greatest breadth. They should be above the supramastoid crests.

Frontomalare orbitale (fmo) A point on the orbital end of the fronto-zygomatic suture.

Frontotemporale (ft) The most medial point on the incurve of the temporal crest, just above the fronto-zygomatic suture.

Glabella (g) The most forward projecting point in the median sagittal plane between the supraorbital ridges.

Gnathion (gn) The lowest median point on the lower border of the mandible.

Gonion (go) A point on the most lateral part of the angle of the mandible. In the case of a rounded angle, determine the limit between the body and the ramus by bisecting the gonial angle.

Intradentale (it) The highest point on the alveolar margin of the mandible in the median line, between the two medial incisors.

Lambda (l) The meeting place of the sagittal and lambdoidal sutures.

Maxillofrontale (mf) The point of intersection of the anterior lacrimal crest with the fronto-maxillary suture. In practice this crest has to be prolonged to round out the medial edge of the orbit.

Nasion (n) The upper end of the internasal suture, where it meets the frontal bone.

Nasospinale (ns) A point, usually within the bone, where a line tangent to the two lateral curves of the lower margins of the piriform aperture crosses the median line and a line tangent to the alveolar processes in the median sagittal plane.

Opisthion (o) The median point of the posterior margin of the foramen magnum.

Opisthocranion (op) The posterior terminus of the maximum length of the braincase from glabella in the median sagittal plane.

Porion (po) The uppermost point in the margin of the external auditory meatus. The point can usually be found by following around the lower side of the suprameatal triangle to a line which bisects the opening.

Prosthion (pr) The most anterior point of the intermaxillary suture on the alveolar margin between the two medial incisors.

Zygion (zy) The most lateral point on the zygomatic arch. It is determined by trial measurement.

Zygomaxillare inferior (zmi) The lowest point of the zygo-maxillary suture.

Zygomaxillare superior (zms) The highest point of the zygo-maxillary suture at the edge of the orbit.

[a] From Neumann (n.d.) unless otherwise noted.

TABLE 7
Previously Undefined Cranial Measurements

Mastoid length 1 (MDL) The length of the mastoid process below and perpendicular to a plane passing through the poria and the inferior borders of the articular tubercles of the temporal bones. Position the calibrated bar of the sliding caliper just behind the mastoid process, so that the fixed arm is tangent to the superior border of the external auditory meatus (porion) and the inferior border of the articular tubercle. Position the moveable arm at the inferior tip of the mastoid process, perpendicular to the plane established by the fixed arm. Take this measurement on the left side.

Mastoid length 2 (MLN) A chord, taken with the sliding caliper, from the inferior anterior margin of the parietal notch to the most inferior point of the mastoid process. If a parietal notch bone is present, locate the superior measuring point midway between the superior and inferior borders of the parietal notch bone. Take this measurement on the left side.

Mastoid breadth (MDB) A chord from porion to the most anterior edge of the superior terminus of the digastric groove. Take this measurement on the left side.

Length of occipital condyle (LCD) Maximum length of the left occipital condyle along the long axis of the condyle, measured from the edges of the articular surface.

Breadth of occipital condyle (BCD) Maximum breadth of the left occipital condyle, measured perpendicular to the length axis from the edges of the articular surface.

rounded to the nearest millimeter or degree. Readings which were exactly midway between two whole numbers were rounded to the nearest even whole number. Bilateral measurements were taken on the left side. When the left side was absent or otherwise unmeasurable, these measurements were taken on the right side. All incomplete crania were reconstructed as far as possible prior to measurement. As a general rule, no attempt was made to estimate measurements when one of the landmarks was missing or when the skull showed evidence of postmortem distortion. Exceptions were made in a small number of instances where damage or distortion was minimal and the error introduced by estimating a measurement was judged to be less than the error which would be contributed by the substitution of a predicted value for a missing variable. In the case of a skull lacking one maxilla, for example, the existing maxilla was measured from the median palatine suture to ectomolare, and this reading was doubled to obtain an estimate of maxillo-alveolar breadth.

The data were recorded on 80 column forms, so as to facilitate transcription to punch cards. All punched data were machine verified in order to detect and eliminate punching errors. As an additional check, 10% of the punched data were checked manually against the original data sheets. At the end of each day of data collection, all measurements were examined for obvious reading and recording errors. After the data were transferred to punch cards, SPSS subprogram CONDESCRIPTIVE (Nie, Hull, Jenkins, Steinbrenner, and Bent 1975) was used to compute the range of values for each measurement. Extreme values were checked.

Measurement Replicability

Fifty complete skulls from the Schild Mississippian series were subjected to two measurement trials for the purpose of estimating intraobserver measurement error. The two measurement sessions were separated by a period of approximately one month. The difference between the measurements obtained in the two measurement trials was attributed to intraobserver measurement error. The average percentage difference between the measurement values obtained in trial 1 and the measurement values obtained in trial 2 was calculated for each measurement, using the following formula:

$$\text{Percentage Error} = \frac{\sum_{i=1}^{N} |x_{i1} - x_{i2}| \,/\, N}{(\overline{X}_1 + \overline{X}_2) \,/\, 2} \cdot 100$$

where

$|x_{i1} - x_{i2}|$ = absolute difference between a measurement value obtained at trial 1 and a measurement value obtained at trial 2

$\overline{X}_1$ = the mean value obtained for a measurement at trial 1

$\overline{X}_2$ = the mean value obtained for a measurement at trial 2

N = number of cases

The percentage errors for each measurement are presented in Table 8. In general, measurement error appears to have been low. The average percentage error was 1.11%, ranging from 0.08% for total facial breadth (TFB) to 4.35% for mastoid length 1 (MDL). As expected, measurement error was relatively greater for short measurements than for longer measurements. Measurement error also tended to be higher for those measurements which proved difficult to take. Measurement errors of less than 3% were regarded as being within an acceptable range of error. Choice of this 3% level was arbitrary. Six of the total of 61 measurements yielded percentage errors in excess of 3%.

The relatively high percentage error (4.35%, or 1.5 mm) for MDL was not surprising in view of the great difficulty experienced in taking this measurement. Although subject to variations in parietal notch morphology, the alternative mastoid length measurement (MLN) was sub-

TABLE 8

Measurement Replicability as Reflected by Percentage Difference in Cranial Measurements from Two Measurement Trials (N=50)

Measurement	Percent error	Measurement	Percent error
Glabello-occipital length	0.23	Orbital height	0.76
Maximum cranial breadth	0.40	Nasal height	0.66
Minimum frontal breadth	0.43	Nasal breadth	3.11
Maximum frontal breadth	0.55	Dacryal chord	1.01
Basion-bregma height	0.13	Minimum breadth nasals	2.23
Porion-apex height	0.58	Breadth nasal bridge	0.58
Length cranial base	0.47	Height nasal bridge	1.30
Biasterionic breadth	0.63	Malar length, inferior	1.44
Frontal chord	0.20	Malar length, maximum	0.57
Frontal subtense	1.10	Malar subtense	3.31
Frontal subtense fraction	2.13	Cheek height	0.35
Parietal chord	0.51	Maxillo-alveolar length	0.96
Parietal subtense	1.30	Maxillo-alveolar breadth	0.62
Parietal subtense fraction	3.02	Facial length, pr	2.01
Occipital chord	0.42	Facial length, alv. pt.	0.80
Occipital subtense	1.81	Angle total facial prognathism	0.73
Occipital subtense fraction	3.75	Angle midfacial prognathism	1.07
Mastoid length 1	4.35	Angle alveolar prognathism	2.09
Mastoid length 2	0.45	Basion-porion height	1.94
Mastoid breadth	2.00	Foramen magnum length	0.91
Total facial breadth	0.08	Length occipital condyle	0.87
Midfacial breadth	0.47	Breadth occipital condyle	2.29
Total facial height	0.76	Height mandibular symphysis	0.99
Upper facial height	0.42	Biangular breadth	0.18
Internal biorbital breadth	0.41	Breadth ascending ramus	0.48
Subtense to internal biorbital breadth	3.13	Bicondylar breadth	0.35
		Coronial breadth	0.46
Biorbital breadth	0.16	Maximum condylar length	0.31
Anterior interorbital breadth	1.70	Breadth mental foramen	0.13
Orbital breadth, mf	0.99	Length of mandible	0.58
Orbital breadth, d	0.85	Gonial angle	0.96

ject to much lower measurement error (0.45%); therefore, MDL was deleted from the variable list.

Three other measurements which exceeded the 3% level of measurement error were the occipital and parietal subtense fractions (OCF and PAF) and malar subtense (MLS). Since the measurement battery included two other measurements of occipital and parietal morphology (one a chord measurement and the other a subtense) which were less subject to measurement error, OCF and PAF were removed from the variable list. Malar subtense (MLS), subject to measurement error of 3.31%, was also eliminated from the measurement pool at this point.

In addition to its unsatisfactory level of measurement error, there is some evidence that MLS is not particularly useful for distinguishing among cranial populations. Howells (1973:153) found little intergroup variation in this measurement, leading him to suggest that it is an unsatisfactory measure of malar morphology.

Two facial measurements, subtense to internal biorbital breadth (SIOB) and nasal breadth (NB), were retained although they yielded error estimates of 3.13% and 3.11%, respectively. SIOB was subject to a measurement error of approximately 0.6 mm, while the average measurement error for NB was about 0.8 mm. These errors are not far beyond the range of rounding error. Since they are not highly correlated with other available facial measurements (Tables 24 and 25) it is likely that they contribute information not duplicated by other measurements. In addition, NB and SIOB were only very rarely unobtainable from the crania studied. Error introduced by substitutions for missing data would therefore be minimal for these two measurements.

Statistical Procedures

Multivariate Discriminant Analysis

Multivariate discriminant analysis was selected for use in the present study because it appeared to be the statistical approach most appropriate to the biological distance questions dealt with here. The form of disciminant analysis used here, canonical discriminant factor analysis (Van de Geer 1971:270), is a procedure whereby individuals and population centroids (means) are located relative to one another in multidimensional space. This is accomplished through the derivation of a set of mutually orthogonal discriminant functions (linear equations of weighted measurements) which have the property of maximizing between-group differences relative to within-group differences. The discriminant analysis procedure also serves as the mathematical basis for the derivation of the Mahalanobis estimate (D^2) of generalized biological distance, generally regarded as the most reliable biological distance statistic (Mahalanobis 1936; Hiernaux 1972:103).

Discriminant analysis was introduced by Barnard (1935) and Fisher (1936). Refinements of the discriminant analysis procedure and extension to the multigroup situation were carried out in later years by workers such as Rao and Hotelling. One of the first uses of discriminant analysis in anthropology was to classify individuals of unknown population affiliation into known groups (e.g., Bronowski and Long 1951,

1952; Rao 1948). More recently, this statistical approach has been used to deal with problems of biological differences among populations (e.g., Howells 1966a, 1973; Oxnard 1973; Rightmire 1970a, 1970b). The increasing availability of high speed computers has contributed to the popularity of multivariate discriminant analysis in recent years.

Discriminant functions (sometimes called canonical variates) are linear equations made up of weighted, discriminating variables. Each discriminant function represents an independent axis, or dimension, in multidimensional space. The general form of the discriminant function (Klecka 1975:435) is

$$D_i = d_{i1}Z_1 + d_{i2}Z_2 + \cdots + d_{ip}Z_p$$

where

D_i = the discriminant score on discriminant function i,
d = weighting coefficients,
Z = standardized values of the discriminating variables, and
p = number of discriminating variables

Each of the p discriminating variables (measurements) entered into the analysis is first converted to a standard form. These standardized discriminating variables (Z_p) have equal variances. A set of mutually orthogonal, linear discriminant functions is then derived. The number of discriminant functions in this set is equal to one less than the number of groups analyzed.[1] Each discriminant function in the set describes an independent axis of discrimination in the multidimensional, discriminant space. The set of discriminant functions is hierarchically arranged. That is, the first discriminant function accounts for as much of the between-group variance as possible; the second discriminant function accounts for most of the variance unaccounted for by the first function; the third accounts for the major part of the remaining variance, and so on.

Each discriminating variable in the discriminant functions is associated with a coefficient, or weight (d), which is proportional in absolute size to the discriminatory power of that particular variable in the particular function (or dimension). The set of weights for a particular discriminant function is derived so as to maximize the distance, in discriminant space, between the means of the discriminant scores (d's) for two groups. In other words, the discriminant functions are constructed such that between-group variance is maximized relative to within-group variance and overlap among groups is minimized.

[1] This assumes that the number of discriminating variables is greater than the number of groups. If the reverse is true, the number of possible discriminant functions which can be derived is equal to the number of variables (Klecka 1975:435).

When the standardized measurements for any particular individual skull are substituted in a discriminant function equation, the result is a discriminant score (D), which locates that individual case along the discriminant axis defined by that particular function. Discriminant scores for each case are computed from each discriminant function in the set. Thus each case is associated with a number of discriminant scores equal to one less than the number of groups in the analysis. The discriminant scores for each case can then be used to plot the positions of individual cases in multidimensional space. Similarly, the average discriminant score for each group can be used to locate group centroids. The result is a spatial representation, in terms of absolute distance in discriminant space, of differences among populations of individuals and of differences among individuals within these populations.

A classical problem in discriminant function analysis is to derive a set of classification functions, one for each group. This set of functions is derived from the pooled within-group covariance matrix and the centroids of the discriminating variables. The equation for the ith group may be represented as

$$C_i = c_{i1}V_1 + c_{i2}V_2 + \ldots + c_{ip}V_p + c_{i0}$$

where C_i is the case's score for group i, c_{ij} are classification coefficients computed for each group, c_{i0} is a constant, and V_j are raw scores of the discriminating variables for the given case. A case is classified into the group whose classification function yields the highest score.[2]

Advantages and Disadvantages of Discriminant Analysis

The multivariate approach, and discriminant analysis in particular, has several advantages over univariate analytic techniques used commonly in the past to deal with problems of human microvariability. These advantages have been discussed at length by Howells (1969b, 1972, 1973), Rightmire (1970b), Oxnard (1973), Bronowski and Long (1952), and others. Among the most useful features of multivariate discriminant analysis is its capacity to deal with many variables and populations simultaneously. The ability to handle numerous measurements at once, while taking into account the effects of intercorrelation, permits the treatment of a skull as a single matrix of interdependent morphological

[2] This brief description of discriminant analysis was based primarily on information provided by Klecka (1975), Howells (1972, 1973), and Oxnard (1973). More detailed discussions of discriminant analysis, including the mathematical procedures for derivation of the discriminant functions, can be found in Cooley and Lohnes (1971), Tatsuoka (1971), Goodman (1974), Blackith and Reyment (1971), Morrison (1974), Rao (1952), Van de Geer (1971), and other textbooks devoted to multivariate statistics.

characteristics, rather than as a set of independent measurements. In this way, the multivariate model more closely reflects biological reality than univariate models. In addition to allowing a more adequate representation of individual specimens, populations of individuals can be more realistically dealt with by discriminant analysis. Similarities and differences among several groups are determined simultaneously on the basis of patterns of both within- and between-group variance and covariance. When the univariate approach is followed, similarities and differences are assessed trait by trait, two groups at a time. Thus the information contained in the variance and covariance matrices as a whole is not exploited. Another useful feature of the multivariate discriminant analysis procedure is that the scaled weights derived for individual measurements can be used to identify specifically which aspects of skull morphology are most important in distinguishing between groups.

The use of multivariate discriminant analysis is not without problems, however. Critical discussions of the application of discriminant analysis in anthropology have been provided by Kowalski (1972), Howells (1972), Corruccini (1975), and Oxnard (1973). One of the most frequently cited difficulties with discriminant analysis is that the assumptions of the statistical model (that the discriminating variables have a multivariate normal distribution and that within-group variance and covariance matrices are homogeneous[3]) are not always met by anthropological data. There appears to be no general agreement as to the seriousness of violating these assumptions. While Kowalski (1972:122) expresses serious concern regarding failure to meet the assumptions of the statistical model, Klecka (1975:435) states that "In practice, the technique [of discriminant analysis] is very robust and these assumptions need not be strongly adhered to." A similar opinion has been expressed by Blackith and Reyment (1971:50). It is generally agreed that these assumptions are more likely to be met when similar populations are being compared, as in the case of the present study, than when taxonomically distinct populations are being compared (Corruccini 1975:6).

Several additional cautions in the use of complex multivariate statistical procedures should be mentioned. It should be noted, as Howells (1972:148) points out, that discriminant analysis will *maximally* discriminate between any given groups, and that the nature and degree of

[3] In regard to the equality of covariance assumption, it has been pointed out that this assumption is somewhat unrealistic within the framework of evolutionary biology, since differences in covariance matrices between living populations are frequently of considerable biological significance (Corruccini 1975:5).

discrimination between groups depends upon the makeup of the particular samples and variables being analyzed. It cannot be uncritically assumed, therefore, that statistical distance measures are necessarily accurate reflections of true biological distances. Kowalski (1972) emphasizes the necessity for careful variable selection so as to avoid distortion of the results due to "noise" factors such as age effects and the inclusion of redundant variables. He also stresses the importance of selecting statistics which yield results interpretable within the framework of the research questions. In short, complex statistical techniques are not a substitute for careful decision making and biological insight; "computers should work so people can think" (Thomas 1976:iv).

Discriminant Analyses in the Present Study

Discriminant analyses for the present study were performed using the SPSS subprogram DISCRIMINANT, written by Tuccy and Klecka (Klecka 1975). All computer runs were carried out at the Indiana University Wrubel Computer Center. Subprogram DISCRIMINANT is briefly described below. Klecka (1975) should be consulted for additional detail regarding both theoretical and computational aspects of this program.

Correlation and covariance matrices, as well as means, standard deviations, and univariate *F* ratios for each variable were computed by subprogram DISCRIMINANT prior to the derivation of the discriminant functions. The discriminant functions were derived in a stepwise manner. At the first step, the variable which maximizes the overall, multivariate *F* ratio for the test of difference among the group centroids (and which therefore minimizes Wilks' lambda) was entered into the discriminant function. At the second step, the variable was entered which provides the greatest overall increase in discriminatory power (i.e., maximizes the overall *F* ratio or minimizes Wilks' lambda) in combination with the first variable entered. The selection procedure continued in this manner, entering at each step variables which, in combination with previously selected variables, best discriminate among groups. A variable could also be deleted at any step if, in combination with the other variables in the set, it no longer contributes new discriminatory information. This stepwise selection process continued until there remained no variables which contribute additional discrimination. At each step, the program indicated the degree of change in Wilks' lambda due to the addition of the new variable and provided a test of statistical significance for this change.

In all of the analyses carried out here, the number of discriminant functions derived is equal to one less than the number of groups ($g - 1$). The relative importance of each discriminant function in discriminating among groups was evaluated according to the percentage of variation explained by each function and a chi-square test for statistical significance of the change in Wilks' lambda brought about by the addition of successive discriminant functions. The standardized discriminant function coefficients, or weights, provide a measure of the discriminating power of each variable in the discriminant functions.

The discriminant scores for each case, on each discriminant function, were determined by solving the discriminant functions, namely summing the products of the standardized variables and their coefficients. The program then plotted each case, and the mean for each group, in two dimensions. Scores on the first discriminant function were plotted along the abscissa, and scores on the second discriminant function were plotted along the ordinate. The result is a spatial representation of the biological distances among groups. In the case of the present study, the first two discriminant functions generally explained 70% or more of the between-group variance, and only the first two discriminant functions were statistically significant. The plot of the first two functions is thus a reasonable graphic approximation of intergroup distances, despite the fact that only two of the $g-1$ discriminant axes are represented.

The mean discriminant scores for each group pinpoint the group centroids—the center, in multidimensional space, of the distribution of cases in a particular group. Mahalanobis generalized distance estimates (D^2) were calculated between group centroids using the mean discriminant scores on each function. For each group pair, the differences between the means for the two groups, on each discriminant function, were squared. These squared differences on each function were then summed over all discriminant functions to yield Mahalanobis distances.[4] The program provided a matrix of pairwise F ratios which indicate the statistical significance of the D^2 value between each group pair.[5] The .05 level of probability was selected as the criterion for statistical significance.

[4] Procedure suggested by Paul L. Jamison (personal communication).

[5] By this method of computing D^2, the sample covariance matrix is computed from the data on all groups entered into the DISCRIMINANT subprogram, not just the two groups for which D^2 is computed. Making the assumption that group covariance matrices are equal, the F ratio reported by the subprogram is calculated by the formula

$$F = \frac{T - g - p + 1}{p} \cdot \frac{N_1 N_2}{(N_1 + N_2)(T - g)} \cdot D^2$$

where F has p and $T - g - p + 1$ degrees of freedom; T is the total number of crania from all groups; g is the number of groups; p is the number of variables; N_1 and N_2 are the sample sizes of the two groups for which D^2 is computed. See Anderson (1958:109–110) for the basis of this significance test.

The final analysis carried out by the DISCRIMINANT program was a classification procedure. This involved the derivation, from the pooled within-group covariance matrix and the centroids for the discriminating variables, of a set of classification functions. One function was derived for each group. For each case, raw variables were substituted into the classification functions for each group to yield classification scores for that case. A case was classified into the group whose function yields the highest discriminant score for that case. Probabilities of membership in each group were calculated for each case, based on the classification scores for that case and the assumption that cases have equal a priori probabilities of belonging to any one of the groups. The results of this classification procedure were summarized in the program output by a table indicating the proportion of correctly and incorrectly classified individuals in each group.

Missing Data

The discriminant analysis procedure requires that there be no missing data—every case must have a value for each variable entered into the analysis. In studies utilizing skeletal material from archeological contexts, however, data are virtually always incomplete. Breakage is common, preservation is variable, and pathological or otherwise anomalous conditions sometimes prevent reliable measurement of certain aspects of craniofacial morphology. Deletion of all cases in which one or more variables are missing would pare already small samples down to an unacceptable size, result in the loss of useful data from incomplete skulls (particularly from areas most susceptible to breakage), and bring into question the representativeness of the metrically complete subsample. Similarly, use only of variables for which there are complete data would severely limit the number of usable variables, result in a loss of useful information, and prohibit the selection of variables on a more theoretically meaningful basis. In order to maximize the information available from the cranial samples, therefore, it was necessary to substitute estimates for missing data.

Most investigators faced with this problem have followed one of three alternative procedures for estimating missing data: substitution of group means, substitution of grand means, or prediction of missing measurements by means of multiple regression. The advantages and disadvantages of these alternatives are discussed below.

Substitution of group means for missing data has the effect of decreasing variance within groups. This in turn serves to inflate intergroup distances based on comparisons of within-group and between-group variances. This effect is especially serious for small groups where the sample mean is particularly subject to sampling error.

Substitution of means over all groups (grand means), on the other hand, increases within-group variance, which in turn obscures between-group differences. Working from a null hypothesis of no difference among groups, use of the grand mean is therefore a more conservative procedure than the use of individual group means. In addition, the grand mean will not amplify sampling bias for small groups. In view of these effects, the use of grand means appears preferable to the use of group means, especially when small groups are included in the analysis.

Both group and grand mean substitution present an additional problem, however. The multivariate approach involves consideration of each case as a constellation of interrelated morphological attributes. Proportion as well as gross size is represented by these measurements (Howells 1973:46). Mean values substituted in particularly large or small individuals may therefore be inconsistent in size with existing measurements for this individual, thus describing a skull of abnormal form. For example, if a moderate mean value for cranial breadth is substituted in the variable list of an unusually large individual, that individual will appear to be considerably more long headed than he actually is.

The estimation of missing data through multiple regression is a much more complicated and time-consuming procedure than the substitution of means. There are, however, several advantages to using regression rather than means to estimate missing data. Predicting missing values on the basis of existing variables overcomes the problem of maintaining consistency in the size of cranial dimensions within cases. In addition, regression-based estimates will result in less alteration of within-group variances than results from either group or grand mean estimates.

Like mean estimates, however, the regression predictions can compound sampling error when missing data are predicted for small groups and when relatively few complete individuals are available for use in generating the prediction equations. For this reason, it seems appropriate to generate prediction equations on the basis of a combined group sample when a number of small groups are involved. This procedure will likely result in slightly less accurate predictions for the large groups. Predictions for the smaller groups will probably be somewhat biased in the direction of the larger groups, but less subject to sampling bias than if the equations themselves were derived from the smaller groups individually.

Artificial cranial deformation is a source of potential error for estimates based on either means or regression. If the cranial samples contained large numbers of deformed crania, it would be possible, through the addition of dummy variables, to take deformation into account in the regression equations. In the present study, however, the number of deformed crania was insufficient to derive regression equations which included deformation scores as independent variables.

Although none of the alternatives for providing missing data estimates is completely satisfactory, it appears that estimates based on the regression procedure introduce the least error. In order to test this conclusion in the present study, the accuracy of grand mean predictions for missing data was compared with the accuracy of missing data predictions based on regression. A series of regression equations were generated for predicting the values of each missing measurement from measurements present. (The procedure for derivation of these equations is described in the next section.) Equations were generated separately for males and females, using the total data pool available (all groups) for each sex. Deformed crania were not excluded. The accuracy of predictions resulting from the solution of these equations was then compared to the accuracy of grand mean predictions for 20 male and 20 female Schild Mississippian crania. Since these crania were virtually complete, the actual measurement values were known and could be compared to the estimated values. The average error and standard deviation of this error, for both regression and grand mean estimates, were computed for each variable.

The mean error and standard deviations of regression and mean estimates for each variable are listed in Table 9. For males, the mean error of the grand mean estimates averaged over all variables is 3.16 mm (s = 2.29), while the average mean error of the regression estimates is 2.22 mm (s = 1.65). For females, the mean error of the grand mean estimates averaged over all variables is 2.98 mm (s = 2.25), and the average mean error of the regression estimates is 2.34 mm (s = 1.78).

With few exceptions, the average error of the regression predictions is lower than the average error of the grand mean estimates, for both males and females. The standard deviation of this error is also quite consistently lower for the regression predictions. These results support the assumption that the substitution of grand means for missing values adds more within-group variance than the substitution of regression-based predictions. Over all measurements, the mean error of the regression estimates tends to be slightly greater in the female than in the male group, while the mean error of the grand mean estimates tends to be slightly lower. Since cranial deformation is more common among males than among females in the Schild Mississippian series, the slightly greater contrast between regression and mean estimates in males may

TABLE 9
Accuracy of Regression and Grand Mean Estimates for Missing Data

	Males				Females			
	Regression estimate		Grand mean estimate		Regression estimate		Grand mean estimate	
Variable	Mean error (mm)[a]	*SD*	Mean error (mm)	*SD*	Mean error (mm)	*SD*	Mean error (mm)	*SD*
L	2.92	2.08	4.73	3.61	3.24	2.59	5.60	4.58
B	3.06	2.06	3.95	2.69	3.39	2.66	3.90	3.29
MF	2.74	1.92	3.97	3.37	2.48	2.59	3.51	2.98
FC	2.44	1.62	4.03	3.18	2.53	1.76	2.84	2.46
H	2.50	2.27	3.81	2.69	2.65	2.55	3.26	2.58
PAH	2.46	1.39	4.51	2.52	2.58	2.16	3.39	2.90
BPH	2.20	1.21	2.63	1.61	1.88	1.11	2.15	1.20
LB	2.43	1.84	3.42	2.39	2.43	1.82	3.51	2.51
TFB	1.89	1.22	4.10	3.12	2.42	1.78	4.44	2.94
MFB	3.54	3.18	4.05	3.26	2.57	2.56	3.77	2.30
TFH	2.10	1.61	4.96	2.88	1.93	1.80	4.28	2.95
UFH	2.04	1.58	3.75	2.10	1.87	1.58	2.60	2.04
IOB	1.77	1.30	3.41	2.43	1.34	1.09	2.68	1.93
SIOB	1.24	1.06	1.99	1.53	1.46	1.13	1.60	1.30
BOB	1.01	0.79	3.10	2.23	1.14	1.08	2.75	2.39
AIB	1.23	0.92	1.98	1.28	1.30	1.05	1.82	1.41
LOBM	0.77	0.61	1.28	1.32	0.91	0.80	1.35	1.00
LOBD	0.63	0.46	1.27	0.97	0.67	0.37	1.00	0.68
LOH	1.01	0.79	1.05	0.76	1.46	1.00	1.58	1.14
NH	1.63	0.98	1.71	1.71	1.35	1.25	1.64	1.42
NB	1.10	0.74	1.40	1.06	1.19	1.08	1.78	1.15
DC	1.09	0.96	2.35	1.66	1.12	0.71	2.13	1.27
MN	1.05	0.77	1.40	1.05	1.01	0.86	1.08	0.94
BNB	2.62	1.71	4.63	2.86	2.77	2.08	4.30	3.90
HNB	1.80	1.38	2.25	1.65	2.29	1.67	2.35	2.03
ML	1.82	1.05	2.86	1.75	1.86	1.08	2.27	1.61
MB	2.33	2.03	3.51	2.75	3.04	2.40	4.21	2.68
FL	2.34	1.94	4.10	3.25	2.75	1.45	4.22	2.98
FLA	2.28	2.03	4.20	3.34	2.96	1.77	4.29	2.82
SH	2.20	1.76	3.10	2.42	2.31	2.12	2.61	2.46
BA	5.95	4.63	6.41	5.21	3.61	3.16	4.09	3.37
RL	1.71	1.08	1.88	1.26	1.65	1.24	2.36	1.86
LM	2.61	1.91	3.83	2.80	3.01	2.30	4.33	2.87
BCB	3.73	2.91	5.67	4.15	4.61	2.80	5.20	3.46
G∠	4.57	3.80	5.83	3.78	5.65	4.78	6.63	5.02
FP∠	1.56	1.47	2.15	2.20	2.49	1.95	2.68	1.97
MP∠	2.41	1.82	2.75	2.58	2.49	2.07	3.41	2.46
AP∠	4.01	3.69	4.68	3.32	4.63	3.49	5.03	3.27
ZZ	2.10	1.22	2.21	1.30	1.23	0.95	1.37	1.23
CyL	1.12	0.90	1.48	1.23	1.40	0.95	1.70	1.34
CrCr	3.74	3.75	5.45	4.65	3.16	1.89	3.70	3.10
IML	1.60	0.98	2.41	1.69	1.99	1.43	2.45	2.17
XML	1.54	1.10	2.26	1.95	2.39	1.59	3.03	2.36
WMH	1.43	1.37	2.10	1.39	1.41	1.08	1.84	1.43

(continued)

TABLE 9 *(Cont.)*

	Males				Females			
	Regression estimate		Grand mean estimate		Regression estimate		Grand mean estimate	
Variable	Mean error (mm)	*SD*	Mean error (mm)	*SD*	Mean error (mm)	*SD*	Mean error (mm)	*SD*
FML	2.35	1.51	2.38	1.67	1.37	1.10	1.66	1.10
LCD	1.63	1.00	1.76	0.93	2.20	1.94	2.22	1.89
BCD	1.22	0.67	1.06	0.75	1.51	0.99	1.45	1.04
ASB	3.00	1.84	2.86	1.63	3.28	2.40	3.03	2.65
XFB	2.05	1.21	4.06	2.78	2.61	1.98	3.70	2.61
FRS	1.27	1.04	1.75	1.50	1.14	1.03	1.64	1.37
FRF	2.87	1.87	3.24	1.86	2.90	1.73	2.57	1.69
PAC	2.98	2.22	4.65	3.56	3.16	2.95	3.63	3.58
PAS	1.83	1.03	2.76	1.53	1.76	1.36	2.06	1.22
OCC	3.31	2.74	4.72	3.34	4.68	2.79	4.61	2.84
OCS	1.88	1.37	2.02	1.77	2.28	1.80	2.17	1.81
MDB	1.76	1.07	2.12	1.76	1.89	1.40	2.20	1.59
MLN	3.98	2.67	4.15	2.60	3.75	2.55	3.99	3.08

[a] Linear measurements in millimeters; angles in degrees.

indicate greater accuracy of the regression technique in estimating missing data for crania with artificial cranial deformation.

On the basis of these results, I decided to estimate missing data in the present study through the use of multiple regression.

Multiple Regression Procedure for Estimation of Missing Values

Stepwise multiple regression (SPSS subprogram REGRESSION) was used to derive equations by which a value for each of 57 measurement variables could be predicted when values were missing. The independent variables entered into the analysis consisted of the 35 measurements which have the least number of missing data over all groups. Equations were derived separately for each of the 57 measurements in the measurement battery. Thus each of these 57 variables was in turn treated as the dependent variable. Separate sets of equations were generated for males and females. For each set, the total data pool (all groups combined) was used. The set of equations for males was based on data from approximately 160 individuals, while the equations for females were based on approximately 200 cases. Missing data were deleted pair-wise from the regression analyses.

Kim and Kohout (1975) have provided details as to the statistical model and the computational procedures followed by subprogram REGRESSION. The general form of the regression equation is as follows:

$$Y^1 = a + b_1X_1 + b_2X_2 + \cdots + b_pX_p$$

where Y^1 is the predicted value for the dependent variable Y, a is the Y intercept, the X's are the independent variables, and the b's are the regression coefficients (Kim and Kohout 1975:328).

At Step 1, a single independent variable was selected from the independent variable list and a regression equation was derived by which this independent variable predicts the dependent variable. The variable selected as the independent variable at this step is the independent variable which explains the greatest amount of variance in the dependent variable. The constant (y intercept), regression coefficient for the independent variable, and an F test of significance for the regression coefficient were computed and printed at this step. At Step 2, a second equation, which includes two independent variables, was generated. The two independent variables in the equation included the independent variable selected at Step 1 plus an additional independent variable. This new independent variable is the variable which explains the greatest amount of variance in the dependent variable left unexplained by the first independent variable. Again, the program printed the constant, the two regression coefficients, and F values for the two regression coefficients.

The stepwise procedure continued in this manner, adding a new independent variable to compute a new prediction equation at each step. Each of the independent variables was entered successively into an equation such that at each step the independent variable added to the equation is that variable which explains the greatest amount of variance in the dependent variable, above and beyond the variance explained by the independent variables in the previous equation. In this manner, a maximum of 34 prediction equations were generated for each measurement variable.

The regression equations were solved, and predicted values substituted for missing measurements prior to the selection of cases and variables for the discriminant analyses. The equations used for these predictions were selected so as to include those independent variables having statistically significant (F test, $p < .05$) regression coefficients. It was possible to estimate approximately 60% of the total number of missing values using these regression equations.

Variable and Case Selection

Variables

The original variable list consisted of 61 measurements. As indicated previously, four of these variables were eliminated on the basis of the measurement replicability results. The remaining 57 variable list was further reduced to 33 variables according to the following criteria:

1. *Missing data.* In order to retain a maximum number of individuals in the samples, the variables with the greatest proportion of missing data were deleted. The variables used in the discriminant analyses were present for at least 80% of the cases entered into the analyses.
2. *Redundancy.* I eliminated variables which were highly correlated with another variable in the variable list, in order to reduce the deleterious effects of "noise" variables (Kowalski 1972:121). A variable was deleted if it shared more than 55% of its variance with any other variable in the list. At the same time, I tried to maintain as broad a representation of craniofacial morphology as possible.
3. *Heritability.* An attempt was made to retain measurements having a relatively large inherited component of variation, according to Osborne and DeGeorge's (1959) research.
4. *Error.* Both the level of measurement error (Table 8) and the average error introduced by missing data estimates (Table 9) were considered when choosing variables.

The 33 variables selected according to the above criteria were

1. Glabello-occipital length (L)
2. Minimum frontal breadth (MF)
3. Frontal chord (FC)
4. Midfacial breadth (MFB)
5. Internal biorbital breadth (IOB)
6. Subtense to internal biorbital breadth (SIOB)
7. Anterior interorbital breadth (AIB)
8. Orbital breadth (LOBM)
9. Orbital height (LOH)
10. Nasal height (NH)
11. Nasal breadth (NB)
12. Dacryal chord (DC)
13. Minimum breadth of nasals (MN)
14. Breadth of nasal bridge (BNB)
15. Biangular breadth (BA)

16. Breadth of ascending ramus (RL)
17. Length of mandible (LM)
18. Gonial angle (G∠)
19. Breadth at mental foramen (ZZ)
20. Maximum condylar length (CyL)
21. Malar length, inferior (IML)
22. Malar length, maximum (XML)
23. Cheek height (WMH)
24. Length occipital condyle (LCD)
25. Breadth occipital condyle (BCD)
26. Biasterionic breadth (ASB)
27. Frontal subtense (FRS)
28. Frontal subtense fraction (FRF)
29. Parietal chord (PAC)
30. Parietal subtense (PAS)
31. Occipital chord (OCC)
32. Mastoid length (MLN)
33. Mastoid breadth (MDB)

It has been shown that a relatively low number of variables can effectively discriminate among groups while keeping noise variation to a minimum (Kowalski 1972:121; Oxnard 1973:39). The 33 variable measurement pool was therefore partitioned into four smaller subsets of variables. These subsets were

1. *Face:* MFB, IOB, SIOB, AIB, LOBM, LOH, NH, NB, DC, MN, BNB, IML, XML, WMH
2. *Vault:* L, MF, FC, ASB, FRS, FRF, PAC, PAS, OCC
3. *Mandible:* BA, RL, LM, G∠, ZZ, CyL
4. *Combination:* L, MF, FC, MFB, AIB, LOBM, LOH, NH, RL, IML, WMH, BCD, FRS, PAS

These measurement subsets were selected so as to reflect broadly defined functional components of the skull (Baer and Harris 1969; Moss and Young 1960; Scott 1955). The vault subset represents the area of the cranium associated primarily with neural functions. The set of face measurements, on the other hand, reflects structures associated with visceral functions. The facial set includes measurements from the orbital, nasal, and zygomatic areas, which in life are associated with optical, respiratory/olfactory, and masticatory functions. A third set of variables represents the mandible, which is part of the masticatory functional complex. Measurements from the vault, face, and mandible are combined in the final variable subset.

Discriminant analyses were carried out separately for each variable subset in order to evaluate the stability over different data sets of patterns of intergroup biological distance.

Cases

This study included several small cranial series. Prior to analysis, the minimum group size for discriminant analysis was set at 10 individuals. This number was selected rather arbitrarily, balancing the fact that statistical results based on small samples can be subject to considerable sample error with the fact that additional measurable individuals simply do not exist for the smaller series.

In order to maximize existing data for the small series, it was necessary to include incomplete crania in the samples. Estimates for missing data were derived using multiple regression, as described in the previous section. Following the substitution of these estimates for missing measurements, all individuals having missing data estimates for over 30% of the measurements in the 33 variable data pool were eliminated from the samples. Thus all individuals which were more than 70% complete prior to missing data substitutions were retained. Use of this criterion balanced the advantage of larger sample size against the disadvantage of greater error introduced by the substitution of predicted values for missing data. (As discussed in the previous section, this error probably increased the within-group variation, thus erring in the conservative direction for hypotheses of no difference between groups.) The 70% completeness level marked a peak in the number of individuals gained as trial levels of tolerance were decreased by 5% intervals from 100% completeness to 50%. It also marked the level at which all samples (except Klunk males) retained at least 10 individuals. In the final samples, an average of 2.8 out of 33 measurement variables (7.9%) were estimated values.

Deformed crania were not excluded from the samples used for the biological distance analyses. Procedures for estimating the effects on biological distance estimates of including deformed crania in the samples are described in the next chapter.

5

Artificial Cranial Deformation

A premise of this study is that intergroup differences in cranial morphology reflect genetic differences between groups. However, cranial morphological variation also may be caused by artificial cranial deformation. In this chapter, the literature on artificial cranial deformation in North America is surveyed, cranial deformation in the study series is described, and alternatives are explored for dealing with cranial deformation in biological distance studies.

Cranial Deformation in North America

The practice of altering cranial morphology through the use of various deforming devices is both ancient and widespread. One of the earliest references to the custom of artificially deforming the head is Hippocrates' description, written about 400 B.C., of such practices among people living around the Black Sea (Flower 1881:39):

> They think those the most noble who have the longest heads . . . immediately after the child is born, and while its head is still tender, they fashion it with their hands, and constrain it to assume a lengthened shape by applying bandages and other suitable contrivances, whereby the spherical form of the head is destroyed, and it is made to increase in length.

Dingwall (1931) and Ewing (1950) have provided comprehensive reviews of the early literature on artificial cranial deformation throughout the world, including North America.

The practice of artificially modifying the shape of the head seems to have made its New World appearance in Ecuador during the Formative period, approximately 4000 years ago (Munizaga 1976:690; Stewart 1973:184). From this area, the custom apparently spread to other areas of the New World. By about 800 B.C., cranial deformation was being practiced in North America by the Adena peoples of Ohio and Kentucky (Stewart 1973:184; Webb and Snow 1945:258).

Stewart (1973:185) has pointed out three distinct areas of North America where cranial deformation was practiced.

1. *Northwest Coast.* The practice of cranial deformation along the northwest coast of North America is thought to have been a relatively late development, perhaps the result of independent invention or trans-Pacific contact in late prehistoric times (Stewart 1973:187). At any rate, a great variety of deforming customs were in evidence by the contact period. Early ethnographic accounts of deformation customs among northwest coast tribes are relatively numerous. In addition, considerable research attention has been focused on deformation practices in this area (Barnett 1955; Boas 1891; Cybulski 1975; Dingwall 1931; Dorsey 1897; McNeill and Newton, 1965; Otteking 1930).

2. *Southwest.* There is evidence that cranial deformation was practiced as early as Mogollon times in the American Southwest (Bennett 1973:10), becoming more common in Pueblo cultures after about A.D. 1000. Deforming practices may have spread northward into this area from Mexico (Stewart 1973:188). Cranial deformation in the Southwest was limited to flattening of the occipital and lambdoid areas. It is generally thought that this flattening was unintentional, a result of binding infants to hard cradleboards (Bennett 1973:14; Hrdlička 1939:194). Additional discussion of cranial deformation in the Southwest can be found in Dingwall (1931), Reed (1949, 1963), Hooton (1930), Ewing (1950), Bennett (1973), and Stewart (1973).

3. *Eastern United States.* Cranial deformation was practiced in this area of North America considerably earlier than in the other two areas. As noted above, it is present in Adena cranial series. There is also a greater variety of deformities evident in prehistoric crania from the eastern United States than in crania from other areas. As in the Southwest, Mexican influence is likely (Stewart 1973:189).

Varieties of Deformation

The first extensive system for classifying various types of artificial cranial deformation was published by Gosse in 1885. On the basis of cranial form, Gosse distinguished 16 major types and numerous subtypes of cranial deformity. Later classifications took into account deforming procedures and apparatuses, as well as cranial form. McGibbon (1912:1170), for example, recognized two basic forms of intentional deformation, one resulting from anterior–posterior restriction of the vault and the other from circumferential binding. Additional early classifications were put forward by Lunier (1869), Topinard (1879), Magitot (1884), Nicolucci (1890), and Kohler (1901).

Several classification systems have been developed for the New World. The most widely recognized are those of Hrdlička (1939), Imbelloni (1938), Neumann (1942), and Stewart (1973). The classifications of Hrdlička and Stewart are generally applicable to the New World, while those of Imbelloni and Neumann are more regional in emphasis. Imbelloni's scheme was developed using deformed crania from South America, while Neumann's system applies mainly to the eastern United States. Since Neumann's classification was derived primarily from skeletal data from the Eastern Woodlands, it was considered the scheme most appropriate to this study and was used as the framework for the following description of North American varieties of deformation.

OBELIONIC DEFORMATION

Obelionic deformation was first described by Stewart (1939a, 1939b) in crania from a shell mound near Lake Okeechobee, Florida. Neumann (1942:306) described this form of parietal flattening as follows: "Obelionic deformation occurs between bregma and lambda with compensatory changes such as broadening of the vault in the anterior parietal and temporal regions. The plane of flattening forms approximately an angle of 30 to 40 degrees with the ear-eye plane. Obelionic deformation . . . seems to be confined to southern Florida. . . ." Stewart (1939a:464) has suggested that this form of deformation was intentionally produced by binding the child to a cradleboard so that the head was pressed against an inclined endpiece.

LAMBDOID DEFORMATION

Lambdoid deformation, according to Neumann (1942:308) "occurs only in a mild form as an occasional individual variation in crania with simple occipital deformation in series from the southeastern states. In skulls from the Chaco Canyon region of New Mexico . . . the plane of flattening is inclined at an angle of 50 to 60 degrees to the ear-eye plane. It was first described by G. Retzius in a series of crania from the Mesa Verde." Stewart (1939a:465) noted that in addition to the steeper plane of flattening, lambdoid deformation is located more posteriorly than obelionic deformation, involving the occiput down to about inion. He suggests a similar origin for lambdoid deformation as for obelionic deformation. This type of flattening is generally thought to have been produced unintentionally (Bennett 1973:14; Hrdlička 1939).

Neumann also recognized *natural* lambdoid flattening, which he considered an aspect of natural vault morphology, as distinguished from the artificial obelionic and lambdoid types of deformation. According to Neumann (1942:308), natural lambdoid flattening is characterized by flattening in an "intermediate position between artificial obelionic and lambdoid deformation when considered from the point of view of an angle formed by the plane of flattening and the ear–eye plane."

OCCIPITAL DEFORMATION

Simple occipital deformation, according to Neumann (1942:308), "is essentially at right angles to the ear–eye plane, is probably unintentional, often markedly asymmetrical, and generally does not involve the frontal bone." This form of deformation has also been termed "occipital flattening" (Hrdlička 1939:194), "vertico-occipital" (Stewart 1973:186), and "cradleboard deformity." The flattening of the occiput characteristic of this form is thought to have resulted from the weight of the infant's head on a hard cradleboard. Simple occipital deformation was common among the Pueblos of the Southwest. Hrdlička has reported that among historic tribes such as the Apache, Navaho, Mohave, and Yuma, infants were securely strapped to the cradleboard for long periods of time and were only removed for the purpose of washing (Dingwall 1931:183). This form of deformation is also found in the eastern United States as early as Adena times (Webb and Snow 1945:258). Neumann (1942:308) noted its association with later Mississippian cultures in the Southeast.

BIFRONTO-OCCIPITAL DEFORMATION

Bifronto-occipital deformation has been described by Neumann (1942:308) as "bifrontal flattening that produces a very narrow frontal bone associated with a moderate degree of vertical occipital flattening." Bifronto-occipital deformation has been associated with Middle Woodland "Hopewellian" cultures in the Midwest (Stewart 1940:15). It was also present in earlier Adena cranial series (Webb and Snow 1945:106). Stewart has suggested that this form of deformation resulted from fastening infants' heads to cradleboards such that pressure was exerted on both sides of the forehead. Webb and Snow (1945:106) also regarded it as unintentional deformation, the result of cradleboard practices.

FRONTO-VERTICOÖCCIPITAL DEFORMATION

Fronto-verticoöccipital deformation "is characterized by flattening of the frontal, probably by means of a board, in conjunction with the simple vertical occipital deformation produced by tying the head of the infant to a flat surface [Neumann 1942:309]." Posterior flattening parallels the basion–bregma plane. Compensatory growth is lateral. This form of deformation was called "fronto-occipital" by Hrdlička (1939:194) and "tabular erect" by Imbelloni (1938). Fronto-verticoöccipital deformation was practiced by Mississippian peoples in the eastern United States (Neumann 1942:309). It is also found in Central America (Hrdlička 1922:85), Mexico (Dingwall 1931:154; Gill 1977:102; Stewart 1973:189), and along the western coast of South America (Hrdlička 1922:85). Romero (1970:66) has stated that this form of deformation is the most ancient type of cranial deformity found in the Valley of Mexico, appearing in the Early Preclassic period (1400–1000 B.C.). A similar type of cranial flattening, which Boas (1891) termed "Cowitchin," was practiced by some northwest coast tribes.

FRONTO-PARIETO-OCCIPITAL DEFORMATION

This deformation is characterized by flattening in three planes, nearly at right angles to one another (Neumann 1942:309). The "plane of the flattened occiput is nearly vertical and forms a broad angle near obelion with the flattened parietals, which in turn form a nearly right angle near bregma with the flattened frontal" (Stewart 1939b:10). Fronto-parieto-occipital deformation can be differentiated from fronto-verticoöccipital deformation according to the direction of compensatory growth, which in the case of the former takes place laterally and superiorly. Stewart (1939b) first described fronto-parieto-occipital deformation in late Mississippian and historic Cherokee crania from the Southeast.

PARALLELO-FRONTO-OCCIPITAL DEFORMATION

This "consists of artificial flattening in which the occipital region is affected by placing a pad at the base of the occiput in such a manner as to produce rough parallelism with that of the frontal bone. Compensatory growth is to a large extent lateral . . . [Neumann 1942:310]." Parallelo-fronto-occipital deformation was practiced by the historic Caddo in the American Southeast. This form of cranial deformation, which Imbelloni has termed "tabular oblique," was also practiced in Mexico beginning sometime in the Late Preclassic period, 500–200 B.C. (Romero 1970:66). A similar form of cranial deformity, sometimes termed "Chinook" (Boas 1891), was also practiced by northwest coast tribes such as the Chinook.

ANNULAR DEFORMATION

Annular deformation, also called "circular or Aymara" (Hrdlička 1939:195), "orbicular" (Imbelloni 1938), and "Koskimo" (Boas 1891), was not described by Neumann (1942) since it was not practiced in eastern North

America. Annular deformation was produced by binding the head so as to compress the skull circularly. Frontal pads were sometimes used in combination with the bindings. Annular deformation is characterized by

> a more or less marked, broad, circular flattening or depression passing over the frontal bone, the temporal squammae and the lower parts of the parietals, and over the lower portion of the occipital, while the posterior and superior portion of the parietals and the upper part of the occipital protrudes in a compensatory way upward and backward. Anterior to the coronal suture in these cases there was generally an elevation, while posterior to the suture there resulted a more or less pronounced annular depression [Hrdlička 1939:195].

This form of deformation was practiced by certain South American tribes (Imbelloni 1938, 1950; Pérez-Martínez 1960) and northwest coast tribes such as the Kwakiutl and Nootka (Cybulski 1975).

Deformation Practices

Stewart (1973:187) has suggested that the use of counterpressure in altering the shape of the skull constitutes reliable evidence for intentional deformation. He has described four basic ways in which counterpressure was applied to the head: (*a*) by use of a device, such as a band across the forehead, to force the back of the head against a hard cradle; (*b*) by use of small boards or tablets, one placed against the forehead and the other against the occiput, with the ends on each side tied tightly together; (*c*) by use of a board or tablet held against the forehead by a tight band passing from one end of the board around the back of the head to the other end; and (*d*) by use of a band wrapped tightly around the head so as to pass over the forehead and under the occiput (Stewart 1973:187). A number of these devices have been illustrated by Pérez-Martínez (1960).

Descriptive accounts by early explorers, traders, and ethnographers provide more detailed information as to deformation practices in particular tribes. Some of these sources also suggest reasons for cranial deformation practices among certain tribes, and indicate which segments of the population were deformed. Dingwall (1931) has reviewed many ethnographic accounts of cranial deformation practices among American Indians in early contact times. These early ethnographic accounts are potentially useful as models for deformation practices among earlier, extinct Indian cultures.

The sociocultural dimensions of deforming practices are probably best known in the northwest coast area. It appears that heads were deformed both for aesthetic reasons and to indicate social status (Dingwall 1931:172). Early reports indicate that among the Chinook and Salishan, possession of a deformed head was a sign of freedom because slaves were not permitted to deform the heads of their children (Dingwall 1931:168; Stewart 1973:188). There are reports of sex differences in deforming practices as well, although the significance of these differences is not clear. Lewis and Clark (1814, cited in Dingwall 1931:164) noted that among the Chinook, female children were always subjected to greater deformation than male children, although both sexes were deformed. Biddle (1814, cited in Dingwall 1931:165) stated that certain Columbia River tribes flattened the heads of their female infants only, while more eastern mountain tribes deformed the heads of male children as well.

Since the cranial series dealt with in this study come from the central Mississippi Valley, ethnographic accounts from the eastern United States are of particular interest here. Most of the available early accounts described deformation practices among lower Mississippi tribes, such as the Natchez, whose way of life was essentially Mississippian at the time of initial European contact.

One of the best descriptions of the method of cranial deformation used by the Natchez is found in the anonymous Luxembourg memoir, which Swanton (1911:54) cites:

> They have . . . the head pointed and almost of the shape of a miter. They are not born so; it is a charm which is given them in early years. What a mother does to the head of her infant in order to force its tender bones to assume this shape is almost beyond belief. She lays the infant on a cradle which is nothing more than the end of a board on which is spread a piece of the skin of an animal; one extremity of this board has a hole where the head is placed and it is lower than the rest. The infant being laid down entirely naked she pushes back its head into this hole and applies to it on the forehead and under the head a mass of clay which she binds with all her strength between two little boards. The infant cries, turns completely black, and the strain which it is made to suffer is such that a white, slimy fluid is seen to come out of its nose and ears at the time when the mother presses on its forehead. It sleeps thus every night until its skull has taken on the shape which custom wishes it to receive.

The use of cradleboards as deforming devices has been reported for a number of other southeastern tribes as well. The Tunica of the lower Mississippi were reported by Gravier (1859) to have used cradleboards to flatten the heads of their infants (Dingwall 1931:183). The Choctaw were reported by several early sources to have flattened their infants' heads with bags of sand on the forehead with the head resting on a wooden cradleboard. Schoolcraft noted that some of the Creek tribes followed this custom as well (Dingwall 1931:188). Among the Choctaw, only the heads of male infants were deformed.

Possible reasons for deformation have also been suggested in early ethnographic writings. For example, Butel-Dumont (1753) wrote that among certain tribes in Louisiana, care was taken to crush and flatten the upper part of the forehead of newborn children with a board so that they might be able to bear loads better (Dingwall 1931:187). Lawson's (1709) account of cranial deformation among the Waxhaw tribes in the Gulf coast area suggests other reasons for cranial deformation (Dingwall 1931:186):

> these Indians lay the hinder part of their children's heads upon bags of sand. . . . They use a roll also which is placed upon the child's forehead, the supporting surface for the infant being a flat board upon which it is tied. It is said that this method makes the limbs of the children straight as an arrow. . . . As the child's head is flattened its eyes 'stand a prodigious way asunder,' and the hair hangs over the forehead in a manner, which to Lawson, seemed like the eaves of a house and appeared 'very frightful.' On inquiry the Indians stated that through the deformation their sight was much strengthened and they were able, thereby, better to discern game at a distance during the chase. . . .

Cradleboards were also used among some more northern tribes. Michaelson (1918–1919) reports a Fox woman as saying that she kept her child in the cradle for a long time so that it would not grow up with a long head or be hump-backed or have bow legs. She also said that children were confined to cradleboards for nearly one year (Dingwall 1931:185).

Archeological evidence for deforming devices and procedures is scarce. Only in the arid areas of South America, where mummies have been found in well-preserved form, is there direct evidence of particular kinds of deforming apparatuses associated with particular forms of cranial deformation (Stewart 1950:44). There is, apparently, no comparable evidence of deforming practices in North America.

The question of which segments of the population were subjected to cranial deformation can be approached through the examination of skeletal series. For example, a particular sex or status group may be overrepresented in deformed subgroups of skeletal series. Sex differences in the incidence of deformation may in turn suggest differential treatment of male and female infants according to such cultural dictates as aesthetic standards, social status, or adult sex roles. The reasons why certain elements of the population were deformed whereas others were not are not easily deduced from the archeological record, however.

Gill (1977:102) found no relationship between sex and form of deformation in Postclassic crania from northwestern Mexico. Hrdlička, on the other hand, reported an overrepresentation of females in crania with fronto-verticoöccipital deformation from San Juan Teotihaucan (Dingwall 1931:153). In the eastern United States, Webb and Snow (1945:106) reported a slightly higher incidence of simple occipital deformation in females than in males from the Adena series, while the incidence of bifronto-occipital deformation in that series was higher in males.

In the Illinois Valley, Neumann observed that the incidence of occipital flattening in females was approximately double the incidence in male crania from the Dickson Mississippian series (Blakely 1973:56; Harn 1971b:63). The fact that only one or two of the individuals in mass graves were deformed suggested to Harn (1971b:63) that if deformation was a status marker, all members of the same family or clan did not share equal status, assuming that related individuals were buried together in the mass graves. On the other hand, there were indications that children buried with deformed females tended to be deformed also.

Cranial Deformation in the Study Series

Artificial cranial deformation is present in several of the study series. The Schild Mississippian series contains the highest frequency of deformed crania. The frequency of deformation is much lower in the Mississippian series from the Yokem site.

In general, the Late Woodland series showed very little cranial deformation. Deformation was not scored in the Ledders series because preliminary examination indicated that it is effectively absent. Exceptions are the two earliest Late Woodland series, Koster and Klunk.

On the whole, the degree of cranial deformation in the study series is mild as compared to, for example, cranial series from South America, the northwest coast, or the American Southwest. Deformation also appears to be less severe in the Schild Mississippian series than that found in the Dickson Mississippian series, according to Harn's (1971b:133) illustrations of the range of cranial deformation in the latter series. None of the Schild Mississippian crania was as severely deformed as the most deformed cranium illustrated by Harn.

In terms of Neumann's (1942) classification, the following forms of deformation were observed in the study series: simple occipital, fronto-verticoöccipital, bifronto-occipital, and lambdoid flattening. It seems likely that most of the observed lambdoid flattening, which is common in all of the study series, is an aspect of natural vault morphology. The cases in which lambdoid flattening is associated with frontal or bifrontal flattening, however, are probably the result of artificial deformation, and can probably be regarded as variations of the fronto-verticoöccipital cradleboard type of deformation.

Frontal and bifrontal flattening occasionally occur unassociated with flattening of the posterior vault. If this frontal flattening resulted from binding infants to cradleboards, a posterior counterforce must also have been exerted. It is possible that cradleboard-related alterations of the posterior vault were so slight that they were not detectable in these adult crania. On the other hand, frontal flattening which occurs with no discernable posterior flattening could have resulted from the use, by very young children, of tumplines—forehead bands used to support loads carried on the back. It seems unlikely, however, that bifrontal flattening would have resulted from the use of tumplines.

Scoring Procedures

Crania were not classified as to type of deformation because anterior flattening was not clearly associated with posterior flattening in all cases. Furthermore, the severity of frontal and posterior components of deformation, when they occurred together, was frequently unequal. It was decided, therefore, to score posterior and anterior aspects of deformation separately. Four kinds of cranial flattening were scored: frontal, bifrontal, occipital, and lambdoid.

All sufficiently complete adult crania were scored according to rank scales of deformation severity. These scales were developed using the Schild Mississippian series because crania in this series were the most numerous, best preserved, and most deformed. Scales were developed independently for each of the four kinds of flattening. All four scales were developed in the same manner. Derivation of the scale for frontal flattening is described below as an example.

All of the adult Schild Mississippian crania which were complete enough to be scored were arranged in a continuum, ranging from no frontal flattening to most frontal flattening. Frontal flattening was judged both by sight and by feel. Crania which appeared to have approximately equal degrees of flattening were grouped together. The resulting groupings were then collapsed into four ranked groups, consisting of crania with no frontal flattening, slight flattening, medium flattening, and marked frontal flattening. These groups, numbered 0 to 3, were agreed upon by a second observer.

The replicability of this ranking system was tested approximately one week later. All of the Schild Mississippian crania were again ranked, following the procedure described above, and these ranks were compared with the ranks assigned in Trial 1. Approximately 87% of the crania were assigned the same rank in Trial 2 as in Trial 1.

Scales for bifrontal, occipital, and lambdoid flattening were derived in the same manner as the scale for frontal flattening. The Schild Mississippian series was used as a reference series in all cases. As with frontal flattening, replicability of the deformation scales was assessed by comparing ranks assigned in two scoring trials. The results for the bifrontal, occipital, and lambdoid scales were, respectively, 75%, 82%, and 74% correct assignment. The scales for bifrontal and occipital flattening ranged from 0 to 3. The scale for lambdoid flattening ranged from 0 to 4.

Following the derivation of the deformation scales using the Schild Mississippian series, each cranium from the other series was scored according to each of these scales. To facilitate scoring, reference skulls were selected from the Schild Mississippian series to represent the upper limits, lower limits, and mode of each category, for each of the four deformation scales. Skulls which were misclassified in the replicability procedures were frequently selected to mark upper or lower limits of various ranks. These Schild Mississippian reference crania were used to score crania from the other series. Table 10 lists the Schild Mississippian reference crania; Figures 8–11 illustrate some of these crania. These photographs illustrate the range of deformation encompassed by the four deformation scales.

Cultural Associations

The incidence of the four kinds of cranial flattening scored in the study series is summarized in Table 11. It is apparent that all forms of deformation are not present in equal proportions in all series. Frontal flattening was found in over one-third of the Schild Mississippian crania, but occurred with low frequency in the other series. The Schild Mississippian series also contains the highest incidence of occipital flattening. On the other hand, bifrontal deformation, while present in approximately 20% of the Schild Mississippian crania, is most frequent in the Klunk (32% incidence) and Koster (25% incidence) Late Woodland series. Lambdoid flattening is common in all of the study series.

Fisher exact tests were carried out to determine the statistical significance of intergroup differences in the incidence of the four kinds of cranial flattening. Deformation scores of 0 indicated absence, while

TABLE 10
Reference Crania for Scoring Cranial Deformation

Type of deformation	Score	Upper limit	Modal cranium	Lower limit
Frontal	0	—	SB-194[a]	—
	1	—	SB-235	SA–96a
	2	SB-186	SA-156	SB–267
	3	—	SA-52	—
Bifrontal	0	SA-138	—	—
	1	SA-154	SA-49	—
	2	—	SB-270	—
	3	—	SB-255	SA-103
Occipital	0	SB-250	—	—
	1	SB-194	SB-231	—
	2	—	SA-83a	—
	3	—	—	SA-84
Lambdoid	0	SB-178	—	—
	1	SA-65	SB-250	—
	2	SB-201	SB-251	—
	3	—	SB-235	—
			SB-238	
	4	—	SB-285	SA-48

[a] SB-194 refers to Schild Mississippian, Knoll B, Burial 194. SA refers to Schild Mississippian, Knoll A.

scores of 1 or greater indicated presence of deformation. A program written by David Asch for a Monroe 1860 programmable calculator was used to compute the probabilities. The results are presented in Table 12.

The Schild Mississippian series has a significantly ($2p < .05$, two-sided test) higher incidence of frontal flattening than any of the other study series. The difference is most marked when the incidence of frontal deformation in the Schild Mississippian series is compared to the incidence in Late Woodland series from the Schild, Yokem, and Koster sites. These results suggest a Late Woodland–Mississippian difference in the incidence of frontal flattening. The Klunk Late Woodland series represents an exception to this generalization.

The incidence of bifrontal flattening also differs between groups. The Klunk and Koster series, which are the two earliest Late Woodland series examined, have significantly ($2p < .05$) higher incidences of bifrontal deformation than all of the other series except Schild Mississippian. Possibly the presence of this form of cranial deformity indicates a carryover from Middle Woodland to early Late Woodland times of the apparatus (perhaps a type of cradleboard) which produced this type of deformity. An alternate explanation is that the Koster and Klunk series contain Middle Woodland material unrecognized as such during excavation. The incidence of bifrontal deformation is very low in the later Late Woodland series from the Schild and Yokem sites. It is also low in the Yokem Mississippian series. The proportion of bifrontal flattening is significantly greater in the Schild Mississippian series than in the Schild Late Woodland series.

The incidence of occipital flattening is relatively low in all series, and no significant between-group differences were found. The highest incidences of occipital flattening occur in the Schild Mississippian, Koster Late Woodland, and Yokem Mississippian series. This finding is consistent with the fact that these series also have the highest incidences of frontal and/or bifrontal flattening, since anterior deformation suggests a deforming apparatus which exerted both force and counterforce.

Lambdoid flattening is common in all series. No significant differences between groups were indicated. As with occipital flattening, however, the series with the highest incidence of lambdoid flattening also have the highest incidence of frontal or bifrontal flattening. This supports the suggestion made earlier that some of the lambdoid flattening may represent a variation of fronto-verticoöccipital or bifronto-occipital forms of cranial deformation. It seems likely, nevertheless, that much of the lambdoid flattening observed was natural morphology.

The above results pertain to the incidence (presence or absence) of cranial deformation in the study series. The degree of cranial deformation, i.e., the number of crania assigned to each rank of the deformation scales, was also compared between series. Crania with scores of 0 for a particular form of deformation were excluded from comparisons involving that form of deformation. Chi-square tests, using SPSS subprogram CROSSTABS (Nie *et al.* 1975), were carried out separately for each type of deformation and for each group pair. None of the chi-square values obtained was statistically significant at the .05 level. These results indicate that, although there are between-group differences in the incidence of the various forms of deformation, severity of deformation does not vary significantly between groups.

Sex Associations

Fisher exact tests were also used to test for statistically significant differences between males and females in both the incidence and the degree of cranial flattening. The results are reported in Table 13. Differences between males and females in the incidence of all four forms of deformation were not statistically significant in any series except Schild Mississippian. In the Schild Mississippian series, the frequency

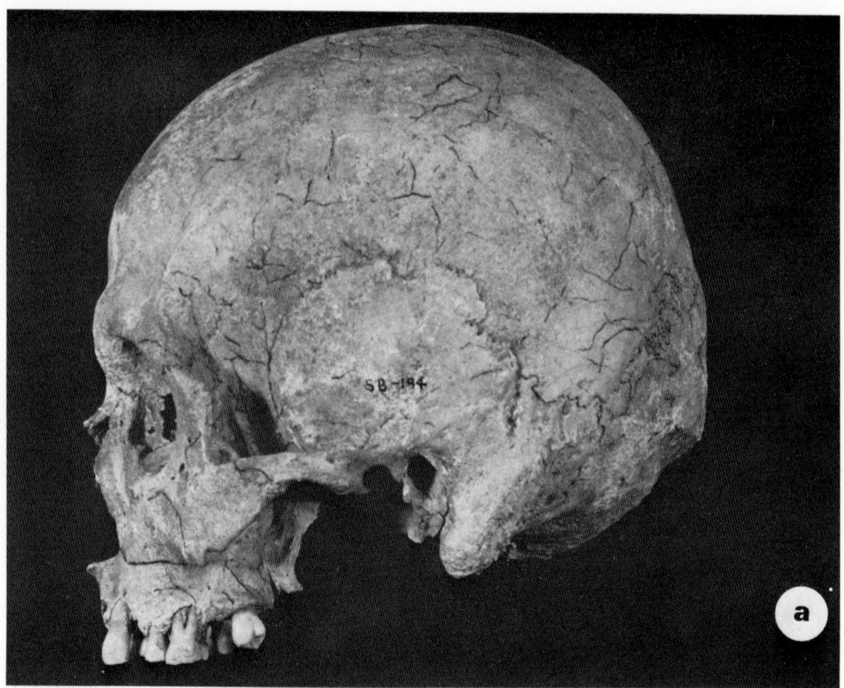

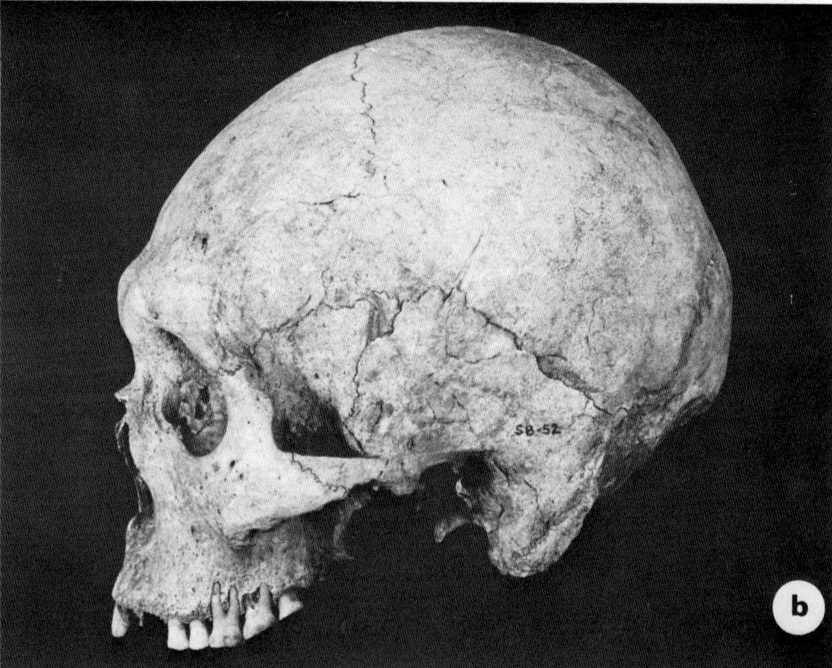

FIGURE 8. Schild Mississippian crania illustrating the range of frontal flattening in the study series. (a) Frontal flattening absent, scored 0; Knoll B, Burial 194. (b) Maximum frontal flattening, scored 3; Knoll A, Burial 52.

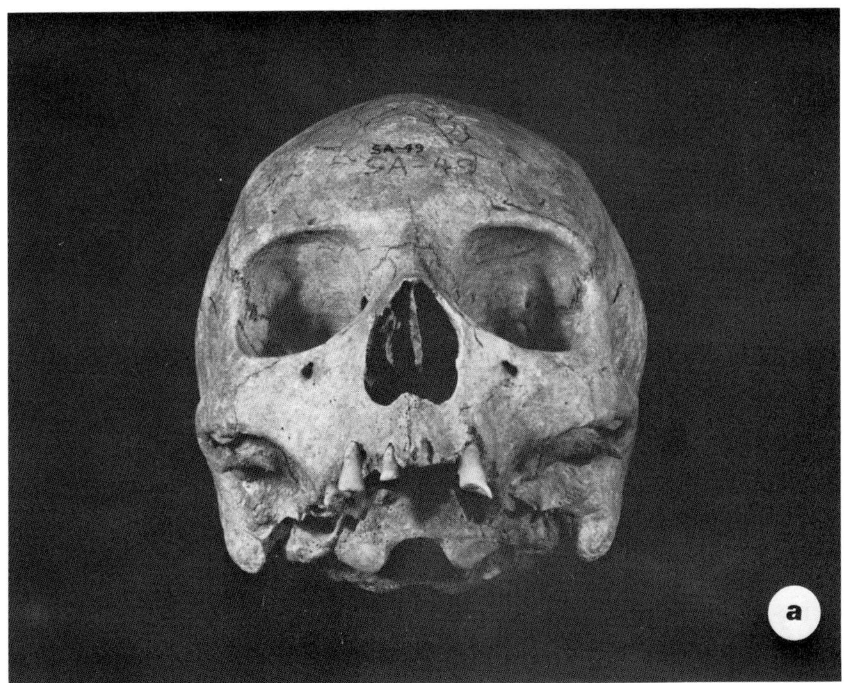

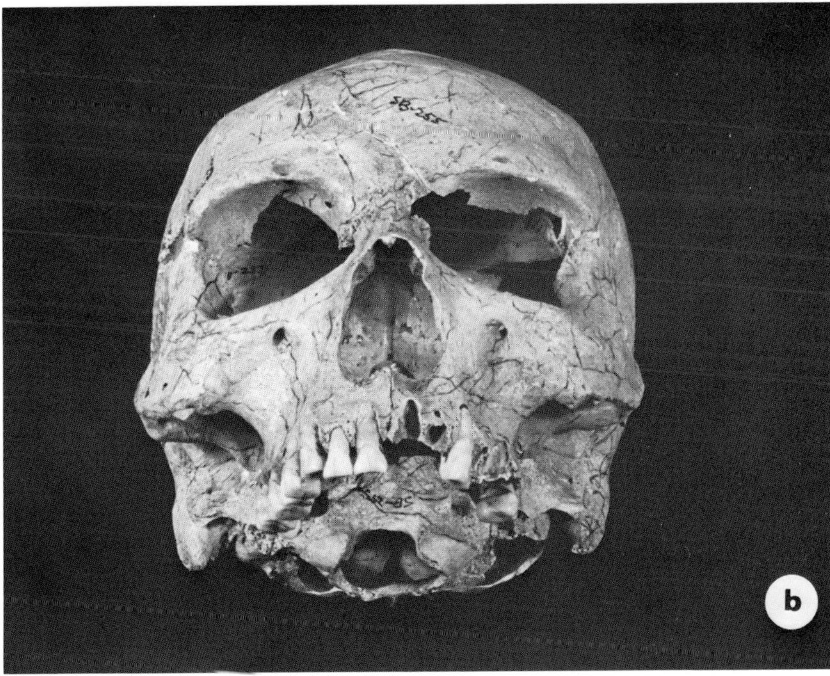

FIGURE 9. Schild Mississippian crania illustrating the range of bifrontal flattening in the study series. (a) Slight bifrontal flattening, scored 1; Knoll A, Burial 49. (b) Maximum bifrontal flattening, scored 3; Knoll B, Burial 255.

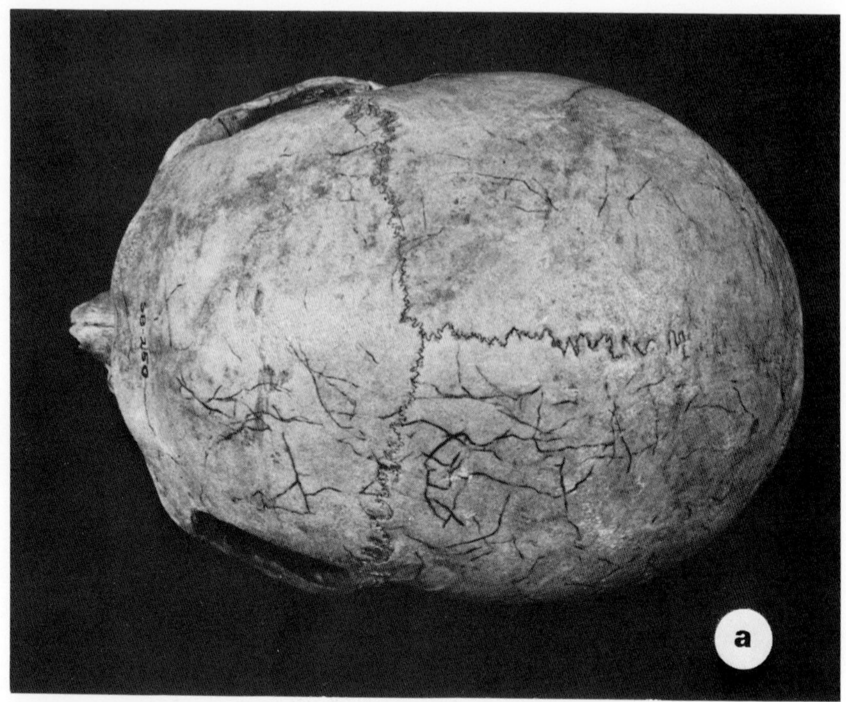

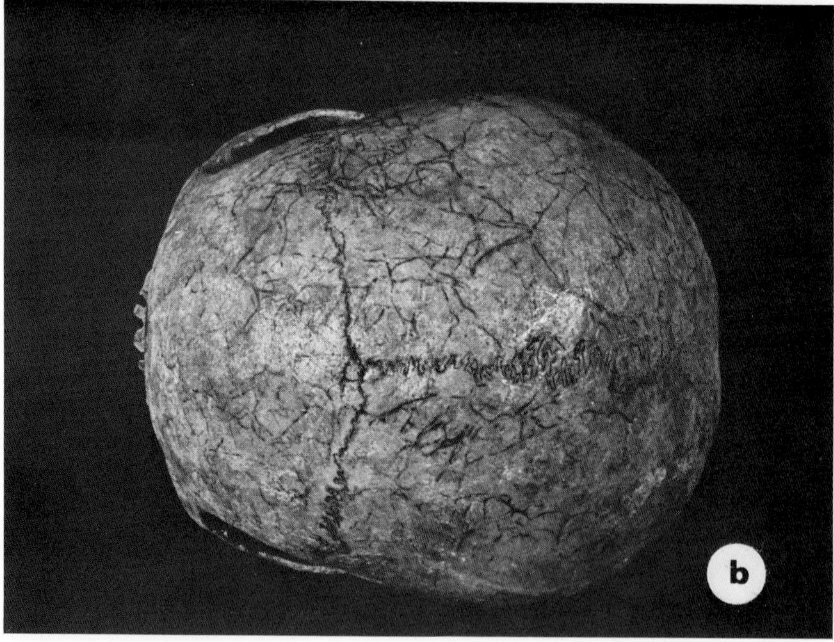

FIGURE 10. Schild Mississippian crania illustrating the range of occipital flattening in the study series. (a) Occipital flattening absent, scored 0; Knoll B, Burial 250. (b) Slight occipital flattening, scored 1; Knoll B, Burial 231. (c) Medium occipital flattening, scored 2; Knoll A, Burial 83a. (d) Marked occipital flattening, scored 3; Knoll A, Burial 84.

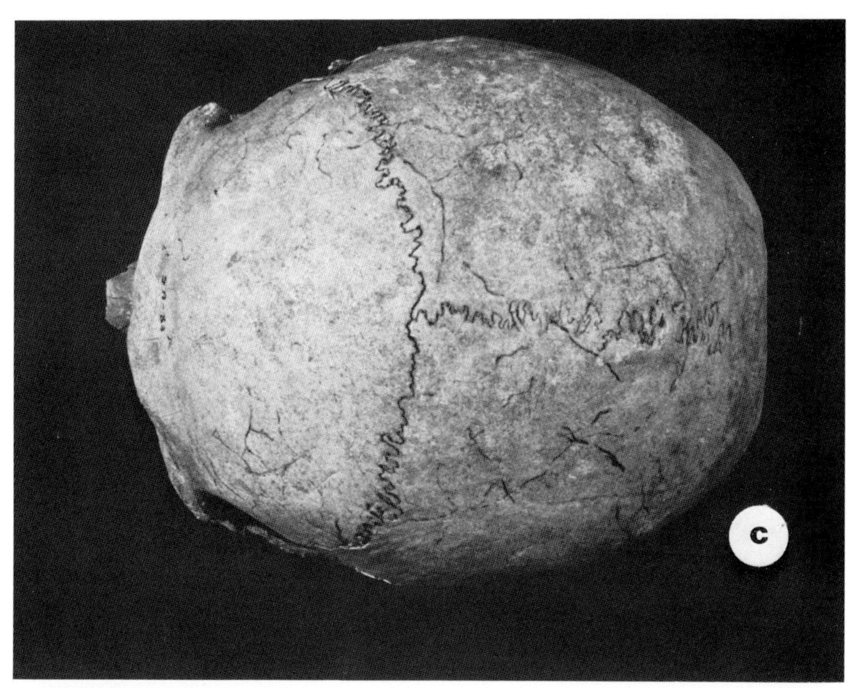
c

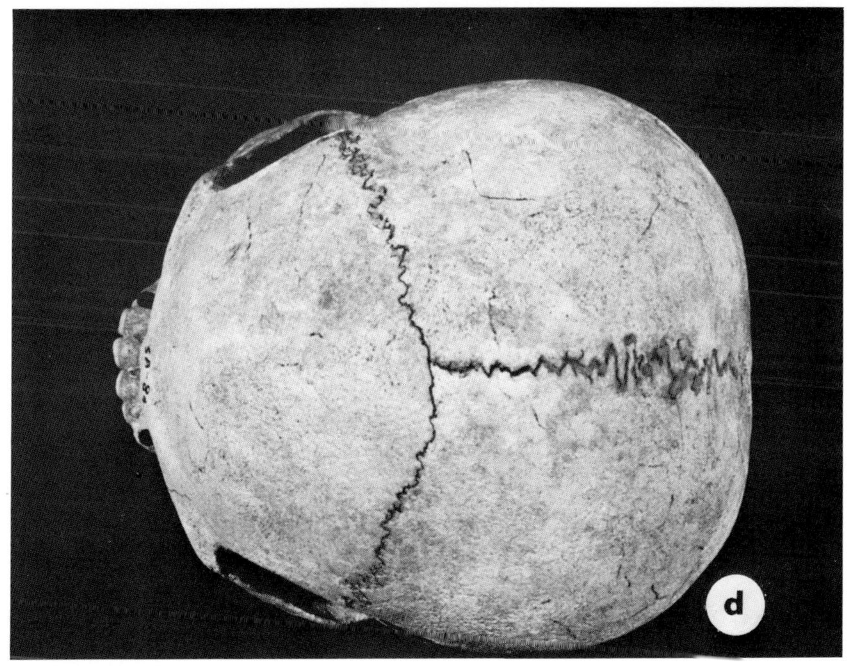
d

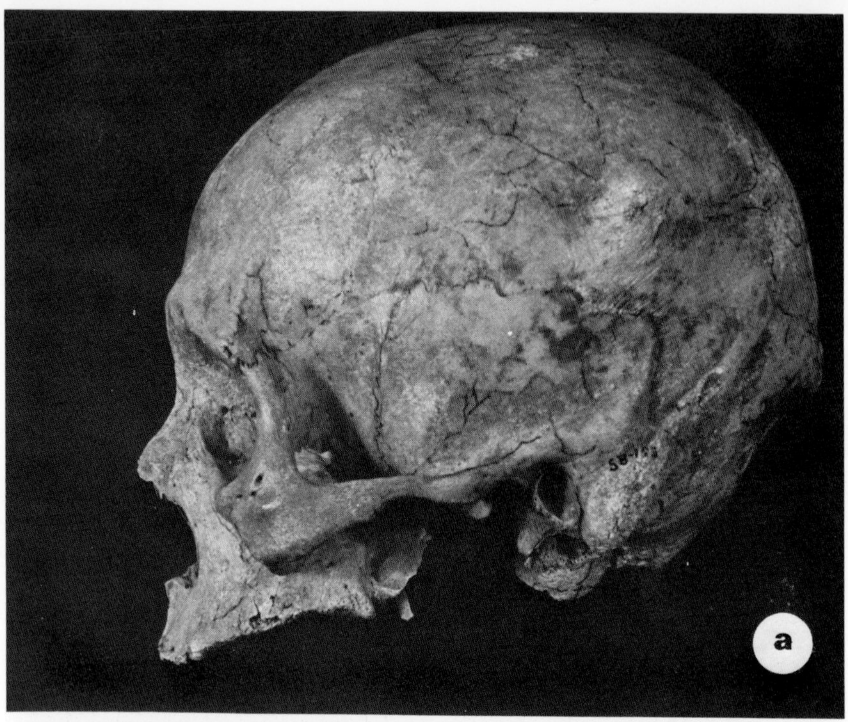

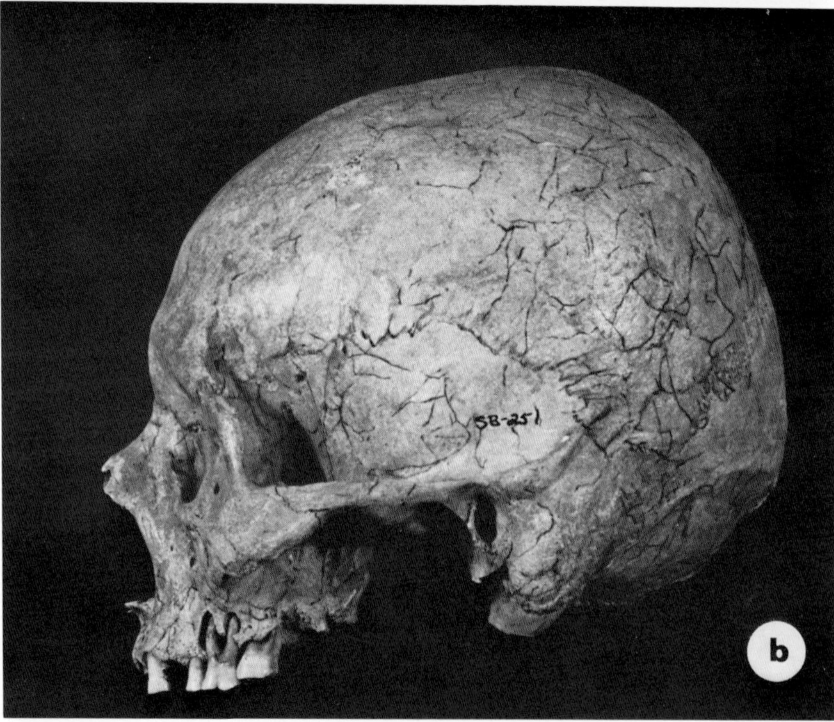

FIGURE 11. Schild Mississippian crania illustrating the range of lambdoid flattening in the study series. (a) Lambdoid flattening absent, scored 0; Knoll B, Burial 178. (b) Slight lambdoid flattening, scored 2; Knoll B, Burial 251. (c) Medium lambdoid flattening, scored 3; Knoll B, Burial 235. (d) Marked lambdoid flattening, scored 4; Knoll B, Burial 285.

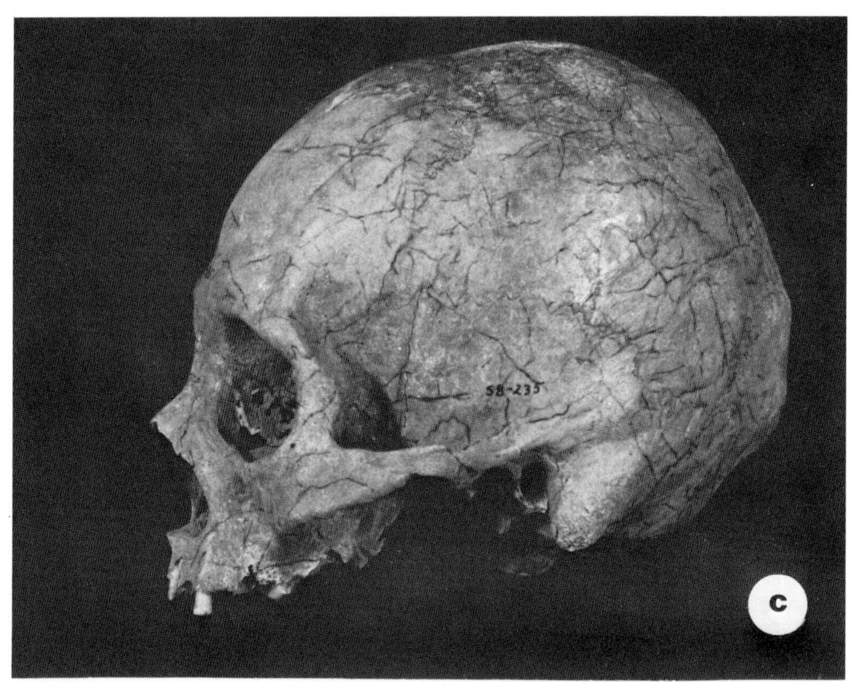
SB-235
c

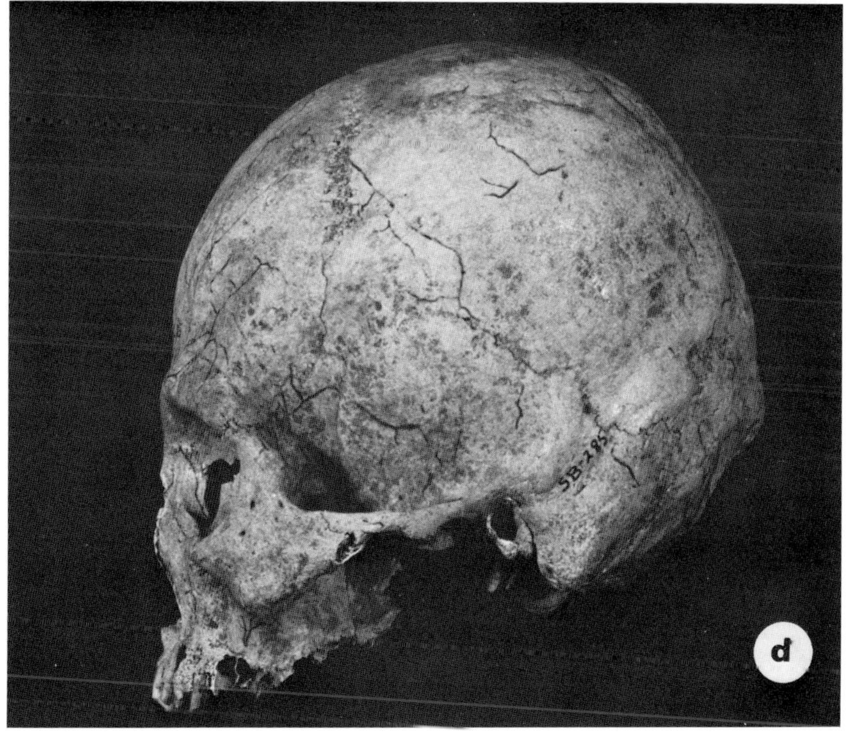
d

TABLE 11
Incidence of Deformation

	Frontal		Bifrontal		Occipital		Lambdoid	
Series	*N*	%	*N*	%	*N*	%	*N*	%
Koster LW								
Male	3	8.1	10	27.0	3	7.9	29	78.4
Female	2	4.7	10	23.3	4	12.9	25	80.6
Total	5	6.2	20	25.0	7	10.1	54	79.4
Klunk LW								
Male	2	20.0	5	50.0	1	11.1	8	88.9
Female	0	0.0	2	16.7	0	0.0	11	91.7
Total	2	9.1	7	31.8	1	4.8	19	90.5
Schild LW								
Male	0	0.0	2	10.0	0	0.0	14	70.0
Female	0	0.0	0	0.0	1	5.3	13	65.0
Total	0	0.0	2	4.7	1	2.6	27	67.5
Yokem LW								
Male	1	4.5	3	13.6	1	6.2	13	72.2
Female	0	0.0	1	2.9	3	10.7	19	65.5
Total	1	1.8	4	7.0	4	9.1	32	68.1
Schild Miss								
Male	25	51.0	11	22.4	11	21.6	40	76.9
Female	14	23.7	10	16.9	3	4.9	52	85.2
Total	39	36.1	21	19.4	14	12.5	92	81.4
Yokem Miss								
Male	1	6.7	1	6.7	2	13.3	8	57.1
Female	3	12.0	2	8.0	2	8.0	21	84.0
Total	4	10.0	3	7.5	4	10.0	29	74.4

of frontal and occipital flattening was significantly higher in males than in females. No significant differences in the degree of deformation were found. That is, when deformation was present, it did not tend to be more marked in one sex than in the other.

The higher incidence of frontal and occipital flattening in males from the Schild Mississippian series suggest that male infants were in some way treated differently than female infants. One can only speculate as to the reasons for this differential treatment. Differences between sexes in aesthetic ideals or social status are possible explanations. Whatever the reasons for the sex differences in cranial deformation practices among the Schild Mississippians, the pattern of sex differences appears not to have been a general Mississippian trait in the central Illinois–Mississippi Valley area. The tendency in the Schild Mississippian series for males to have a higher incidence of frontal and occipital deformation than females is not evident in the Yokem Mississippian series (Table 13). Nor is the Schild pattern found in the Dickson Mississippian series. In contrast to the higher incidence of deformation in

TABLE 12
Tests for Significance of Intergroup Differences in Cranial Deformation, Sexes Combined

	Fisher exact tests, single-tail probabilities				
	Koster LW	Klunk LW	Schild LW	Yokem LW	Schild Miss
Frontal flattening					
Klunk LW	.4700	—	—	—	—
Schild LW	.1068	.1077	—	—	—
Yokem LW	.2033	.1860	.5644	—	—
Schild Miss	<.0001*	.0088*	<.0001*	<.0001*	—
Yokem Miss	.3460	.6413	.0474	.0910	.0011*
Bifrontal flattening					
Klunk LW	.3484	—	—	—	—
Schild LW	.0032*	.0053*	—	—	—
Yokem LW	.0048*	.0086*	.4807	—	—
Schild Miss	.2311	.1576	.0155*	.0255	—
Yokem Miss	.0163*	.0182*	.4653	.6122	.0612
Occipital flattening					
Klunk LW	.4002	—	—	—	—
Schild LW	.1433	.5814	—	—	—
Yokem LW	.5635	.4766	.2197	—	—
Schild Miss	.4103	.2725	.0607	.3857	—
Yokem Miss	.6277	.4332	.1873	.5884	.4605
Lambdoid flattening					
Klunk LW	.2077	—	—	—	—
Schild LW	.1255	.0433	—	—	—
Yokem LW	.1240	.0427	.5673	—	—
Schild Miss	.4420	.2524	.0576	.0535	—
Yokem Miss	.3519	.1234	.3365	.3461	.2348

* $2p < .05$, two-sided test.

TABLE 13
Tests for Significance of Differences in Deformation between Males and Females

	Fisher exact tests, single-tail probabilities			
	Frontal	Bifrontal	Occipital	Lambdoid
Koster LW	.4281	.4473	.3851	.5303
Klunk LW	.1948	.1130	.4286	.6857
Schild LW	(*a*)	.2109	.4872	.5000
Yokem LW	.3860	.1550	.5369	.4413
Schild Miss	.0030*	.3165	.0085*	.1864
Yokem Miss	.5159	.6883	.4841	.0737

* $2p < .05$, two-sided test.
[a] Frontal flattening not present among males and females.

males than in females in the Schild series, Neumann observed that the incidence of cranial deformation in females was approximately double that in males in the Dickson Mississippian series (Blakely 1973:56).

Cranial Deformation and Biological Distance

The confounding effects of artificial cranial deformation on biological distance estimates have been dealt with in several different ways by past workers. For the most part, one of the following general approaches to this problem, or a combination of these approaches, has been adopted:

1. Mathematical correction for the effects of deformation on cranial measurements.
2. Deletion of deformed crania from samples used to derive biological distance estimates.
3. Selection of measurements thought to be unaffected, or minimally affected, by artificial deformation.

The first approach was suggested by Shapiro (1928), who developed regression formulas to be applied to the means of three measurements in series of deformed male crania. These regression formulas were used to estimate values of cranial vault measurements had the crania not been deformed. Shapiro's formulas estimated maximum head length on the basis of length of the cranial base (basion–nasion), maximum cranial width on the basis of cranial module, and cranial height on the basis of breadth-height index.

There are several problems with this approach. First, Shapiro's formulas cannot be used to estimate individual measurement values; only average values can be predicted. This limitation prohibits the use of biological distance statistics, such as Mahalanobis D^2, which are computed from individual measurement values. A second problem arises from the assumption that the predictor variables are relatively free from the effects of deformation. Later research has suggested that this assumption is probably not tenable. It has been shown by several workers (Björk and Björk 1964:356; Newman 1947:14; Stewart 1943:167), for example, that deformation in series of Peruvian crania affected the length of the cranial base, which Shapiro used to predict head length.

Buikstra (1976:47) has noted two additional assumptions which must be made if Shapiro's approach is followed. First, one must assume that the undeformed crania are representative of the sample. This assumption would not be justified if social factors were a determining factor in which individuals were deformed and the degree to which they were deformed. Second, it must be assumed that the difference between undeformed and deformed crania is sufficiently clear to the observer that the sample can be divided into deformed and undeformed subsamples. My own experience supports Buikstra's (1976:47) contention that midwestern series containing deformed crania are generally not clearly divisible in this manner. Deformation is a continuously distributed condition, rather than a discrete trait which is clearly absent or present. In addition, it is frequently difficult to distinguish artificial deformity from natural cranial morphology. This problem has been encountered in studies of the living as well. Hooton and Dupertuis (1951:104) recognized natural lambdoid flattening in the majority of the Irish males in their sample. Occipital flattening was present in approximately 21% of the sample. Hooton and Dupertuis expressed uncertainty as to whether this flattening was an aspect of natural morphology or whether it was artificial, the product of cradleboard use. Similarly, it is frequently difficult to distinguish artificial bifrontal deformation from natural sagittal keeling.

A second approach to the problem of cranial deformation in biodistance studies—the deletion of deformed crania from the samples used for intergroup craniometric comparisons—has been followed by many workers including Giles and Bleibtreu (1961), Howells (1973), Neumann (1952), and Long (1966). Some of the problems discussed above are also encountered in this approach. First, undeformed crania must be reliably distinguished from artificially deformed crania and, as mentioned previously, it is extremely difficult and probably impossible to distinguish slight effects of the deforming process from natural morphology. Also, variation in application of the deforming apparatus, in the length of time infants were subjected to deforming pressures, and in the timing of the deformation experience relative to individual growth factors all contributed to considerable variability in the form and degree of artificial deformity visible in the adult skull. When an undeformed subsample is selected for comparative purposes, therefore, the possibility that undetected artificial deformation remains in the sample cannot be discarded. This problem has been pointed out previously by Buikstra (1976:47), Brothwell (1975:75), Newman (1947:19), and Hrdlička (1939:195).

Another objection concerns a point raised earlier in the discussion of the use of corrective formulas—the assumption that undeformed crania represent the morphology of groups which contain both deformed and undeformed individuals (Buikstra 1976:47), or conversely, that the deformed individuals eliminated from the sample are not a biased segment of the gene pool. This would not be the case if the practice of deformation were associated with certain social classes which tended toward endogamy.

As noted earlier, a third procedure commonly followed when comparing groups which include deformed crania is to use measurements believed to be unaffected, or relatively unaffected, by deformation. Neumann sought to minimize the effects of artificial deformation in the Dickson Mississippian series by omitting "affected measurements in crania exhibiting moderate and marked deformation" (Blakely 1973:134). Similarly, El-Najjar (1978:153) omitted the measurements he considered most susceptible to deformation effects (cranial length, cranial breadth, and basion–bregma height) from his variable list in a study of biological distance among American Southwest cranial series containing deformed individuals. Brothwell (1965:72) has also suggested that deformed crania are useful for intergroup comparisons if variables are carefully selected. He regarded the following measurements as those least likely to be affected by deformation: basi-bregmatic height, upper facial height, palatal length, palatal breadth, length of the foramen magnum, breadth of the foramen magnum, simotic chord, bi-dacryonic arc, bi-dacryonic chord, minimum ramus breadth, and symphysial height. Likewise, Hughes (1968:42) has suggested that many facial and basal measurements are nearly unaffected by distortion of the vault. The use of facial measurements to minimize the effects of deformity in moderately deformed crania has also been favored by Hrdlička (1931:92, 1939:196), Falkenburger (1938:21), Ewing (1950:59), and Corruccini (1972:377).

As in the first two procedures, selecting measurements so as to minimize deformation effects is not without problems. There is considerable evidence to suggest that deformation affects the face and base as well as the cranial vault. McNeill and Newton (1965:249), in their study of Northwest Coast crania with anteroposterior and annular deformation, have shown that both types of deformation are associated with cranial base alterations. These effects, although similar in crania with both types of deformity, were more marked in crania with annular deformation than in crania with anteroposterior deformation. Moss (1958) has also shown that these forms of deformation affect base morphology, although his results suggested different patterns of effects associated with each type of deformation. Cybulski (1975:66–68), also working with Northwest Coast crania, has described alterations in facial morphology due to artificial cranial deformation, noting that alteration of facial as well as vault morphology was intended by the people who practiced deformation, according to ethnographic reports. Blackwood and Danby (1955:189), in a study of circumferentially deformed crania from New Britain, also state that cranial base and face morphology is altered by the stresses of deforming apparatuses on the vault.

Although the effects of deformation are clearly not limited to the cranial vault, facial morphology is probably least affected by deformation. Blakely's (1973:142) assessment of the effects of deformation on his biological distance estimates supports this position. Blakely omitted the measurements taken in areas of the skull directly subjected to the deforming apparatus and traditionally regarded as being affected by deformation (L, B, H, LB, and possibly LM and BCB). He used primarily facial measurements in his comparison of Late Woodland and Mississippian series from the Dickson site. He then carried out a discriminant analysis based on 16 measurements and indices from deformed and undeformed subgroups of the Dickson Mississippian series. The distance between deformed and undeformed subgroups was not statistically significant at the .05 level. Blakely concluded that while these 16 facial dimensions may not have been free of the effects of deformation, the effects of deformation on the distance estimates were minimal.

Deformation Effects in the Present Study

At the outset of this investigation, I considered selecting for the biological distance analysis measurements which were not significantly associated with cranial deformation. This procedure proved to be impractical for several reasons. First, a review of previous research suggested that no area of the skull is completely free of deformation effects Second, the number of deformed crania in the samples proved to be insufficient to generate stable measures of association between metrics and deformation in the study series. Third, it proved to be impossible to select variables on the basis of deformation effects and, at the same time, to maximize the data available from small samples. Deformation effects were therefore examined following the biological distance analyses rather than at the variable selection stage.

Cranial deformation alters natural vault morphology. One can reasonably expect, therefore, that the more marked the cranial deformity, the greater the deviation from average cranial morphology in groups, such as the study series, where only a minority of crania are deformed. Deformed crania will tend to be located in discriminant space at a greater distance from the group centroid than undeformed crania. Thus the association between degree of cranial deformation and distance from group centroid can be used as an indirect indication of the overall effects of cranial deformation on the set of measurements used to perform the discriminant analysis.

As described in the previous chapter, four data sets, representing the face, vault, mandible, and a combination of these areas, were selected from an original battery of 55 measurements. The relative susceptibility of each data set to deformation effects was examined by measuring the association between degree of cranial deformation and distance of cases from group centroids derived from the different data sets. Using the SPSS subprogram DISCRIMINANT (Nie *et al.* 1975), discriminant analyses were carried out for each of the four data sets. For each case, the program calculated Mahalanobis D^2 values, which are estimates of generalized distance between a particular case and its group centroid. These D^2 values were used as the measure of deviation from average group morphology. Deformation was measured by ranks on the four deformation scales described earlier. Kendall rank–order coefficients of correlation (τ) between D^2 values and deformation scores were used to measure the association between deformation and degree of deviation from typical group morphology. These correlations were computed using the SPSS subprogram NONPAR CORR (Nie *et al.* 1975). The Schild Mississippian and Koster series were used for this correlation analysis because they provide the largest samples and they contain deformed crania. Sets of correlations, including coefficients for each kind of deformation, were computed separately for D^2 values obtained from each of the four different sets of measurements. These correlations were then compared with one another to determine if deformation effects vary according to the data set used to compute the D^2 estimates.

Table 14 presents coefficients of correlation between the four kinds of deformation and the D^2 values obtained from the four different variable subsets. Frontal, occipital, and lambdoid flattening explain a significant ($p < .05$) portion of the variation in the D^2 values derived from vault dimensions, especially in the two Schild series, where the incidences of frontal and occipital deformation are highest. The correlations between deformation and D^2 values based on the face and combination measurement subsets are lower, and fewer are statistically significant than when the D^2 values were derived from the vault measurement subset. The D^2 values computed from the mandible measurements are least correlated with deformation, suggesting that they are relatively unaffected by the four kinds of cranial flattening.

In order to obtain a more general measure of the effects of deformation on measurement variability, a summary deformation score was obtained by summing, for each case, the scores on the four individual deformation scales. Kendall rank–order correlations were again calculated, using the SPSS subprogram NONPAR CORR (Nie *et al.* 1975), between deformation and distance from group centroid as measured by Mahalanobis D^2. The results are given in Table 15.

TABLE 14

Correlation between Distance from Group Centroid (D^2) and Deformation Score, for Each Type of Cranial Flattening and Each Measurement Subset

	Kendall rank-order coefficients of correlation, τ			
	Frontal flattening	Bifrontal flattening	Occipital flattening	Lambdoid flattening
Vault variable subset				
Schild Miss males ($N=53$)	.2554*	.0777	.3058*	.2163*
Schild Miss females ($N=58$)	.2455*	.0614	.2313*	.1286
Koster LW males ($N=31$)	−.0826	.0079	−.0268	.3043*
Koster LW females ($N=35$)	.2000	.1777	.0308	.2516*
Face variable subset				
Schild Miss males	.0413	.1003	−.1853	−.0837
Schild Miss females	.3909*	.1291	.1239	−.0616
Koster LW males	.0048	−.0039	.0642	−.1244
Koster LW females	.1539	.0000	.2650*	.0189
Mandible variable subset				
Schild Miss males	.0739	.1158	−.0632	.0191
Schild Miss females	.0226	−.0626	−.1776	.0320
Koster LW males	−.2470	.0629	.1070	.0695
Koster LW females	.0615	−.0317	.1418	.0755
Combination variable subset				
Schild Miss males	.1239	−.0099	.1134	.0527
Schild Miss females	.2703*	.0626	.1817	−.0145
Koster LW males	−.0339	−.0039	.0802	−.0841
Koster LW females	.2462*	.0889	.1541	.0755

* $p < .05$, one-sided test.

TABLE 15

Correlation between Distance from Group Centroid (D^2) and Summary Cranial Deformation Score, for Each Measurement Subset

	Kendall rank-order coefficients of correlation, τ			
	Schild Mississippian		Koster Late Woodland	
Variable subset	Males, $N=53$	Females, $N=58$	Males, $N=31$	Females, $N=35$
Vault	.3303*	.2932*	.2259	.1555
Face	.0152	.1937*	−.0599	.0470
Mandible	.1367	.0023	.0684	.0687
Combination	.1367	.2287*	−.0684	.0904

* $p < .05$, one-sided test.

In general, the results reflect those obtained when the four deformation scores were entered separately. The association between deformation and D^2 is strongest when vault measurements are used to compute the distance estimates. The summary deformation score explains a significant ($p < .05$) portion of the variation in D^2 values based on vault measurements in the Schild Mississippian series. The corresponding correlations for the Koster series are also relatively high, although they fall short of statistical significance. The associations between deformation and D^2 scores based on the face, mandible, and combined morphological subsets are generally lower than those based on the vault subset, and they are statistically significant in only two cases. Both instances occur in the Schild Mississippian female series, where deformation and D^2 based on both face and combination measurement subsets are significantly correlated. The associations between deformation and D^2 are somewhat weaker when D^2 values are derived from face measurements than when they are obtained from the combined measurement subset. The correlations using D^2 values derived from mandible measurements are the lowest of all the measurement subsets.

To summarize, these results indicate that the presence of deformed individuals in cranial samples is more likely to distort biological distance estimates based on vault measurements than estimates derived from face measurements. The results obtained here are thus consistent with previous research, which suggested that the cranial vault is most susceptible and the facial skeleton least susceptible to the effects of artificial cranial deformation.

6

Adult Age and Cranial Morphology

The majority of studies of adult age changes indicate that alterations in both neurocranial and viscerocranial dimensions occur in adulthood. Most of this research has been carried out on living populations. Although soft tissue changes undoubtedly account for some of the observed age changes in the living, most investigators have concluded that changes in adult head dimensions are partly due to continued appositional bone growth in adult life.

The questions addressed here are first, whether cranial measurements change with increase in adult age in the west–central Illinois study series, and, second, if so, are the changes similar to the adult age changes described in the literature?

The object of this analysis is not to examine growth per se, which is best studied in the living where precise age determinations are possible and a longitudinal research design can provide information on individual variations in growth rates. Rather, the major purpose is to estimate the contribution of intragroup age differences to intragroup morphological variation. This information will be used to assess the influence of developmental variation on patterns of biological distance among the study series.

Previous Research

Cross-Sectional Studies

One of the earliest investigations of continued growth in the adult cranium was Hellman's (1927) analysis of developmental change in the human face, using American Indian skeletal material. Hellman concluded that the face continues to grow in height and width at a slow rate until old age. He recognized a reverse trend during old age, when face size decreases. Unfortunately, Hellman was unable to age his material precisely. He based his age estimates on dental attrition; "old age" individuals were those in whom the grooves on the molar occlusal surfaces were obliterated.

M. S. Goldstein (1936) compared head and face measurements between samples of old and young Jewish males. Each sample numbered 50 individuals. The age range for his "young" group was 20.5 to 21.5 years, while his "old" group ranged in age from 60 to 106 years. Goldstein (1936:86) concluded that, "The effects of old age are: all dimensions of the head except minimum frontal diminish somewhat; all face lengths [heights], except nose, decrease appreciably, primarily as a result of loss of teeth; all face widths are slightly greater. . . ."

Hrdlička's (1936) research on "Old American" whites and American Indians also suggested that growth in both length and breadth of the head and face, especially the mouth, nose, and ears, continues at a slow rate in adulthood to at least the fourth decade. Hrdlička also found that while some elements continue to grow until the sixth decade, head size begins to diminish with senility.

A cross-sectional study by Hooton and Dupertuis (1951) of age changes in a very large sample of adult Irish males also indicated an increase in facial dimensions with age. The following age changes were noted: total facial height and upper facial height increased until the fourth decade, followed by a decrease in the case of total facial height; head breadth increased until the fifth decade, when it began to decrease slightly; head length, bizygomatic diameter, bigonial diameter, and nose height increased in size into the sixth decade, with a slight decline in bizygomatic diameter and bigonial diameter in old age; nasal breadth increased slowly throughout life; head height declined through life; minimum frontal diameter remained stable until the middle of the sixth decade, when it began to decline.

Lasker (1953) carried out a cross-sectional study of male and female series from two adult Mexican populations. He found little tendency for head length to change with age except for an increase with age in one female series. Head breadth and head height increased significantly with age in both female series; a similar tendency was also noted in the male series. Minimum frontal diameter and interocular width did not change with age. In the face, bizygomatic diameter and bigonial diameter tended to increase with age in both series and both sexes. Total facial height increased with old age in one male and one female series. Upper facial height also increased in this female series, but in the corresponding male series all facial heights tended to decrease in old age. Lasker attributed this result to greater tooth loss and consequent resorption of alveolar bone and facial shortening in this male group. Nasal height showed a tendency to increase with age in one male and one female series. Nasal breadth increased significantly with age in all series. Lasker (1953:61) concluded that his results were generally consistent with those of previous studies, suggesting that increase in face size with age is to some extent due to appositional bone growth.

Baer (1956) has reported the results of a cross-sectional study of age changes in the head and face in the third decade of life. Large samples of both sexes were obtained from the 1946 Army Anthropometric Survey data. Subjects ranged in age from 19 to 33 years. Like previous research, Baer's work indicated that the human face continues to increase in size after adulthood is reached. For males, Baer's growth curves suggested that face breadth increases more slowly, but over a longer time period, than total facial height. In contrast to findings of Hooton and Dupertuis' (1951) Irish study, head length and breadth showed no significant increase during the third decade. In the case of head length, Baer's findings are compatible with Lasker's (1953) results. In the female series, Baer found that total facial height did not show a size increase in the third decade comparable to that in males. He interpreted this result as indicative of developmental sex differences.

Howells and Bleibtreu (1970), in a study of growth in large male and female samples of Huttcrites aged 15–29, also found age changes in adult crania. They reported a tendency for head breadth, face breadth, jaw breadth, ear size, and nasal breadth to increase with age. The trend was generally more positive in males than females.

At least three factors—summarized by Baer (1956:570)—have been proposed in these studies to account for changes in adult head and face dimensions:

1. Secular change, which would result in size differences between different age groups in the same population.
2. Selective survival, which would eliminate individuals of less favorable body size or body proportions at a relatively younger age, with resultant size and shape differences within populations when the members are arranged by age. (This explanation was considered most fully by Hooton and Dupertuis.)
3. Ontogenetic development, which would include changes due to both soft tissue alterations in morphology with age (such as gains in fatty tissue) and to actual bone growth.

Longitudinal Studies

The studies reviewed thus far were cross-sectional, involving single observations of individuals of different ages. A longitudinal research design, involving multiple observations of the same individuals at different ages, eliminates secular change and selective survival as explanations of change in adult cranial size, thereby allowing the growth factor to be measured more directly. Ideally, we would like to have data on a large number of individuals observed repeatedly from late adolescence to senility. As Hooton and Dupertuis (1951) point out, however, this type of study could only be carried out by successive generations of workers dedicated to the same project and maintaining constant methodology, or by a Methuselah. There are, however, a small number of studies in which the same adult individuals were observed twice. Four of these longitudinal studies are described below.

The work of Büchi (1950) represents one of the first attempts at a longitudinal approach to the problem of postadolescent changes in head and face morphology. Büchi obtained two sets of measurements, with the second set collected nine years after the first, from series of approximately 200 male and female Swiss adults. He noted a continuous increase in head and face size in adulthood in both sexes, with some difference between sexes in the timing and ceasing of this increase. Head size increased into the eighth decade. Like Baer (1956), Büchi found that total facial height in males increased into the fifth decade, while face breadth increased more slowly but for a longer period of time, with significant increases into the seventh decade. In females, face height increased into the fourth decade. Büchi's results generally supported the findings of the cross-sectional studies described above.

Israel (1968), in a longitudinal study of 43 males and 53 females, found further evidence of continuing cranial growth in adulthood. Israel obtained measurements of cranial thickness, diameter, and intersutural distances from lateral radiographs. Skull diameters were measured both endocranially and ectocranially, in the sagittal plane. Both inner and outer intersutural distances were measured from nasion to bregma and from bregma to lambda. Israel (1968:134) concluded that "continuing growth in the skull occurs in adults with an increase in both thickness, diameter and intersutural distance over an extended period of time."

Several years later, Israel (1973a) reported additional analyses of longitudinal data consisting of 41 measurements from lateral radiographs of 26 adult white females. Two radiographs were measured for each individual; the mean age for the first observation was 35.4 years, and the mean age for the second observation was 54.9 years. In addition to supporting his previous conclusion that the cranium thickens and both endocranial and ectocranial skull diameters increase with age, Israel demonstrated continued growth in visceral cranial structures. This enlargement of both vault and face represented an overall expansion of about 3–5%, which appeared to be of similar magnitude in all areas except for skull thickness, sella turcica, and frontal sinus; the latter dimensions showed a relatively greater increase. He concluded that the craniofacial complex is in a state of growth throughout life. Additional longitudinal research (Israel, 1977) likewise indicated continued growth in the craniofacial skeleton in both males and females, and reaffirmed differences in the magnitude of this expansion for different areas of the skull. For both males and females, Israel (1977:47) found that remodeling of the sella turcica, frontal sinus, and skull tables took place at a rate approximately twice that for skull length.

A longitudinal study reported by Tallgren (1974) does not support the suggestions of Israel and others that the human skull continues to grow in adulthood. Tallgren took 33 neurocranial measurements from lateral radiographs of 32 Finnish females, all denture wearers, ranging in age from 20 to 73 years. Two series of measurements were taken 15 years apart. Results indicated no significant changes in neurocranial size, skull thickness, or dimensions of the cranial base over the 15-year observation period. Tallgren suggested, therefore, that no continuous growth of the calvarium or cranial base had occurred with increasing age. Israel's failure to use a headholder in his earliest observations, with consequent differences in roentgenographic enlargement at the two stages of observation, is offered by Tallgren as a possible explanation of the noncorrespondence with Israel's results. Israel (1977) has subsequently presented evidence to refute this suggestion. Another possible explanation for the differences in results may be, at least in part, differences in the dental status of the two populations studied. Tallgren's sample was edentulous, while Israel's sample included both dentulous and edentulous individuals.

Summary

Cross-sectional studies suggest that growth of the human skull continues at a slow rate in adulthood. Several head and face dimensions have been shown to increase slowly well into the sixth decade. A decrease in overall head size in senescence has been noted by several workers. The results pertaining to individual measurements are not entirely uniform. The relatively small increase being measured, environmental variation both within and between samples, methodological differences, and microevolutionary differences among samples are three factors which may account for some of the discrepancies.

Longitudinal studies, which are not as susceptible to environmental effects, are few. The longitudinal research of Büchi (1950) and Israel (1968, 1973a, 1977) suggests that growth of the craniofacial complex continues into adulthood, thus supporting the results of the cross-sectional studies. Tallgren's (1974) research, on the other hand, does not show evidence of adult age changes in the neurocranium. The reasons for the noncorrespondence of Tallgren's results with those of previous research are unclear; methodological and sampling factors may be involved.

Age Effects in the Study Series

As described in Chapter 3, individuals in the study series were assigned to young, middle-aged, or old adult age categories. Using the Student t statistic, mean values of cranial measurements were compared between adjacent age categories to see if cranial dimensions vary with advancing age. It was necessary to combine six of the study series in order to obtain adequate samples for this analysis. Sexes were analyzed separately. Two-tailed probability levels were used to test for statistical significance, which was set at the .05 probability level. In the few instances where the two samples being compared had significantly different variances (F statistic significant at the .05 level), an approximate t was computed using separate variance estimates rather than a pooled variance estimate. The SPSS subprogram T-TEST (Nie *et al.* 1975) was used for the computations.

Results of t-Tests

The means of cranial measurements for each age category, the standard deviations, and the t test results are given for males in Table 16 and for females in Table 17. These results are discussed below for the various areas of the cranium.

Vault length. In males, there is a consistent but nonsignificant trend toward increasing skull length until old adulthood, and then a decrease. Female cranial length increases with age without declining at old adulthood. These trends are consistent with most past research.

Vault breadth. The skull breadth of west–central Illinois males is slightly less among middle-aged adults than among young or old adults.

The differences are not statistically significant. In contrast, most other investigators have found head breadth to increase until the fifth decade or later and then to decrease slightly. Female skull breadths show a weak, statistically nonsignificant increase from young to old adulthood. The trend conforms with past research.

Vault height. Changes in skull height with age are nonsignificant in both male and female study series. Male cranial height decreases with age, then remains constant. Female cranial height increases very slightly with age. These trends are consistent with most previous research, except that Lasker (1953) found a tendency among males for increasing head height with age.

Cranial base. Cranial base dimensions in the male study series do not show a clear overall trend either to increase or decrease with age. The only statistically significant difference occurs in the breadth of the occipital condyle, which increases from young to middle-aged adults. The trend is reversed with old age but not at a statistically significant level. Comparative data from studies of the living are not available.

In the female series, cranial base dimensions tend to increase with age. The only statistically significant change is an increase in the length of the cranial base from young to middle adulthood, a trend which continues nonsignificantly among old adults. Israel (1973) reported similar results for length of the cranial base.

Face height. Among males and females, face height measurements generally decrease with age. For males, the decline is especially marked in old age, and it is statistically significant for two measurements, upper facial height and left orbital height. For females, the age trends are considerably weaker and less consistent than among males. One female measurement, nasal height, increases significantly from middle to old age. The possibility that facial shortening in the study series is partially attributable to dental loss with age is examined later in this chapter.

Face breadth. In the male study series, total facial breadth decreases significantly from young to middle adulthood, then increases nonsignificantly from middle to old age. A weaker trend occurs in old adults toward larger midfacial breadth and larger nasal breadth. The remainder of the facial breadth measurements either remain approximately constant or decrease slightly with age. The decrease in minimum breadth of nasals from middle to old adults is statistically significant. The decreases with age are contrary to the research reviewed earlier, most of

TABLE 16

Adult Male Cranial Measurements, by Age

	Young, $N=54$[b]		Middle, $N=58$[b]		Old, $N=39$[b]		*t*-tests for comparisons[c]			
							Young/middle		Middle/old	
Measurement[a]	Mean	*SD*	Mean	*SD*	Mean	*SD*	*t*	*df*	*t*	*df*
Vault length										
L	180.90	6.32	182.53	7.11	180.38	5.95	−1.23	102	1.52	90
FC	113.13	4.70	113.70	4.51	112.83	3.49	−0.72	133	1.12	119
PAC	110.91	6.32	111.56	6.00	109.84	5.86	−0.57	114	1.47	104
FRF	51.33	3.65	51.75	3.92	50.70	3.20	−0.60	121	1.45	104
Vault breadth										
B	138.45	5.56	137.11	5.80	138.53	4.51	1.12	88	−1.19	78
MF	94.60	4.19	93.30	4.67	93.33	4.44	1.66	129	−0.03	116
XFB	116.20	4.66	114.98	4.10	114.76	4.70	1.37	95	0.22	83
ASB	107.68	4.48	107.11	4.23	107.40	5.61	0.68	104	−0.28	76
Vault height										
H	142.32	5.41	140.26	5.28	140.41	4.30	1.64	71	−0.13	65
PAH	120.05	5.82	119.05	3.97	119.03	3.31	0.87	73	0.02	66
Cranial base										
LB	104.62	4.40	103.60	5.38	104.03	4.15	0.89	72	−0.36	63
FML	38.33	2.71	38.98	2.85	38.57	2.75	−1.04	80	0.60	68
LCD	26.29	2.41	26.50	2.00	26.97	1.86	−0.48	105	−1.15	91
BCD	13.93	1.26	14.59	1.43	14.06	1.39	−2.63*	112	1.78	92
BPH	24.28	2.76	24.18	4.15	23.70	2.92	0.12	57	0.50	59
Face height										
TFH	122.94	5.78	122.10	6.75	122.10	4.20	0.63	87	−0.00	55
UFH	74.37	3.91	74.60	4.58	72.32	5.80	−0.31	121	2.33*	101
SH	37.07	2.96	37.05	3.83	36.58	3.46	0.03	139	0.69	121
LOH	34.69	1.45	34.77	1.59	33.80	2.21	−0.26	117	2.27*	55
NH	53.33	2.18	52.94	2.87	52.72	2.81	0.87	117	0.37	102
WMH	23.65	2.21	23.99	2.43	23.64	2.22	−0.89	148	0.82	127
Face breadth										
TFB	139.00	5.14	136.74	3.86	138.53	5.12	2.00*	64	−1.55	59
MFB	99.83	5.15	99.85	4.77	100.28	4.78	−0.01	141	−0.48	116
IOB	98.69	3.74	98.39	3.69	98.30	3.73	0.46	128	0.13	111

BOB	98.55	3.26	98.81	3.51	98.69	3.28	−0.37	97	0.17	84
AIB	19.94	2.12	19.55	2.06	19.47	1.73	1.01	113	0.19	94
DC	21.22	2.30	20.89	2.20	20.60	2.43	0.75	104	0.59	89
MN	9.34	1.91	9.08	1.72	8.32	1.30	0.79	117	2.36*	102
LOBM	42.67	1.79	42.87	1.75	42.54	1.50	−0.62	121	0.96	97
NB	25.58	1.54	25.75	1.82	26.13	1.56	−0.60	133	−1.15	112
BNB	60.01	4.53	60.09	4.62	61.22	4.46	−0.09	138	−1.30	113
MB	66.81	3.80	66.08	4.54	64.76	4.90	1.03	138	1.45	110
BA	105.69	6.53	103.77	7.62	106.42	7.74	1.44	114	−1.66	98
BCB	122.16	6.88	121.94	7.54	122.15	6.30	0.15	97	−0.13	81
CrCr	100.80	6.46	99.57	5.31	101.18	4.71	1.00	89	−1.40	77
ZZ	46.57	2.58	46.40	2.68	47.02	2.61	0.38	136	−1.22	115
CyL	21.18	1.96	20.98	1.81	21.30	1.79	0.57	123	−0.89	104
Face depth										
FLA	98.89	4.65	97.69	4.88	98.90	6.57	1.05	67	−0.82	59
RL	33.84	2.31	33.77	2.53	33.96	2.63	0.16	147	−0.39	122
LM	107.87	5.15	107.16	5.16	108.57	6.34	0.73	112	−1.19	95
SIOB	18.85	2.20	18.45	2.89	18.50	2.02	0.87	116	−0.11	104
HNB	24.18	2.54	23.64	3.03	23.85	2.44	0.82	73	−0.30	67
ML	55.23	2.54	55.19	3.33	54.64	3.71	0.08	131	0.82	112
IML	33.46	2.78	33.16	2.96	34.00	3.00	0.61	141	−1.50	118
XML	53.24	3.68	53.52	3.48	53.70	3.13	−0.48	137	−0.28	114
Other										
G∠	119.01	7.16	118.84	6.01	120.65	6.14	0.15	138	−1.54	111
FP∠	82.89	2.92	83.45	2.87	82.66	3.47	−0.83	73	1.02	65
MP∠	88.49	3.04	89.05	2.84	87.66	3.75	−0.83	72	1.72	64
AP∠	67.14	6.66	66.03	6.21	67.14	5.69	0.74	72	−0.74	63
OCC	99.38	5.90	100.21	5.74	101.63	6.19	−0.71	98	−1.10	86
FRS	22.13	2.41	22.48	2.40	22.16	2.26	−0.79	121	0.68	104
PAS	24.51	3.21	23.52	2.84	23.23	2.56	1.74	112	0.55	103
OCS	25.24	3.14	26.44	2.78	26.09	3.71	−1.99*	94	0.50	83
MDB	33.18	3.29	32.85	3.18	34.20	3.14	0.66	160	−2.54*	143
MLN	46.75	5.24	46.22	4.52	46.70	4.14	0.70	159	−0.66	143

* $p<.05$.
[a] Linear measurements in millimeters; angles in degrees.
[b] Average sample size. Sample size varies with different measurements.
[c] Two-sided tests.

TABLE 17

Adult Female Cranial Measurements, by Age

Measurement[a]	Young, $N=72^b$		Middle, $N=58^b$		Old, $N=51^b$		*t*-tests for comparisons[c]			
							Young/middle		Middle/old	
	Mean	*SD*	Mean	*SD*	Mean	*SD*	*t*	*df*	*t*	*df*
Vault length										
L	172.96	5.90	173.58	5.12	174.16	6.68	−0.60	114	−0.52	107
FC	108.77	4.28	108.62	4.10	109.33	4.59	0.22	156	−0.95	133
PAC	107.48	5.16	107.47	4.59	108.21	6.05	0.01	143	−0.76	103
FRF	47.59	4.06	48.03	3.21	48.72	3.24	−0.74	147	−1.21	125
Vault breadth										
B	134.00	4.25	134.65	4.51	135.07	6.60	−0.76	103	−0.36	78
MF	90.56	4.43	90.18	4.26	91.03	4.04	0.53	148	−1.14	123
XFB	111.30	4.81	111.55	3.94	111.73	5.20	−0.31	124	−0.20	93
ASB	103.74	4.15	104.30	3.97	104.51	4.48	−0.76	118	−0.26	103
Vault height										
H	136.48	4.20	137.51	5.16	137.28	4.80	−1.03	85	0.20	73
PAH	115.11	3.39	115.49	4.99	116.42	4.92	−0.42	73	−0.86	81
Cranial base										
LB	99.71	4.13	101.62	4.48	101.86	4.08	−2.09*	87	−0.24	75
FML	36.26	2.14	36.49	2.04	36.55	2.21	−0.53	95	−0.13	77
LCD	24.60	2.56	24.77	2.04	24.96	1.96	−0.41	126	−0.49	103
BCD	13.99	1.32	14.08	1.41	14.02	1.49	−0.41	136	0.24	111
BPH	23.36	2.91	23.47	2.55	22.82	3.46	−0.18	77	0.88	66
Face height										
TFH	114.51	5.99	112.60	5.83	114.44	7.17	1.51	92	−1.01	51
UFH	70.21	3.88	69.72	3.97	69.39	4.84	0.72	130	0.40	110
SH	34.74	2.64	34.57	3.63	33.57	3.79	0.32	116	1.53	126
LOH	34.18	2.07	34.03	1.56	34.09	2.00	0.48	135	−0.19	123
NH	49.84	2.74	50.08	2.38	51.57	3.24	−0.54	135	−2.83*	100
WMH	22.01	1.92	21.80	2.23	21.76	1.92	0.67	173	0.11	141
Face breadth										
TFB	127.95	5.44	128.39	4.49	130.93	5.73	−0.36	68	−1.91	58
MFB	96.36	4.15	95.50	5.15	97.15	4.35	1.04	159	−1.86	133
IOB	94.39	3.68	94.39	4.07	96.00	3.38	0.01	152	−2.46*	130

BOB	95.38	3.26	95.60	4.03	97.43	3.26	−0.34	120	−2.47*	98
AIB	19.27	2.09	19.20	1.87	19.40	1.91	0.21	128	−0.56	112
DC	20.38	2.26	20.79	2.36	20.19	1.79	−1.00	124	1.50	108
MN	9.26	1.64	9.17	1.81	9.13	1.71	0.29	140	0.31	123
LOBM	40.69	1.84	41.15	1.96	42.00	1.73	−1.45	143	−2.54*	122
NB	25.17	1.92	26.12	2.18	25.78	1.99	−2.81*	145	0.92	121
BNB	58.10	5.11	57.86	5.53	59.85	4.77	0.29	157	−2.17*	128
MB	63.71	3.75	61.32	4.73	60.83	6.01	3.37*	127	0.51	119
BA	96.95	5.88	94.02	5.14	96.06	5.76	2.88*	125	−1.88	99
BCB	115.19	6.26	114.55	5.44	117.00	5.94	0.56	110	−2.01*	85
CrCr	93.59	5.38	94.04	5.74	94.81	4.47	−0.43	107	−0.69	86
ZZ	45.36	2.24	44.63	2.54	44.55	2.38	1.89	152	0.19	127
CyL	18.81	1.76	18.80	1.72	19.04	1.88	0.03	150	−0.72	116
Face depth										
FLA	95.21	3.90	97.26	4.46	95.76	4.65	−2.19*	78	1.39	70
RL	32.36	2.74	31.88	2.73	32.31	2.04	1.14	174	−1.06	139
LM	103.14	4.16	105.19	6.30	105.04	4.59	−1.98	72	0.13	84
SIOB	16.90	2.53	16.82	2.01	16.89	2.21	0.21	140	−0.19	116
HNB	20.91	2.91	20.14	2.94	21.45	2.63	1.21	87	−1.89	64
ML	53.70	2.77	53.85	3.68	53.04	3.14	−0.27	110	1.28	114
IML	31.20	2.41	31.34	2.76	31.22	2.85	−0.34	152	0.25	123
XML	50.13	3.14	50.00	3.03	50.15	3.46	0.26	148	−0.26	118
Other										
G∠	123.33	5.76	124.77	6.25	123.10	6.13	−1.35	154	1.53	126
FP∠	81.24	3.37	81.79	3.54	82.87	4.24	−0.72	81	−1.21	75
MP∠	86.42	3.86	87.33	2.66	87.55	4.04	−1.27	78	−0.28	68
AP∠	66.56	4.79	65.79	6.68	67.95	7.45	0.59	66	−1.33	74
OCC	97.84	5.16	99.00	5.47	98.21	5.22	−1.13	108	0.73	96
FRS	22.75	2.39	22.18	2.42	22.23	2.91	1.42	147	−0.10	125
PAS	23.20	2.42	22.85	2.57	23.22	3.22	0.82	134	−0.70	119
OCS	24.83	2.84	24.87	2.99	24.73	3.38	−0.07	103	0.21	96
MDB	30.28	3.30	29.95	2.65	30.92	2.95	0.76	186	−2.11*	148
MLN	42.63	4.29	41.96	4.10	42.58	4.74	1.06	182	−0.85	149

* $p < .05$.
[a] Linear measurements in millimeters; angles in degrees.
[b] Average sample size. Sample size varies with different measurements.
[c] Two-sided tests.

which found that facial breadth dimensions increased in adulthood until senility, after which they began to decline. On the other hand, the increase with age of nasal breadth, breadth of the nasal bridge, and, to a lesser extent, midfacial breadth in the study series reflects the findings of previous workers.

Female facial breadth dimensions tend to increase with age in the west–central Illinois series. For middle-aged to old adults statistically significant increases occur for internal orbital breadth, biorbital breadth, orbital breadth, and breadth of the nasal bridge. For young to old adults the increase in nasal breadth is also statistically significant. These findings accord with previously reported results.

In both male and female series, maxillary breadth and maxillary length decrease with age. The decrease from young adults to middle adults is statistically significant in females. This reduction is likely a reflection of increased dental loss, and consequent alveolar bone loss, with age, an explanation which is evaluated in the next section.

In both male and female west–central Illinois series mandibular breadths tend to decrease slightly from young adulthood to middle adulthood (unlike findings of other investigations), and then to increase slightly from middle to old adulthood (consistent with previous research). The trends are not statistically significant in males. In females, the decrease in bigonial diameter from young to middle-aged adults is statistically significant, as is the increase in bicondylar breadth from middle to old age.

Face depth. Measurements of facial depth in the male study series tend to decrease somewhat from young to middle adulthood, and then to increase slightly. These trends are weak and nonsignificant. In the female series, facial length shows an opposite trend. It increases significantly from young to middle adulthood and then decreases slightly in old adulthood. The remaining measurements of facial depth remain relatively constant in females or increase slightly with age.

Other measurements. In males, measurements of facial prognathism do not change consistently with age, nor do the measurements themselves show parallel trends. Among females, facial angles tend to increase with age; that is, facial prognathism diminishes with age. Changes are nonsignificant for both sexes.

The gonial angle in males tends to increase from middle to old adulthood. In females, the gonial angle shows a tendency to increase from young to middle adulthood and then to decrease in old adulthood. These trends are nonsignificant. Previous research (Carlsson and Persson 1967; Israel 1973a, 1973b) also noted no significant age trends.

In both male and female study series, mastoid breadth and mastoid length are larger in old adults than in middle-aged adults. For mastoid breadth, the differences are statistically significant. Both dimensions decrease slightly from young to middle adulthood.

Males show a statistically significant increase in height of the occiput from the lambda-opisthion plane from young to middle adulthood. Females remain relatively constant through adulthood.

Discussion

The results presented here indicate tendencies for cranial dimensions to change with age in adult series from the west–central Illinois region. Table 18 summarizes the trends. Although few of the changes are statistically significant in either males or females, the age trends tend to reflect previous research. A relatively greater number of facial measurements vary significantly with age, especially in the female series, than measurements from other areas of the cranium. Since the facial measurements include measures of structures related to masticatory functions, the effects of age are perhaps a reflection, in part, of skeletal remodeling related to loss of teeth with advancing age.

Studies of the living indicate a tendency toward general size increase in cranial dimensions with age. The west–central Illinois female series likewise shows a rather consistent trend toward overall size increase.

TABLE 18
Summary of Age Trends in Adult Crania from West–Central Illinois, Dental Loss Uncontrolled

	Males		Females	
Dimension	Young to middle	Middle to old	Young to middle	Middle to old
Vault length	increase	decrease	(increase)	increase
Vault breadth	decrease	increase	increase	increase
Vault height	decrease	constant	increase	(increase)
Cranial base	unclear	unclear	increase	(increase)
Face height	(decrease)	decrease	(decrease)	unclear
Face breadth	(decrease)	unclear	(increase)	increase
Maxilla length and breadth	decrease	decrease	decrease	decrease
Mandible breadth	decrease	increase	decrease	increase
Face depth	(decrease)	(increase)	increase	(decrease)
Facial angles	(increase)	(decrease)	increase	increase
Gonial angle	constant	increase	increase	decrease
Mastoid size	(decrease)	increase	decrease	increase

Note: Parentheses indicate very slight trends.

Of the 55 measurements considered, 67% were larger in old adult females than in young adult females. My findings thus support the results of most previous research on living females; they do not support Tallgren's (1974) conclusion that there are no significant age changes in adult female crania.

Previously noted tendencies for cranial dimensions to increase with age are not clearly present in the male study series. This is not unexpected in light of several potentially confounding factors. These factors derive both from differences in samples and differences in research method.

First, differences in the nature of the samples studied could account for some of the observed differences. Most of the studies of adult age changes have been carried out on living populations where the sample represents a limited number of generations living within a relatively constant environment. In contrast, the west–central Illinois sample represents several populations living in the area over a period of approximately 600 years. Within this time, major subsistence changes took place, and changes through time in subadult growth patterns suggest that these shifts in adaptive strategy had biological consequences (D. C. Cook 1975b). The west–central Illinois sample, therefore, is cross-sectional not only in being made up of more than one growth cohort, but in the much broader sense that it is a sample of populations living in the area through several centuries and in various ecological situations.

Second, the study series is made up of individuals who have *died* at various ages. Insofar as presenility deaths were associated with factors which altered growth patterns (chronic disease, nutritional deficiency), the middle adult, and, especially, the young adult samples are not strictly comparable to samples of people *living* at these ages.

Third, the age categories used here are not entirely consistent with the age categories of other studies. The old age group in particular varies from one study to another. For example, Hellman (1927) defined old age as the age at which grooves on the molars were obliterated, while the mean age of M.S. Goldstein's (1936) "old men" group was 74 years. Individuals classified as old adults in the present study may have been older than the individuals in Hellman's old age group, since the molar grooves are often obliterated by middle age in the west–central Illinois series. On the other hand, the old adults (age 50+) in the study samples are very likely younger, on the average, than Goldstein's "old men."

Fourth, the measurements taken on the living are affected by soft tissue morphology, and are not strictly comparable to measurements taken from skulls. For example, nasal breadth in the living is a measurement of the maximum breadth of the external nasal structure, whereas nasal breadth in skulls is a measurement of the bony nasal aperture. Thus not all of the age changes noted in the study series may be analogous to age changes found in the living.

Fifth, some of the crania in the study samples have been artificially deformed. The application of deforming processes in infancy is thought to alter vectors of cranial growth, and thus to affect adult cranial morphology (Moss 1958). Deformed individuals in the study series may therefore not represent individuals with normal growth curves. This factor probably does not affect one adult age group more than another, since severity of deformation is not associated with age in any of the series. However, the incidence of some forms of deformation does appear to be associated with sex. For the Schild series, statistical tests indicated a significantly higher incidence of deformation in males than in females (see Chapter 5). Since the samples used to examine age changes contain a disproportionate number of Schild crania, the association of deformation with sex may in part explain why the female age trends, more than the male series trends, conform to the patterns of age changes found in previous research.

Finally, differences in the extent of antemortem dental loss may account for some of the differences in patterns of adult age changes in the study series and in series studied by previous workers. Tallgren's (1974) study, for example, was carried out on a sample of denture wearers, while the majority of the individuals in the study series were dentulous. Antemortem tooth loss and its effects on cranial age changes are discussed below.

Dental Loss and Age Changes in Morphology

The changes in cranial morphology discussed in the previous section cannot be attributed to cranial growth in adulthood without a consideration of the effects of dental loss on cranial morphology.

While the dental status of the samples used in the various aging studies is often not clearly indicated, most investigators have given some consideration to dental loss and its effects on cranial morphology. Lasker (1953:51), for example, did not measure facial heights in some individuals because of loss of teeth. Similarly, M. S. Goldstein (1936:52) attributed the reduced facial heights (except nose height) in old adults to loss of teeth and alveolar absorption, noting that all but 10 of the old men in his series had dentures which were removed during the period of examination. Hooton and Dupertuis (1951:23) suggested that the decrease in head breadth observed in old Irish males may have been in part attributable to temporal muscle thinning as a consequence of dental loss and masticatory atrophy. Decrease in facial height with age was likewise attributed to dental loss, which they described as "severe" in over half of the Irish males by age 50. Howells and Bleibtreu (1970:97) also acknowledged the effects of dental loss on facial height measurements and suggested that wear and loss of teeth may be a cause of differences in the results of adult age change studies (Howells and Bleibtreu 1970:121). Tallgren (1974:286) reported that most of his subjects were edentulous and all were denture wearers. He does not discuss the possible effects of dental loss on his results, however. Israel (1968, 1971, 1973a, 1973b, 1977), whose samples included individuals both with and without teeth, examined the effects of dental status on the relationship between age and mandibular morphology. Israel (1971:135) concluded that loss of teeth did not severely affect the mandible except in the alveolar ridge area.

In order to clarify the associations between cranial morphology and age in the study series, the relationship between cranial morphology and age was studied while taking into account the effects of dental loss.

Associations between number of teeth lost antemortem and age is, as expected, highly correlated in the study series. Pearson's correlation coefficient is 0.4342 ($df = 121$, $p < .001$) for males and 0.5527 ($df = 124$, $p < .001$) for females.

The average numbers of teeth lost prior to death for males and females in the three age categories are compared in Table 19. Two-tailed *t* tests[1] of the differences between age categories were carried out separately for male and female series, using the SPSS subprogram T-TEST (Nie *et al.* 1975). The results are given in Table 19. The increase in lost teeth is highly significant from young adulthood to middle adulthood in both males and females, and from middle to old adulthood in females.

On the whole, females show more antemortem tooth loss than males. Combining all series and all age categories, females had lost an average of 6.69 teeth at the time of death, while males had lost 5.04 teeth. This difference falls short of statistical significance at the .05 level ($p = .103$) when a *t* test is carried out.[2]

[1] The *t* statistics were computed using separate estimates of variance rather than the pooled estimate because variances in the two samples were unequal.

[2] This sex difference is due primarily to the high incidence of teeth lost prior to death in the Schild Mississippian female series, which makes up the greater part of the combined

TABLE 19
Incidence of Antemortem Dental Loss

	Mean number of teeth lost[a]			t-tests for comparisons[b]					
				Young/Middle			Middle/Old		
	Young	Middle	Old	t	df	p	t	df	p
Males	1.38	6.35	9.61	−4.02	60	<0.001	−1.68	49	0.100
Females	2.20	6.48	13.43	−3.03	48	.004	−3.38	68	0.001

[a] Young: N = 47 males, 54 females. Middle: N = 51 males, 33 females. Old: N = 23 males, 37 females.
[b] Two-sided tests.

Partial correlation was used to examine the association between age and cranial dimensions, with the effects of dental loss controlled. Partial correlation coefficients were computed using the SPSS subprogram PARTIAL CORR (Nie *et al.* 1975). These partial coefficients were compared to zero-order correlations between measurements and age in order to estimate how much of the variance can be attributed to the association of age with loss of teeth. A two-tailed test of statistical significance was applied to each zero-order and first-order partial correlation coefficient. The criterion for significance was $p < .05$.

This analysis was carried out separately for male and female series of west–central Illinois crania (sites combined), from which complete dental data were available. Individuals were included only if it was possible to determine whether or not each of the 32 teeth was present at the time of death. Samples consisted of 121 males and 124 females. Missing data were deleted pairwise; that is, an individual was deleted from the computation of a particular correlation coefficient if one of the two variables (or three variables in the case of the partial correlations) was missing, but this same individual was included in the computation of other coefficients if complete data were present.

The resulting pattern of associations between age and cranial measurements (Table 20) is consistent with the t test mean comparisons described in the previous section. Some differences between the t test and correlation results are predictable because the Pearson correlation coefficient is a measure of linear association. The association with age is not linear for all measurements. Some measurements increase up to a certain age and then decrease with age, or vice versa. In addition,

female sample. An average of 11.24 teeth were lost prior to death in the Schild Mississippian female series, while an average of 5.71 teeth were lost antemortem in the Schild male series.

TABLE 20
Effects of Antemortem Dental Loss on Correlation between Cranial Measurements and Age

Measurement	Males			Females		
	N	r_{am}	$r_{am.t}$	N	r_{am}	$r_{am.t}$
Vault length						
Glabello-occipital length	92	.0108	.0401	100	.1213	.1140
Frontal chord	107	−.0230	−.0023	114	.1020	.0677
Parietal chord	97	−.1467	−.1752	106	.0390	−.0297
Frontal subtense fraction	97	.0560	.0315	115	.2030*	.1020
Vault breadth						
Maximum cranial breadth	85	−.1148	−.1306	93	.0699	−.0090
Minimum frontal breadth	108	−.1857	−.1531	110	.0113	−.0087
Maximum frontal breadth	91	−.1802	−.1290	104	−.0192	−.0183
Biasterionic breadth	94	−.0720	−.0963	97	.1468	.1038
Vault height						
Basion-bregma height	78	−.1115	−.1313	83	.1350	−.0077
Porion-apex height	82	−.0214	−.0640	87	.1095	−.0300
Cranial base						
Length of cranial base	77	−.0929	−.0820	82	.3124*	.2329*
Foramen magnum length	82	.1583	.1773	86	.0639	.0990
Length of occipital condyle	94	.0498	.0948	97	.0893	.0506
Breadth of occipital condyle	99	.0200	.0523	100	.1279	.1004
Basion-porion height	73	−.0469	−.0911	78	−.0175	−.0434
Face height						
Total facial height	82	−.0545	.1024	77	−.0318	−.0360
Upper facial height	113	−.1272	.0116	108	−.1263	−.0047
Height of mandibular symphysis	118	−.0895	.0908	121	−.1216	.0219
Orbital height	110	−.1324	−.1375	110	.0689	−.0914
Nasal height	113	−.0257	−.0743	111	.2257*	.1080
Cheek height	118	−.0386	.0486	120	−.0773	−.0385
Face breadth						
Total facial breadth	72	−.0767	−.0795	76	.2071	.1250
Midfacial breadth	117	.0281	.0327	117	.1819*	.1099
Internal biorbital breadth	106	−.0451	−.0596	113	.3031*	.2058*
Biorbital breadth	97	.0086	−.0337	104	.3198*	.1656
Anterior interorbital breadth	107	−.1262	−.0846	108	.0912	.1302
Dacryal chord	102	−.1664	−.0835	103	−.0327	−.0109

(*continued*)

the correlation analysis was based on more restricted samples of the age distribution. The requirement that dental data be complete for a case to be included eliminated a disproportionate number of individuals over 50 years of age. In the male series, 38.8% of the total sample of 121 individuals were 20 to 34.9 years of age, 42.1% were 35 to 49.9 years of age, and 19% were over 50. In the female sample of 124 individuals, 43.5% were 20 to 34.9 years of age, 26.6% were 35 to 49.9 years of age, and 29.8% were over 50.

Table 21 summarizes the effects of controlling for dental loss on age

TABLE 20
Continued

Measurement	Males			Females		
	N	r_{am}	$r_{am.t}$	N	r_{am}	$r_{am.t}$
Minimum breadth of nasals	109	−.2714*	−.2861*	110	−.0281	−.0123
Orbital breadth, mf	111	−.0627	−.0226	111	.3137*	.1683
Nasal breadth	114	.1153	.0890	116	.1411	.0744
Breadth of nasal bridge	117	.0774	.0635	117	.1723	.1129
Maxillo-alveolar breadth	118	−.2398*	−.0535	117	−.2587*	.0247
Biangular breadth	104	.0987	.0983	112	−.0391	−.0418
Bicondylar breadth	92	−.0741	−.0417	98	.2269*	.1303
Coronial breadth	88	.0305	.0177	98	.0750	.0017
Breadth at mental foramen	118	.0104	.0656	123	−.0568	.0012
Maximum condylar length	104	−.1037	−.0568	111	.1257	.1176
Face depth						
Facial length, alv. pt.	76	−.0541	.0523	80	.1092	.2309*
Breadth of ascending ramus	119	−.0980	−.0300	122	.0760	.1445
Length of mandible	102	−.0112	.0079	102	.2446*	.2522*
Subtense to int. biorb. breadth	101	−.1154	−.0443	107	.0028	.0456
Height of nasal bridge	74	.0116	−.0323	80	.0269	.0530
Maxillo-alveolar length	119	−.1106	.0619	117	−.0542	.1281
Malar length, inferior	116	−.0372	−.0271	113	.0591	.0302
Malar length, maximum	114	−.0606	−.0725	110	.0041	−.0157
Other						
Gonial angle	114	.0647	.0759	119	.0274	.0269
Angle total facial prognathism	81	−.0008	−.0362	86	.1915	.0783
Angle midfacial prognathism	80	−.0917	−.0909	87	.1111	.0260
Angle alveolar prognathism	80	.0476	.0687	85	.1289	.0007
Occipital chord	93	.2707*	.2784*	94	.0930	.0354
Frontal subtense	97	.0902	.0871	115	−.0951	−.0065
Parietal subtense	97	−.2316*	−.2574*	103	−.0499	−.1596
Occipital subtense	90	.2788*	.2461*	93	.0993	.1284
Mastoid breadth	118	.0985	.1051	121	.0658	.0196
Mastoid length (MLN)	119	−.0557	−.0583	120	.0039	−.0310

* $p < .05$.

Note: r_{am} is Pearson zero-order coefficient of correlation between adult age a and cranial measurements m; $r_{am.t}$ is first order partial controlling for antemortem dental loss t.

trends in cranial morphology. Certainly, some of the age trends in the study series are partially due to dental loss. This is true in particular for measurements of areas of the face that are closely associated with masticatory functions.

Adult Age Changes and Biological Distance

Of the 55 measurements taken from the west–central Illinois study series, 15 (27.3%) are significantly correlated ($p < .05$) with age in one

TABLE 21
Effects of Dental Loss on Correlation between Cranial Measurements and Age

Dimension	Males	Females
Vault length	No effect	Little effect; possibly weakens positive association between frontal subtense fraction and age
Vault breadth	No effect	Little effect; possibly weakens positive association between cranial breadth and age
Vault height	No effect	Weakens positive association between vault height and age
Cranial base	No effect	No effect
Face height	Weakens negative association between age and total facial height, upper facial height, and height at the mandibular symphysis; little effect on remaining measurements	Weakens negative association between age and both upper facial height and height at the mandibular symphysis; weakens positive association between age and both orbital height and nasal height; no effect on remaining measurements
Face breadth	No effect	Weakens positive association between age and measures of face breadth
Maxilla length and breadth	Weakens negative assoication between age and both maxillo-alveolar length and maxillo-alveolar breadth	Weakens negative association between age and both maxillo-alveolar length and maxillo-alveolar breadth
Mandible breadth	No effect	Weakens positive association between age and bicondylar breadth
Face depth	Weakens negative association between age and facial length; little effect on remaining measurements	Strengthens positive association between age and facial length
Facial angles	No effect	Weakens positive association with age
Gonial angle	No effect	No effect
Mastoid size	No effect	No effect

or both sexes. The statistically significant correlations range from 0.2030 to 0.3198, averaging 0.2588. Thus, age explains an average of 6.7% of the variation in the 14 measurements which are significantly associated with age.

Since the primary objective of this research is to compare inherited morphological variation between the west–central Illinois cranial series, the component of within-group variation attributable to age, although small, constitutes a source of bias in estimates of intergroup biological distances. One means of limiting the effects of age-related morphological variation on biodistance estimates would be to select measurements which are not significantly associated with age in the study series. Unfortunately, data limitations prohibited the selection of variables on this basis in the present study. The four measurement subsets compiled for possible use in the biodistance analysis and the criteria for variable selection have been described previously (Chapter 4). The 9-variable vault subset included three measurements significantly associated with age, the 14-variable face subset included four age-affected measurements, the 6-variable mandible subset included one measurement significantly associated with age, and the 14-variable combined morphology subset included 3 variables shown to be significantly associated with age in the study series.

If the age structures of the cranial samples used for the biodistance analyses were approximately the same, the inclusion of age-related measurements would have little effect on estimates of intergroup biological distance between these groups. Table 22 compares the age

TABLE 22
Age Distribution of Biodistance Samples

	20–34		35–49		50+	
	N	%	*N*	%	*N*	%
Koster Late Woodland						
Males	12	38.7	17	54.8	2	6.5
Females	13	37.1	14	40.0	8	22.9
Klunk Late Woodland						
Males	0	0	5	62.5	3	37.5
Females	5	41.7	5	41.7	2	16.7
Schild Late Woodland						
Males	3	27.3	4	36.4	4	36.4
Females	11	57.9	3	15.8	5	26.3
Yokem Late Woodland						
Males	3	21.4	9	64.3	2	14.3
Females	8	32.0	11	44.0	6	24.0
Ledders Late Woodland						
Males	1	7.1	6	42.9	7	50.0
Females	6	50.0	4	33.3	2	16.7
Schild Mississippian						
Males	25	47.2	15	28.3	13	24.5
Females	23	39.7	15	25.9	20	34.5
Yokem Mississippian						
Males	8	53.3	4	26.7	3	20.0
Females	6	25.0	9	37.5	9	37.5

structures of the male and female samples of adult crania from the seven study series. These samples were used for biological distance analyses.

The age structures of the cranial samples reflect quite closely the demographic profiles for the total adult series (Table 3). Like the total series, the majority of individuals in the cranial samples are young or middle-aged adults, with a tendency for underrepresentation of crania in the 50+ age group. Exceptions to this generalization are the male samples from the Ledders, Klunk, and Schild Late Woodland series, and the female samples from the Yokem and Schild Mississippian series.

Division of the already small cranial samples into the three adult age categories resulted in very low frequencies in some cells, as can be seen in Table 22. For this reason, conclusions arising from the comparison of age structures between samples are tentative. Kolmogorov–Smirnov tests (Blalock 1972:262) were used to determine the statistical significance of differences in adult age structures in the samples. For each sex, tests were carried out for all pairs of samples. None of the between-group differences is statistically significant at the .05 level of probability. When the .10 level was used as the criterion for statistical significance, significant differences are indicated for 4 out of 21 comparisons between male groups: Ledders–Koster, Ledders–Schild Mississippian, Ledders–Yokem Mississippian, and Klunk Late Woodland–Schild Mississippian. None of the differences between female samples is statistically significant at the .10 level.

With these exceptions, then, differences in age structure between samples are no greater than expected by chance. These results suggest that the inclusion of age-related measurements in the discriminant analysis variable lists will have little effect on the estimates of biological distance among female groups and among most of the male groups.

The effects of including age-affected measurements in the distance analysis are considered further in Chapter 7 when the results of the discriminant analyses are examined. The discriminant function weights assigned to the age-related variables are particularly useful in this regard, since these weights provide an indication of the discriminatory power of individual variables. Relatively large weights associated with age-related variables would suggest that the age differences between samples contribute more to the discrimination than the analyses of this chapter would predict. (The age profiles of the samples presented in Table 22 can be used to indicate if the samples in question do in fact differ with regard to age structure.) On the other hand, low weights associated with age-related variables would suggest that age differences between groups was not an important factor in explaining intergroup morphological differences.

7

Late Woodland Biological Distances

At the outset of this investigation, two general problems in west–central Illinois prehistory were defined. The first concerns the structure of biological relationships among Late Woodland communities in the region. The second concerns interactions among Late Woodland and Mississippian peoples. These questions were dealt with using discriminant analysis of cranial measurements, according to the rationale and methodology described in Chapter 4. The present chapter presents the discriminant analysis results pertaining to Late Woodland patterns of biological distance, while the following chapter is addressed to the question of Late–Woodland–Mississippi relationships.

The first set of discriminant analyses was designed to discover if ecological changes from Middle to Late Woodland were accompanied by changes in the structure of biosocial interactions among local communities of west–central Illinois. Buikstra (1976) has shown that Middle Woodland skeletal series from within the region can be distinguished from one another, and that intergroup biological differences generally reflect distance by river. In the present study, Late Woodland patterns of biological distance were compared with this Middle Woodland pattern to see if the mosaic of biosocial interactions which characterized the Middle Woodland period was maintained through Late Woodland times.

This chapter contains four sections. The first presents univariate results consisting of group means, standard deviations, and one-way analyses of variance for 33 cranial measurements. The *F* ratios obtained from the analyses of variance indicate between-group differences for each measurement, independently of other measurements in the variable subset. The second section describes the results of the multivariate discriminant analyses based on face measurements, and discusses these findings in terms of alternative models of Late Woodland intergroup relationships. The results of distance analyses based on alternative data sets are presented in the third section. The final section summarizes the findings regarding biological relationships among Late Woodland groups of west–central Illinois.

Univariate Results

Each of the 33 measurements was compared across series in order to identify morphological differences among Late Woodland groups. These groups included four male series (Koster, Schild, Yokem, Ledders) and five female series (Koster, Klunk, Schild, Yokem, Ledders). The Klunk male series was excluded because of its small size. One-way analyses of variance were carried out separately for male and female series. The SPSS subprogram DISCRIMINANT (Nie *et al.* 1975) was used to perform the computations.

The resulting *F* ratios are a measure of the degree of within-group variation as compared to the between-group variation in each measurement. The .05 level of probability was used as the criterion for statistical significance of the *F* ratios.

Table 23 contains the group means and standard deviations for each of the cranial samples. Pearson coefficients of correlation among the cranial measurements are presented in Tables 24 and 25. Table 26 gives the results of the one-way analysis of variance tests for both male and female series.

Males

Statistically significant *F* ratios were obtained for 7 of the 33 cranial measurements in the male study series (Table 26). Four of the statistically significant measurements—minimum frontal breadth (MF), internal biorbital breadth (IOB), anterior interorbital breadth (AIB), and minimum breadth of nasals (MN)—measure aspects of upper facial breadth. As expected, they are relatively highly correlated with one another (Table 24). Comparison of group means (Table 23) suggests that significant differences in these measurements are due primarily to differences between the Schild series and the three other Late Woodland series. The Schild crania have considerably narrower upper faces than the other Late Woodland series. The means for the remaining facial

TABLE 23

Cranial Measurements by Sex and Series, Males

Variable	Koster LW M	Koster LW SD	Klunk LW M	Klunk LW SD	Schild LW M	Schild LW SD	Yokem LW M	Yokem LW SD	Ledders LW M	Ledders LW SD	Schild Miss M	Schild Miss SD	Yokem Miss M	Yokem Miss SD
L	182.42	6.48	179.00	3.35	182.00	7.69	182.86	6.30	183.29	5.22	179.70	6.72	182.20	3.21
MF	94.16	3.68	90.90	6.14	90.64	3.83	94.50	3.13	94.64	4.96	93.85	4.79	95.40	4.50
FC	113.87	3.51	111.30	3.27	113.82	4.90	115.71	5.03	114.36	3.00	112.32	4.69	113.33	4.05
MFB	99.58	4.61	98.75	2.49	98.73	2.83	101.07	5.98	99.93	4.75	99.62	5.09	103.13	3.91
IOB	97.61	3.03	97.70	2.71	95.36	2.50	98.79	4.34	98.93	3.38	99.21	3.70	99.47	4.02
SIOB	19.39	2.40	18.10	2.28	17.18	2.36	18.14	2.38	18.07	3.05	19.08	2.04	19.20	2.11
AIB	20.29	1.95	18.60	1.65	18.27	1.85	19.64	2.02	20.29	1.98	19.30	1.90	20.33	1.68
LOBM	42.32	1.66	42.88	1.46	41.73	1.42	42.57	1.65	42.50	1.56	43.23	1.89	43.07	1.58
LOH	34.84	1.75	34.38	2.56	34.18	1.66	35.07	1.27	34.21	0.70	34.21	1.78	34.60	1.30
NH	52.42	2.73	53.88	2.80	52.55	2.54	54.64	1.95	52.21	3.26	52.79	2.38	54.27	2.02
NB	26.23	1.63	24.78	1.43	25.82	1.60	26.43	2.03	26.07	1.33	25.38	1.61	26.13	1.51
DC	21.23	2.09	20.50	1.60	20.36	2.11	21.43	1.22	22.29	2.52	20.11	2.31	21.20	1.32
MN	9.29	1.79	9.22	1.64	7.55	1.37	8.64	1.91	9.50	1.74	8.83	1.57	9.47	1.30
BNB	59.90	4.41	59.67	3.46	59.91	3.67	60.57	4.60	61.29	4.10	60.30	5.25	60.60	4.00
BA	104.42	5.97	102.25	7.92	103.36	8.95	108.64	5.31	102.79	5.89	105.25	7.36	105.33	6.69
RL	33.16	2.21	33.46	3.30	32.00	1.79	34.64	3.03	33.57	1.95	34.47	2.56	34.67	2.19
LM	107.90	5.57	109.90	5.49	106.82	4.83	108.14	5.25	108.50	4.82	106.89	5.08	108.13	4.87
G∠	120.77	8.01	120.20	9.26	120.27	4.47	118.64	5.34	118.29	4.21	118.47	6.13	117.33	7.81
ZZ	46.48	2.16	47.09	2.84	45.73	2.94	47.07	2.76	46.64	2.71	45.94	2.35	48.00	3.02
CyL	20.97	1.45	21.00	1.50	20.18	2.09	21.00	2.88	21.79	2.08	21.11	1.60	21.87	1.46
IML	32.87	3.01	33.38	2.13	31.91	2.34	34.29	2.52	32.93	3.22	34.49	2.92	33.40	2.77
XML	52.71	3.31	53.12	1.88	51.91	2.07	54.50	2.90	52.64	3.08	54.55	3.35	53.47	3.94
WMH	23.23	1.91	24.62	1.68	23.00	2.19	24.50	2.07	24.07	1.77	23.98	2.11	23.93	2.05
LCD	26.29	1.53	26.73	2.28	28.00	2.45	27.29	1.73	27.50	1.87	25.96	2.09	26.60	1.84
BCD	14.61	0.92	14.09	2.02	14.64	0.81	14.86	1.23	14.07	1.21	13.77	1.30	13.47	0.74
ASB	107.97	4.35	106.50	4.38	106.09	5.66	108.36	5.03	107.14	5.17	106.47	3.87	108.13	3.62
FRS	23.35	1.82	20.80	2.78	23.36	2.46	23.64	2.53	22.43	1.60	21.53	2.22	22.73	2.25
FRF	51.19	3.42	51.90	2.47	50.45	2.58	52.64	3.63	51.00	3.40	51.13	3.75	51.20	3.19
PAC	111.58	5.88	110.33	4.82	106.55	6.12	113.43	5.81	110.07	5.08	110.40	5.86	111.40	5.23
PAS	23.71	2.19	24.11	3.22	21.82	2.89	23.64	2.53	22.29	2.76	25.04	2.65	23.40	2.50
OCC	99.35	6.41	101.33	6.30	101.55	6.44	99.93	4.53	101.86	4.07	99.91	4.98	101.47	6.25
MDB	33.45	2.86	34.00	3.07	32.00	3.00	33.86	3.11	33.00	2.32	34.08	2.78	34.13	3.70
MLN	46.58	5.00	46.70	2.98	43.91	3.42	48.29	4.89	45.64	3.20	46.87	4.54	47.27	4.95

(continued)

TABLE 23 (*Continued*)

Cranial Measurements by Sex and Series, Females

Variable	Koster LW		Klunk LW		Schild LW		Yokem LW		Ledders LW		Schild Miss		Yokem Miss	
	M	*SD*	*M*	*SD*	*M*	*SD*	*M*	*SD*	*M*	*SD*	*M*	*SD*	*M*	*SD*
L	173.49	6.41	174.08	2.15	176.47	5.49	172.92	5.64	173.67	4.74	173.67	6.26	173.62	4.13
MF	89.77	3.57	89.50	5.00	89.63	3.81	90.44	4.05	90.08	2.39	91.22	4.55	92.38	4.03
FC	108.06	4.64	106.42	2.84	109.95	3.81	108.84	4.71	109.50	2.81	108.98	4.65	110.00	3.49
MFB	95.09	4.91	93.75	2.86	96.47	4.29	96.92	5.29	96.00	3.95	96.91	4.06	96.58	4.27
IOB	94.57	3.34	93.50	3.09	92.68	3.48	94.36	4.01	93.92	4.12	96.00	3.22	96.42	3.12
SIOB	16.94	2.39	16.50	2.32	17.53	2.09	17.04	2.15	16.92	1.78	16.62	1.95	17.04	1.52
AIB	19.20	1.92	18.33	1.37	19.11	1.79	19.84	1.75	19.75	2.34	18.86	2.03	19.88	1.90
LOBM	41.14	1.94	40.50	1.62	40.79	2.02	40.08	1.66	40.50	1.51	42.03	1.89	41.54	1.67
LOH	33.77	1.75	32.67	1.07	34.00	1.37	33.68	2.46	34.42	2.07	34.50	1.98	34.38	1.28
NH	50.74	2.55	48.83	2.12	50.37	1.86	49.72	2.72	50.42	2.47	50.72	3.40	50.67	2.16
NB	25.63	1.80	25.25	1.66	26.26	2.26	25.88	2.19	25.75	2.45	25.66	1.93	25.17	1.46
DC	20.00	2.53	21.17	1.95	20.37	1.50	21.44	1.78	21.08	2.15	20.02	2.15	20.67	1.81
MN	8.94	1.78	8.92	1.98	8.79	2.12	9.44	1.66	10.08	1.88	9.17	1.53	9.71	1.37
BNB	57.66	5.11	57.25	5.55	58.00	4.47	59.24	5.90	57.42	4.27	58.81	5.07	59.08	5.47
BA	95.86	6.33	97.33	5.33	94.63	4.89	96.64	6.30	93.58	5.05	96.33	5.02	96.50	4.10
RL	31.63	2.13	32.75	2.45	31.16	2.36	32.36	2.00	31.33	2.06	32.86	2.48	32.50	2.11
LM	104.14	4.19	104.08	6.24	103.42	2.71	103.80	4.56	104.00	3.02	104.45	5.73	105.08	4.02
G∠	124.31	6.76	124.58	6.35	126.11	5.84	123.16	5.44	125.50	6.10	121.67	6.58	123.29	6.69
ZZ	44.29	2.30	45.50	2.20	44.58	2.09	44.88	2.54	44.92	1.78	45.16	1.94	45.75	2.74
CyL	18.63	1.66	18.58	1.38	18.11	1.49	19.12	1.56	18.08	1.56	19.34	1.79	19.46	1.38
IML	31.29	2.83	31.67	2.71	29.63	1.77	31.36	2.43	30.00	2.86	31.79	2.57	32.12	2.21
XML	50.51	2.64	50.42	2.57	48.68	2.63	49.88	2.85	49.33	3.58	50.72	3.31	50.83	3.51
WMH	21.66	2.13	22.00	1.35	21.37	2.11	22.64	2.10	21.75	2.18	21.97	2.07	21.33	1.71
LCD	24.74	1.82	24.42	2.02	24.58	1.43	24.96	2.05	24.42	1.51	24.72	2.34	25.04	2.49
BCD	13.83	1.07	14.75	1.60	14.26	1.05	13.52	1.05	13.83	1.19	14.34	1.61	13.67	1.09
ASB	104.17	3.89	103.83	3.64	103.63	3.71	104.00	3.94	103.08	2.68	104.21	3.84	104.00	3.06
FRS	22.17	2.08	23.17	2.37	23.00	1.80	23.32	1.97	22.33	2.39	21.88	2.82	22.62	2.26
FRF	47.49	3.81	46.83	3.88	48.11	2.90	48.44	3.50	47.58	2.81	48.21	3.38	49.29	3.13
PAC	107.31	4.70	107.50	4.50	108.05	4.97	107.96	5.13	105.42	6.16	107.83	5.49	107.29	4.48
PAS	22.71	2.19	23.08	2.75	22.32	1.80	23.36	3.20	21.92	3.15	23.90	2.70	22.46	2.69
OCC	97.60	4.76	95.92	4.70	97.21	3.12	97.64	3.35	98.92	4.06	99.22	5.75	98.79	4.41
MDB	30.34	2.84	31.08	1.62	28.05	2.72	31.52	3.22	30.33	4.10	31.40	2.82	30.42	3.12
MLN	41.83	4.64	43.58	4.60	40.26	5.46	42.52	3.55	41.75	5.24	42.79	4.22	43.08	3.73

TABLE 24

Correlation Coefficients for 33 Cranial Measurements, Males

	L	MF	FC	MFB	IOB	SIOB	AIB	LOBM	LOH	NH	NB	DC	MN	BNB	BA	RL
MF	.161															
FC	.405	.351														
MFB	.087	.182	.045													
IOB	.288	.619	.237	.488												
SIOB	.313	.378	.269	−.126	.284											
AIB	.300	.357	.193	.119	.423	.388										
LOBM	.286	.423	.256	.270	.598	.292	−.021									
LOH	−.033	.006	.061	−.139	.094	.164	.018	.100								
NH	.291	.229	.225	−.003	.199	.329	.116	.282	.225							
NB	.153	.145	.102	.387	.302	.006	.298	.197	−.044	.089						
DC	.209	.322	.078	.166	.418	.275	.732	.088	.034	.015	.438					
MN	.183	.312	.091	.131	.241	.233	.521	.040	−.036	.076	.249	.406				
BNB	.287	.223	.160	.484	.341	.131	.307	.258	.026	.118	.300	.217	.194			
BA	.101	.138	−.010	.261	.299	−.085	−.087	.248	−.073	.056	.164	.058	−.053	.178		
RL	.164	.149	.047	.311	.243	.028	.192	.136	−.170	.134	.218	.121	.072	.195	.164	
LM	.264	.138	.165	.170	.233	.151	.125	.191	−.052	.214	.170	.159	.054	.155	.160	.224
G∠	−.054	−.013	.047	−.155	−.086	.069	.018	−.048	−.006	−.053	.044	−.019	.083	.011	.002	−.260
ZZ	.154	.156	.160	.413	.359	−.045	.081	.224	−.086	.133	.303	.095	−.113	.181	.295	.279
CyL	.135	.203	−.013	.297	.244	.111	.187	.153	.035	.320	.208	.229	.091	.165	.166	.282
IML	.254	.130	.097	−.001	.231	.192	.314	.147	−.005	.181	.223	.218	.089	.010	.247	.389
XML	.162	.170	.097	.210	.291	.179	.165	.195	−.078	.164	.166	.102	.116	−.249	.154	.341
WMH	.188	.105	.245	433	.333	−.079	.092	.186	−.133	.218	.080	.045	.055	.141	.062	.423
LCD	.230	−.108	.075	.139	.062	.116	.022	.051	−.203	.081	−.103	−.038	−.065	.028	.256	.258
BCD	.005	−.092	.004	−.113	−.187	−.044	−.022	−.159	.071	−.146	−.015	.112	−.107	−.029	−.092	−.058
ASB	.179	.200	.207	.242	.337	.032	.155	.186	.053	.184	.131	.174	.113	.159	.278	.134
FRS	.130	.263	.532	.014	.082	−.109	−.031	.133	.065	.031	.033	−.054	.010	.075	.029	−.090
FRF	.122	.071	.462	.044	.167	.108	.163	.144	.126	.046	.165	.087	.162	.033	−.102	−.019
PAC	.475	.096	.242	−.019	.152	.106	.144	.108	−.071	.069	−.076	.070	.115	.032	.139	.090
PAS	−.078	.033	.019	.124	.075	−.076	.101	−.080	−.124	−.049	−.029	.016	.061	−.141	.100	.098
OCC	.411	.096	.166	.093	.259	.176	.111	.172	−.062	.212	.070	.120	.019	.205	.152	−.024
MDB	−.018	.329	.171	.238	.321	.053	.176	.129	−.110	.070	.174	.166	.005	.227	.150	.307
MLN	.095	.191	.180	.230	.194	.084	.036	.096	−.133	−.041	−.015	−.028	−.039	.126	−.099	.151

(*continued*)

TABLE 24
Continued

	LM	G∠	ZZ	CyL	IML	XML	WMH	LCD	BCD	ASB	FRS	FRF	PAC	PAS	OCC	MDB
G∠	.442															
ZZ	.318	−.098														
CyL	.148	−.250	.178													
IML	.218	−.046	.142	.171												
XML	.158	−.125	.193	.254	.693											
WMH	.155	−.316	.384	.386	.129	.303										
LCD	.291	.084	.159	.050	.220	.225	.209									
BCD	.148	.316	.020	−.157	−.162	−.125	−.237	.108								
ASB	.092	−.197	.192	.247	.122	.131	.234	.128	.077							
FRS	.055	.212	−.076	−.113	−.015	−.049	−.089	−.070	.126	.072						
FRF	.138	.088	.098	−.067	.099	.188	.132	−.116	−.045	.100	.119					
PAC	.114	−.042	−.063	−.046	.244	.123	−.063	.150	−.025	.081	.255	.015				
PAS	.025	.016	.031	−.053	.172	.245	−.036	.035	−.076	.027	.125	.067	.586			
OCC	.079	−.119	.265	.058	.092	.057	.200	.166	−.133	.222	−.080	.028	−.188	−.472		
MDB	.111	−.010	.200	.132	.074	.087	.284	−.009	−.130	.208	.032	.084	.081	.129	−.021	
MLN	−.093	−.158	.195	.080	−.099	.054	.227	.092	−.024	.108	−.007	−.070	.162	.167	.026	.340

Note: Correlations based on all crania in biodistance sample, $N = 138$.

TABLE 25

Correlation Coefficients for 33 Cranial Measurements, Females

	L	MF	FC	MFB	IOB	SIOB	AIB	LOBM	LOH	NH	NB	DC	MN	BNB	BA	RL
MF	.284															
FC	.505	.344														
MFB	.296	.290	.230													
IOB	.286	.573	.251	.438												
SIOB	.288	.233	.180	.206	.293											
AIB	.196	.346	.060	.213	.456	.286										
LOBM	.260	.309	.255	.398	.657	.202	−.017									
LOH	.148	.201	.133	.133	.283	.178	.053	.237								
NH	.217	.135	.207	.332	.328	.195	.142	.300	.455							
NB	.162	.154	.159	.272	.368	.126	.402	.207	.098	.203						
DC	.155	.247	.056	.137	.387	.194	.724	.038	.072	.044	.375					
MN	.106	.246	.011	.109	.241	.236	.554	.011	.140	.130	.276	.383				
BNB	.210	.391	.222	.453	.493	.347	.343	.430	.280	.187	.450	.345	.169			
BA	.154	.199	.289	.223	.304	.186	.096	.207	.140	.146	.145	.009	−.012	.174		
RL	.024	.196	−.112	.211	.135	.101	.079	.080	−.101	−.010	−.107	.046	.096	−.040	.077	
LM	.315	.103	.270	.361	.206	.045	−.006	.220	.153	.327	.185	.050	.031	.105	.145	.170
G∠	.141	−.025	.161	.027	.001	−.035	.050	−.010	.128	.104	.213	.074	−.008	.146	.186	−.359
ZZ	.117	.100	.056	.373	.132	.126	.131	.033	.081	.056	.022	.091	.171	.109	.256	.185
CyL	.086	.110	.111	.397	.417	.111	.061	.342	.062	.188	.158	.095	.020	.225	.151	.253
IML	.251	.289	.169	−.012	.451	.189	.281	.216	.164	.140	.106	.254	.224	.073	.091	.220
XML	.180	.132	.116	.108	.257	.135	.071	.133	−.040	.178	−.041	−.013	.086	−.348	.102	.342
WMH	.135	.156	.216	.417	.215	.183	.144	.094	−.043	.263	.010	.052	.170	.038	.138	.337
LCD	.173	.106	.062	.088	.244	.131	.032	.213	.181	.128	.001	.065	.016	.055	.295	.033
BCD	.285	.106	.054	208	.215	.113	.081	.166	.181	.057	.043	.031	.081	.140	.131	.137
ASB	.129	.173	.247	.068	.185	.096	−.004	.206	.117	.098	.057	.025	−.016	.062	.173	−.047
FRS	.277	.292	.499	.050	−.011	−.017	−.048	−.037	−.104	−.061	.023	−.050	−.117	.084	.060	−.130
FRF	.182	.211	.542	.100	.166	.099	.204	.074	.123	.219	.123	.145	.019	.119	.266	−.050
PAC	.561	.220	.318	.181	.190	.088	.165	.093	.099	.039	.142	.058	.104	.023	.203	.076
PAS	.044	.127	.194	−.002	.105	.132	.061	−.008	.059	.008	.056	−.058	−.001	−.078	.213	.041
OCC	.317	.158	.140	.049	.205	−.030	.016	.193	.054	.070	.054	.064	.006	.075	.111	−.093
MDB	.091	.204	.145	.190	.376	.207	.065	.304	−.019	.073	.079	.026	−.043	.188	.348	.152
MLN	.185	.193	.180	.018	.297	.216	−.016	.280	.050	.120	.030	.007	−.008	.156	.207	.053

TABLE 25
Continued

	LM	G∠	ZZ	CyL	IML	XML	WMH	LCD	BCD	ASB	FRS	FRF	PAC	PAS	OCC	MDB
G∠	.351															
ZZ	.310	.021														
CyL	.266	−.179	.224													
IML	.160	−.097	.186	.335												
XML	.086	−.289	.142	.277	.632											
WMH	.162	−.141	.152	.317	.118	.351										
LCD	.125	.149	.050	.100	.101	.117	−.016									
BCD	.186	.088	.061	.091	.123	.055	.033	.114								
ASB	−.073	−.055	.058	.124	.089	.130	.015	.030	−.025							
FRS	.018	.178	−.063	−.218	−.077	−.081	−.058	−.108	−.114	−.017						
FRF	.105	.104	−.022	.034	.063	.089	.136	.094	−.014	.187	.138					
PAC	.219	.115	.160	.073	.283	.244	.064	.071	.223	.044	.217	.119				
PAS	.019	.041	.097	.062	.229	.233	.009	.074	.011	−.000	.103	.101	.672			
OCC	.158	.010	.074	.128	.098	−.034	−.058	.223	.055	.204	−.073	.103	−.011	−.223		
MDB	.119	−.101	.206	.191	.226	.216	.171	.288	.100	.063	−.038	−.024	.027	.055	.180	
MLN	−.061	−.163	.002	.065	.233	.128	.094	.173	.084	.144	.051	.097	.096	.098	.162	.374

Note: Correlations based on all crania in biodistance sample, $N = 185$.

TABLE 26
One-way Analysis of Variance among Late Woodland Series

Variable	*F* ratio[a]	
	Male	Female
L	0.10	1.27
MF	2.88*	0.20
FC	0.76	1.63
MFB	0.55	1.27
IOB	2.94*	0.97
SIOB	2.48	0.43
AIB	3.19*	1.60
LOBM	0.67	1.33
LOH	1.29	1.48
NH	2.65	1.68
NB	0.31	0.53
DC	1.86	2.14
MN	3.36*	1.25
BNB	0.38	0.50
BA	2.38	1.00
RL	2.87*	1.59
LM	0.23	0.10
G∠	0.67	0.70
ZZ	0.60	0.75
CyL	1.30	1.49
IML	1.49	2.21
XML	1.77	1.54
WMH	1.97	1.28
LCD	3.20*	0.30
BCD	1.47	2.82*
ASB	0.56	0.22
FRS	0.96	1.46
FRF	1.03	0.56
PAC	3.24*	0.63
PAS	2.31	0.84
OCC	0.83	0.85
MDB	1.01	3.97*
MLN	2.12	1.11

* $p<.05$.
[a] Males, $df = 3,66$; females, $df = 4,98$.

measurements (which do not vary significantly among groups) indicate that Schild males have smaller faces overall than the other series.

Three other measurements—breadth of ascending ramus (RL), length of occipital condyle (LCD), and parietal chord (PAC)—also differ significantly. Again, these mainly reflect differences between Schild and the other series. The ascending mandibular ramus is considerably narrower in Schild than in the other series. It is widest in the Yokem Late Woodland series. Length of the occipital condyle is greatest in the Schild series, and the parietal chord is markedly shorter than in the other series.

These differences appear to be a reflection of the overall smaller size of the Schild crania. Twenty-one of the 33 measurements (approximately 64%) have lowest means within the Schild series.

It appears unlikely that the smaller Schild crania can be accounted for by age differences with respect to the other Late Woodland series. Kolmogorov–Smirnov tests did not indicate statistically significant differences in age structures. Furthermore, *t* tests reported in Table 16 indicate that measurements which differ significantly among male groups do *not* vary significantly with age. The only exception to this generalization is minimum breadth of nasals (MN), which is significantly smaller in old males than in middle-aged males. However, the relatively smaller nasals of the Schild male series are not accounted for by age effects, since this series does not have a marked excess of old adults (see Table 22). It seems reasonable, therefore, to regard the narrow nasals in the Schild group as an aspect of the general tendency in that group toward smaller, narrower faces.

Females

The Late Woodland female series are considerably more similar in cranial morphology than the Late Woodland male series. Only 2 of the 33 measurements—breadth of the occipital condyle (BCD) and mastoid breadth (MDB)—differ significantly among series (Table 26).

Comparison of group means (Table 23) indicates that the Klunk and, to a lesser extent, the Schild Late Woodland series have a broader occipital condyle (BCD) than other series. The occipital condyle is not found to vary significantly with age in the female study series (Table 17).

The second measurement associated with a statistically significant *F* ratio in females, MDB, is most divergent (smallest) in the Schild series. Although MDB is associated with age in females, this association probably does not account for the smaller Schild MDB. According to the *t* tests reported in Table 17, MDB is significantly greater in old adults than in middle-aged adults. Since middle-aged adults are somewhat underrepresented in the Schild female series (Table 22), the Schild age profile would, if anything, tend to increase the mean MDB rather than decrease it.

Unlike the Schild male crania, the Schild female crania are not markedly smaller than crania from the other Late Woodland series. Compared to the remaining Late Woodland female series, the Schild series has the smallest mean for 8 (24%) and the largest mean for 6 (18%) of the 33 measurements in the variable list.

Multivariate Distance Results Based on Face Measurements

The biological distance results based on the variable subset composed of face measurements (described in Chapter 4) are discussed here in greater detail than the distance results for the other variable subsets. Several factors suggest that the subset of face variables provides more reliable estimates of biological distance than the alternate data sets.

First, fewer data are missing in the face variable subset. Approximately 5.5% of the face measurement data set are missing, while 9.9%, 9.7%, and 6.2% of the vault, mandible, and combined measurement data sets, respectively, are missing.

Second, the effects of artificial cranial deformation on face-derived distance estimates tend to be considerably less than for vault-based distances and slightly less than for distances obtained from the combined variable subset (see Chapter 5).

Third, face measurements are more variable between groups, on the whole, than are other measurements. The sensitivity of facial morphology to population differentiation has also been noted by other workers (Friedlaender 1975:117; Howells 1969a:453). Although the distances based on mandibular measurements are less associated with deformation than those based on face measurements, mandible measurements do not vary appreciably between groups. Mandibular morphology is therefore considerably less effective in discriminating among groups than facial morphology.

As noted previously, the first set of discriminant analyses was directed toward examining the structure of biological relationships among local Late Woodland communities in west–central Illinois. Three alternative models were evaluated according to their capacity to explain the resulting pattern of biological distances. These models are—

1. Unlike the populations of the preceding Middle Woodland period, Late Woodland communities were characterized by biological homogeneity on a regional level. Intergroup biological distances can be best explained as microevolutionary differentiation through *time* among subgroups of a relatively homogeneous regional population.
2. Like preceding Middle Woodland groups, Late Woodland communities were not biologically homogeneous. The pattern of biological relationships among Late Woodland cranial series reflects intersite distance by *river*, indicating a continuation into Late Woodland of the Middle Woodland pattern of biological interaction.
3. Late Woodland communities, like preceding Middle Woodland

groups, were not biologically homogeneous. However, the pattern of intersite relationships differs from that of the preceding Middle Woodland period. Along with decreasing orientation to the rivers and increased exploitation of upland resource zones, the Late Woodland pattern of biological distances becomes less river-oriented, corresponding better to intersite distance by *land* than to intersite distance by river.

Males

Using the subset of 14 face measurements, discriminant analyses were carried out for four Late Woodland male series—Koster, Schild, Yokem, and Ledders. Next, the eight crania from the small Klunk series were submitted as unclassified cases, to be classified with reference to the other four series.

Before discussing the biodistance results in terms of the models just described, consideration is given to possible environmental effects due to artificial cranial deformation or to differences in age structure among series.

DEFORMATION EFFECTS

Artificial cranial deformation is virtually absent from the Late Woodland series except for Koster and Klunk which have a significantly higher incidence of bifrontal flattening (see Tables 11 and 12). Deformation in the Klunk series will not bias the biodistance estimates for males, since Klunk crania were excluded from the discriminant analysis. For the Koster series, the effects of deformation on the set of face measurements are minimal (Tables 14 and 15). Bifrontal deformation does not correlate significantly with the distance of individuals from the group centroid (D^2).

AGE EFFECTS

A rather marked difference was noted (Table 22) between the age profiles of two of the Late Woodland male series, Koster and Ledders. The possibility of bias in the biodistance results due to age structure differences must therefore be considered.

Two of the 14 male face measurements, orbital height (LOH) and minimum breadth of nasals (MN), are significantly smaller in old than in middle-aged adult males (Table 16). The standardized discriminant function coefficients resulting from discriminant analysis (Table 27) indicate the relative contribution of each of the 14 face measurements to each of the three discriminant functions. The coefficients thus reflect

TABLE 27
Standardized Discriminant Function Coefficients Resulting from Analysis of Face Measurements, Late Woodland Male Series

Variable	Discriminant function		
	I	II	III
MFB	.21271	−.17335	.53670
IOB	−.01580	.87694	−.26741
SIOB	.69741	−.30930	.29531
AIB	1.07997	−.26093	.11776
LOBM	.57666	−.04981	.14197
LOH	.20814	−.14682	.61545
NH	−.87057	.07978	.34642
NB	.27746	−.34708	.07171
DC	−1.06235	.46744	−.19430
MN	.41904	.59668	−.03331
BNB	−.76611	−.15533	−.18549
IML	.09927	.34547	.37258
XML	−.84970	−.49237	.11450
WMH	−.02655	.22621	.05428

the relative usefulness of each measurement for discriminating among the cranial samples. Neither LOH nor MN is heavily weighted in the first discriminant function, which explains the major part (64%) of the total between-group variance. Comparison of the group centroids associated with the first discriminant function (Table 28) indicates that the first function primarily discriminates the Koster series from the other Late Woodland series. Since age-related variables are not heavily weighted in the first function, the difference between Koster and the other series can be attributed to factors other than age.

The second function (Table 28), which explains 19.5% of the total between-group variance, distinguishes primarily between the Schild and Ledders series. The second most heavily weighted variable in the function is MN, which earlier was shown to be significantly smaller in

TABLE 28
Centroids of Male Late Woodland Groups in Reduced Space, Analysis Based on Face Measurements

Series	Discriminant funtion		
	I	II	III
Koster	.90238	−.14759	.11707
Schild	−.96399	−.76574	−.54464
Yokem	−1.08323	.15003	.66958
Ledders	−.15746	.77843	−.50086

old males than in middle-aged males. The group means (Table 23) indicate that MN is considerably larger in the Ledders crania than in the Schild Late Woodland crania. However, this is not an age-related difference since Ledders and Schild have an approximately equal ratio of middle to old adults in these two series (see Table 22).

The third discriminant function explains the remaining 16.5% of the total between-group variance and serves primarily to distinguish the Yokem series from the Schild and Ledders series. The most heavily weighted variable in this function, orbital height (LOH), is significantly smaller in old adult males than in middle-aged males. The Yokem crania have higher orbits than either the Schild or Ledders crania (Table 23). Since the ratio of middle to old adults is considerably greater in the Yokem series than in the Schild or Ledders series, it is likely that some of the intergroup variation is attributable to age differences.

BIOLOGICAL DISTANCE

Table 29 summarizes the group membership predictions made according to the discriminant scores for each case. Of the total number of cases, 67% were correctly classified; that is, they were assigned to the series in which they actually belonged. The correct assignment of approximately two-thirds of the crania suggests that there are systematic differences in facial morphology among the Late Woodland male series.

Figure 12 gives Mahalanobis sample distances (D^2) for all male group pairs and indicates distances with statistically significant ($p < .05$) F ratios. The D^2 values are placed on a map to facilitate the comparison of biological and spatial distances. The intergroup biological distances, on the whole, are not large. Two of the six, however, are statistically significant suggesting that Late Woodland communities living in the region were not biologically homogeneous. It is noteworthy that the Yokem–Schild and Yokem–Ledders distances, which probably reflect

TABLE 29
Group Membership Predictions Based on Face Measurements, Late Woodland Male Series

Actual group	Predicted membership				
	Koster	Schild	Yokem	Ledders	*N*
Koster	*21*	3	3	4	31
Schild	0	*8*	1	2	11
Yokem	1	3	*8*	2	14
Ledders	2	2	1	*9*	14
Klunk	1	2	1	4	8

Note: Frequencies in italics are correct classifications.

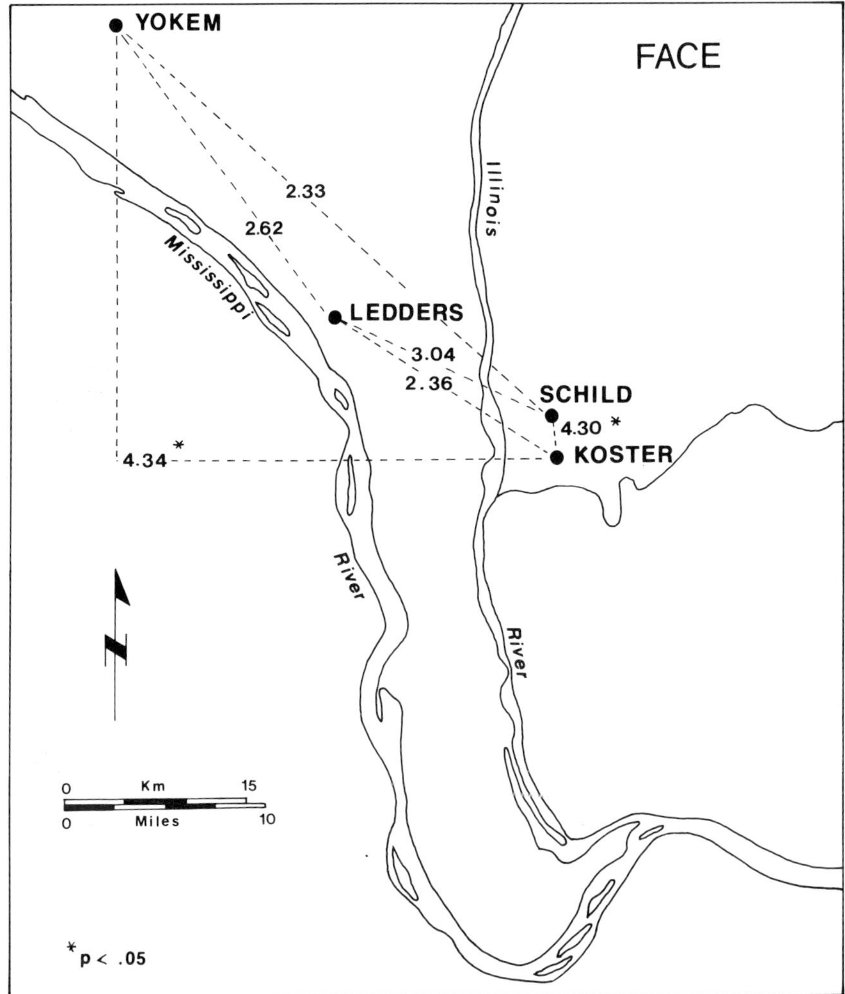

FIGURE 12. Geographical distances and biological distances (D^2) based on face measurements, male Late Woodland series.

between-group differences in age structure as well as epigenetic differences, are comparatively small and not statistically significant. This result suggests that the distance estimates are not significantly distorted by age effects.

In spite of the significant intergroup differences, the first model of intraregional homogeneity would be supported if intergroup variability were explainable by microevolutionary differentiation through time. The two largest intergroup distances involve the Koster series, which differs significantly from the Schild and Yokem Late Woodland series. Since Koster is the earliest series (see Table 1), these significant differences suggest a correspondence between temporal and biological divergence. The relatively small distance between the Schild and Yokem series, which are relatively close temporally, would also support the first model.

The remaining distance results, however, do not reflect temporal relationships among sites. Biological distance between the earliest series (Koster) and the latest series (Ledders) is relatively small. Similarly, the biological distance between Schild and Ledders is relatively low considering the temporal difference between these series.

In addition, predictions of group membership for the Klunk crania (Table 29) do not reflect the temporal relationships. Half of the Klunk crania are most similar to the Ledders series, which is temporally most distant from Klunk. Only one of the eight Klunk individuals is most similar to the Koster series, which is closest to Klunk in time. (It should be noted here that the Koster and Klunk series share a relatively high incidence of bifrontal deformation. The tendency for Klunk crania to be assigned to series other than Koster supports the earlier conclusion that facial morphology is not seriously affected by deformation.)

On the whole, then, the pattern of biological distances among the male Late Woodland series cannot be adequately explained by temporal differences among sites. These results do not, therefore, support the first model of a homogeneous intraregional population, with intergroup differences due to microevolutionary divergence over time.

The remaining two models predict correspondence between spatial and biological dimensions (Figure 12). If the rivers were the main avenue of biosocial interaction as the second model predicts, one would predict relatively large intergroup biological distances between the Illinois River sites (Schild and Koster) and the Mississippi River sites (Yokem and Ledders). Of the four biological distances between Illinois and Mississippi River sites, only one (Yokem–Koster) is relatively high and statistically significant. On the whole, the uplands separating the two rivers do not appear to have been a major barrier to gene flow. Although the intraregional heterogeneity characteristic of the Middle Woodland period is also evident among Late Woodland series, Late Woodland interseries biological distances, unlike Middle Woodland distances, do not generally reflect intersite distances by river. In other words, the results do not support the second model.

Results from male Late Woodland series best support the third model. This model predicts intraregional heterogeneity and a tendency for biological distances to correspond better to intersite distance by land than to distance by river. The most geographically separated sites, Yokem and Koster, are also the most distant biologically. Although biological distances among the remaining sites do not correspond exactly with intersite geographical distances, the relatively small biological distance between Illinois and Mississippi river series suggests that biological interactions were associated more closely with intersite proximity via land than proximity via river.

Group membership predictions for the Klunk crania (Table 29) also support this conclusion. Half of the Klunk individuals were classified as Ledders, the nearest series geographically. Two Klunk crania were classified as Schild, the next closest site; and one Klunk individual was assigned to both Yokem and Koster, the most distant sites.

The biological distance between Schild and Koster, which are situated very near one another in the Illinois Valley, is greater than expected according to the third model. It is possible that the Koster series contains some Middle Woodland material which was unnoticed at the time of its excavation. As noted previously (see pages 100–101), the Koster series shows a Middle Woodland-like form of cranial deformation. On the other hand, the Koster–Schild distance may reflect environmental (e.g., nutritional and/or disease status) differences. The Koster series is larger than the Schild series in all but 2 of 14 face measurements included in the discriminant analyses. For even the two remaining measurements (NH and BNB), the Schild mean is approximately equal to, or only very slightly greater than, the Koster mean. Thus the main differences in Schild and Koster facial morphology are effects of overall size.

Females

For females, the Klunk series was included with the other Late Woodland series for biological distance analysis. Consideration is given first to possible environmental effects on the female distance results.

DEFORMATION EFFECTS

The incidence of bifrontal flattening in the Klunk and Koster series (sexes combined) is significantly higher than in the other Late Woodland series (Tables 11 and 12). It is of approximately equal incidence at Koster among females and males. For Koster females, as among the males, the association between degree of bifrontal flattening and distance of an individual from the group centroid (D^2) based on face measurements is low and not statistically significant.

Occipital deformation is more frequent among Koster females (12.9%)

than among Koster males (7.9%), and for females the association between distance of individuals from the group centroid and degree of occipital deformation is statistically significant. It is possible, therefore, that some of the intergroup variability between Koster and the other Late Woodland female groups is attributable to deformation.

The incidence of bifrontal deformation among Klunk females (16.7%) is considerably lower than among Klunk males (50%). Two of the 12 Klunk female crania show some degree of bifrontal deformation; frontal and occipital deformation are absent. Analyses reported in Chapter 5 (page 115) suggest that bifrontal deformation does not significantly affect distance estimates based on face measurements. It is unlikely, therefore, that bifrontal flattening has severely inflated biological distances between Klunk females and the other Late Woodland series.

AGE EFFECTS

Five of the face measurements used in the female distance analysis vary significantly between adult age groups (see Table 17). These are internal biorbital breadth (IOB), orbital breadth (LOBM), nasal height (NH), nasal breadth (NB), and breadth of nasal bridge (BNB). All except NB are significantly larger in old adult females than in middle-aged females. NB is significantly larger in middle-aged than in young adults.

The relative contribution of particular face measurements to each discriminant function is reflected by the standardized coefficients associated with each measurement (Table 30). Two of the age-related

TABLE 30
Standardized Discriminant Function Coefficients Resulting from Analysis of Face Measurements, Late Woodland Female Series

Variable	Discriminant function I	II	III	IV
MFB	−.04933	.63537	.42456	−.35471
IOB	.47021	.02448	−.60377	.16676
SIOB	−.04828	.14593	.61031	−.16003
AIB	−.92039	.39320	−.70880	−.75176
LOBM	−.69105	−.38925	.23256	.27112
LOH	−.26119	.73017	−.35174	.29114
NH	−.42398	−.54296	−.05388	−.15886
NB	−.22852	−.02264	.66445	−.21808
DC	.67938	.13427	.28151	.74437
MN	.24386	.10681	−.18906	.83856
BNB	.40356	−.27533	−.59292	−.02420
IML	.56319	−.24896	.79655	−.97332
XML	−.05932	−.22324	−.90694	.59388
WMH	.35578	.18541	.00929	−.39572

variables, LOBM and NH, are among the most discriminatory variables in the discriminant functions.

Orbital breadth (LOBM) is the second most heavily weighted variable in the first discriminant function, which explains 48.4% of the between-group variation in facial morphology. This function serves primarily to distinguish the Klunk series from the remaining series (Table 31). The Klunk and Yokem means for LOBM are very slightly lower than means for the other Late Woodland groups (Table 23). The maximum between-group difference in mean LOBM is only 1.08 mm. The frequency of old adults in the Klunk female series is low compared to the other Late Woodland series, while the frequency of middle-aged adults in the Yokem series is relatively high (Table 22). It is possible, therefore, that the relatively low mean LOBM in both of these series is, in part, a consequence of the age distribution of the samples. However, Kolmogorov-Smirnov tests (Chapter 6) did not detect statistically significant differences. This fact, together with the observation that Klunk and Yokem means do not vary markedly from the other group means, suggests that age effects on LOBM do not constitute a serious source of bias.

The second variable which must be examined for age effects is nasal height (NH). It is weighted third highest in the second discriminant function (Table 30), which explains an additional 26.1% of the total intergroup variation and serves primarily to distinguish the Klunk and Ledders series from one another and from the other Late Woodland series (Table 31). It is unlikely that the variation in NH between the Klunk and Ledders series is affected by age factors because their age structures are very similar (Table 22). Since NH increases significantly from middle age to old adulthood, an underrepresentation of old adults would likely have the effect of lowering the mean NH. The frequency of old adults in Ledders is low, but the mean NH for Ledders is rel-

TABLE 31
Centroids of Female Late Woodland Groups in Reduced Space, Analysis Based on Face Measurements

Series	Discriminant function			
	I	II	III	IV
Koster	−.37505	−.47010	−.26152	−.12372
Klunk	1.18145	−.63904	.39325	.37569
Schild	−.74971	.23743	.61495	−.03924
Yokem	.67296	.50041	−.10012	−.30089
Ledders	−.30250	.59171	−.39557	.67412

atively high. There is no evidence, therefore, that age effects are important in distinguishing Ledders from the other series. On the other hand, some of the variation of NH between Klunk and the other Late Woodland series (Ledders excluded) may be attributable to age factors. The mean NH for Klunk is smaller than for any of the other female series, possibly reflecting the relatively low frequency of old Klunk adults.

In conclusion, there is some evidence for age effects on the biological distance estimates, especially between Klunk and the other series. It is unlikely, however, that they are an important source of bias. Measurements that vary with age in females generally are not weighted heavily in the discriminant functions (Table 30). Furthermore, Kolmogorov–Smirnov tests (see Chapter 6) indicated no significant differences in age structure among the Late Woodland female series.

BIOLOGICAL DISTANCE

Table 32 summarizes the group membership predictions for each case. Of the total number of female crania, 50.5% were assigned to the group to which they actually belong. The correct assignment of slightly over half of the female crania suggests that the Late Woodland female series differ systematically in their facial morphology. Correct assignment was achieved 16.5% less frequently in the female series than in the male series, however, indicating relatively greater morphological overlap among the female series.

Figure 13 gives Mahalanobis sample distances for all female group pairs, and indicates distances with statistically significant ($p < .05$) F ratios. Two of the 10 are statistically significant, further indication that Late Woodland populations were not biologically homogeneous.

The first model of interregional relationships proposes a relatively homogeneous Late Woodland population, with no more intergroup

TABLE 32
Group Membership Predictions Based on Face Measurements, Late Woodland Female Series

Actual group	Predicted membership					N
	Koster	Klunk	Schild	Yokem	Ledders	
Koster	*14*	3	7	7	4	35
Klunk	1	*9*	0	2	0	12
Schild	3	0	*10*	3	3	19
Yokem	4	3	3	*12*	3	25
Ledders	1	2	0	2	*7*	12

Note: Frequencies in italics are correct classifications.

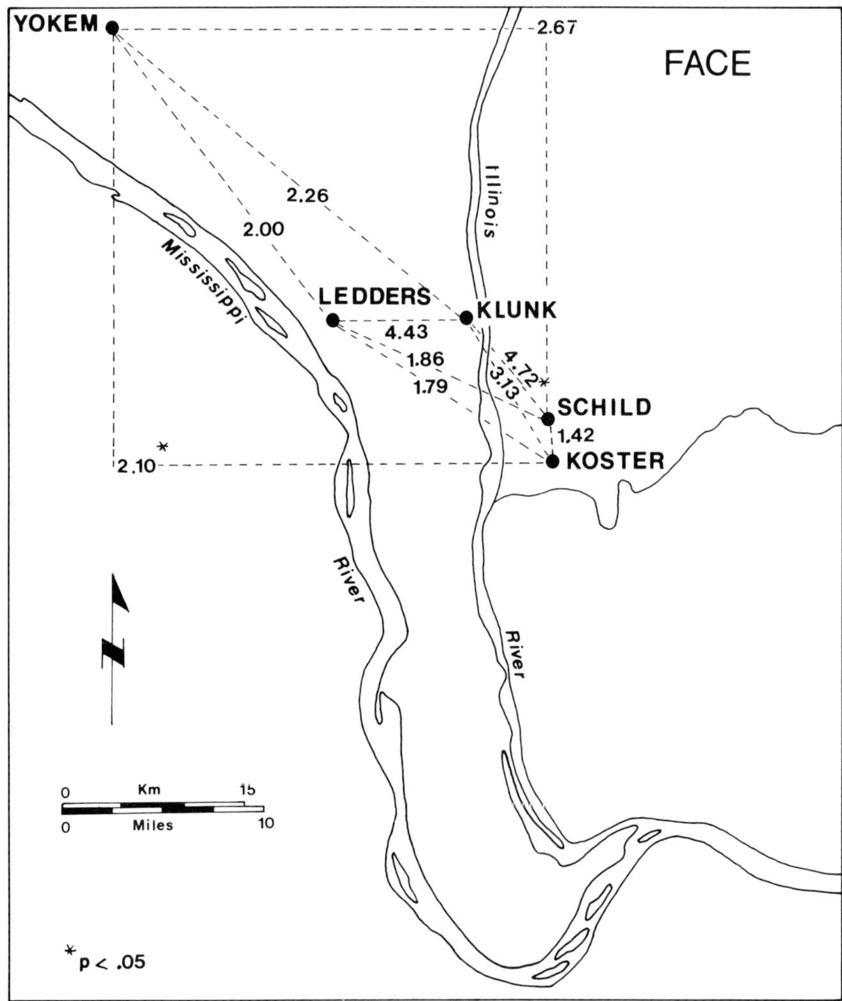

FIGURE 13. Geographical distances and biological distances (D^2) based on face measurements, female Late Woodland series.

divergence than would be expected in light of time differences among series. The relatively large Koster–Yokem, Klunk–Ledders, and Klunk–Yokem distances support such a temporal model, as these group pairs also have a comparatively large temporal separation. The relatively large Koster–Klunk, Klunk–Schild, and Schild–Yokem distances are not consistent with the temporal model, however, since these pairs are close to one another in age. In general, these results do not lend clear support to the first model and are consistent with the results for males.

The second model proposes a continuation into the Late Woodland period of the Middle Woodland pattern of biological relationships—intergroup biological heterogeneity which reflects intersite spatial separation by river. The resulting prediction of relatively high biological distances between Illinois River series and Mississippi River series is not confirmed for females. The Klunk–Schild and Klunk–Koster distances are comparatively high, although these are sites adjacent to the Illinois River. In addition, the Schild–Ledders and Koster–Ledders distances are comparatively low and are nonsignificant, although these series are quite distant from one another by river. Thus, for the second model, only the prediction of Late Woodland heterogeneity is confirmed. In evaluating the second model, male and female results lead to similar conclusions.

The third model predicts differences between series, and a tendency for biological distances to reflect intersite land distances more closely than intersite river distances. When spatial and biological distances are compared (Figure 13), it is apparent that biological distances between the Klunk series and the other Late Woodland female series do not reflect their spatial relationships. The Klunk females are most different morphologically from the series at the two nearest sites, Schild and Ledders. The Klunk–Koster and Klunk–Yokem distances are also quite large.

If the Klunk series is excluded, however, the pattern of biological relationships among the remaining Late Woodland series corresponds very well to the predictions of the third model. The series most distant from one another spatially, Yokem–Koster and Yokem–Schild, are also the most distant from one another biologically. The series from sites closest to one another, Schild and Koster, are the most similar to one another morphologically.

The Klunk series is clearly the most distinct female Late Woodland series. Accordingly, the first discriminant function, which explains nearly half of the total intergroup variation, is constructed so as to primarily distinguish the Klunk series from the other series (Table 31). The standardized discriminant function coefficients (Table 30) indicate that the most important discriminating variables in the first discriminant function are, in order of importance, anterior interorbital breadth (AIB), orbital breadth (LOBM), dacryal chord (DC), and inferior malar length (IML). When group means (Table 23) are compared, the Klunk series is most distinct from the other series in its small value for AIB. AIB is the most heavily weighted variable in the first discriminant function. Klunk also has a larger IML than any of the other series.

As discussed previously, one of the most discriminatory variables,

LOBM, is age-affected. But since the majority of the heavily weighted variables are not age-related, age effects cannot adequately explain the distinctness of the Klunk female series. It is also unlikely, as discussed earlier, that deformation effects can account for the morphological separation of the Klunk series. These findings could be interpreted as evidence that the Klunk people were relatively isolated biologically from other Late Woodland communities in the region. On the other hand, sampling error is always possible when dealing with small samples. It is also possible that the Klunk series contains some Middle Woodland skeletal material unrecognized as such during excavation.

Results from Alternative Data Sets

The results of the preceding section were based on analyses of face measurements. Discriminant analyses were also carried out using three alternative data sets described in Chapter 4. One was made up of vault measurements, another was composed of mandible measurements, and the third was composed of a combination of vault, face, and mandible measurements. This section briefly describes the biological distance results based on these three data sets, and compares them with the results based on face measurements.[1]

To facilitate comparisons among the data sets, the Mahalanobis D^2 values are presented in Figure 14 (males) and Figure 15 (females). These results generally support the findings from face measurements. On the whole, the intergroup biological distances are not large, and few are statistically significant. The Klunk female series is an exception to this generalization. (The Klunk male sample was too small to be included in the discriminant analyses.) Like the results based on the face measurements, the alternative data sets indicate that the Klunk female series is distinct from the other female series. The fact that the vault-derived distances between Klunk and the other series are not markedly greater than those based on the other data sets (Figure 15) suggests that the distinctness of the Klunk series cannot be attributed to cranial deformation.

Biological distances between Yokem and the other series also tend to be larger than other intergroup distances. This tendency, although not as marked as that for the Klunk series, is seen across all data sets in both sexes, indicating that the Yokem series is distinguishable morphologically from the other Late Woodland series.

[1] Tests for congruence among data sets are described in Chapter 8.

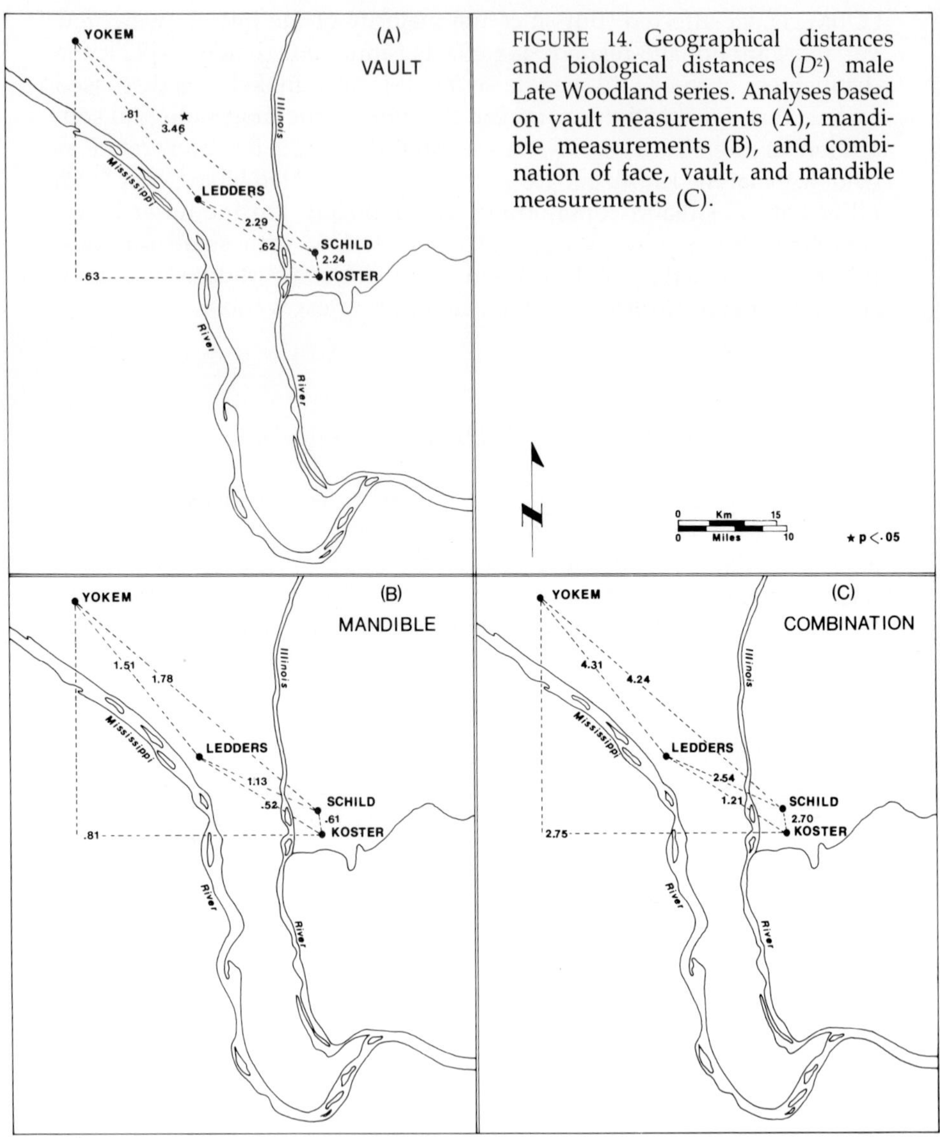

FIGURE 14. Geographical distances and biological distances (D^2) male Late Woodland series. Analyses based on vault measurements (A), mandible measurements (B), and combination of face, vault, and mandible measurements (C).

The results from the three alternative data sets, like those obtained from face measurements, indicate that intergroup biological distances do not correspond well to time differences among sites. The Koster and Ledders series are most separated in time, but estimates of biological distance between them are low to moderate across all data sets and in

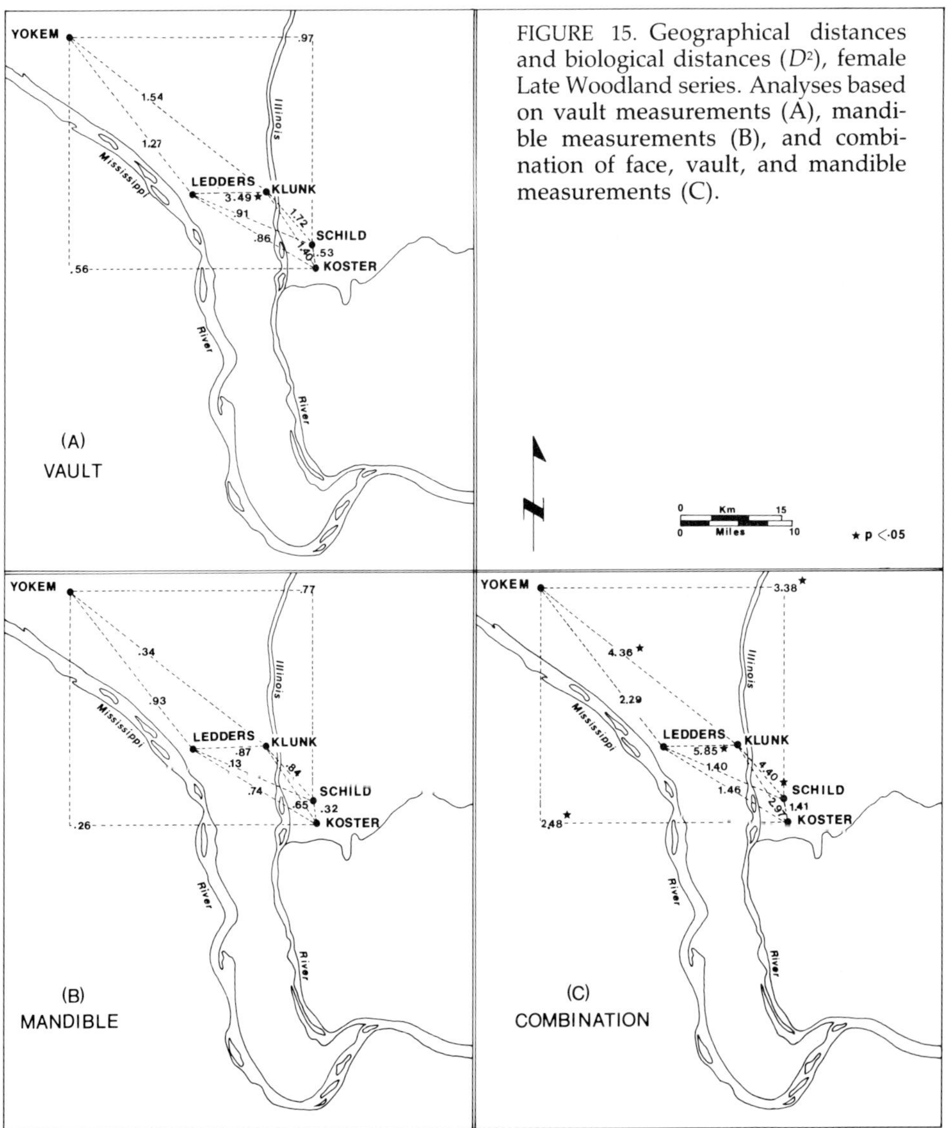

FIGURE 15. Geographical distances and biological distances (D^2), female Late Woodland series. Analyses based on vault measurements (A), mandible measurements (B), and combination of face, vault, and mandible measurements (C).

both sexes. The biological distance between Schild and Ledders is also relatively low considering the temporal difference between these series, and the Schild–Yokem distances are relatively high given the temporal proximity of these series.

The results from the alternative data sets, like those obtained from face measurements, do not indicate a close correspondence between biological distance and intersite distance by river. If the rivers were the primary locus of biosocial interaction, one would predict relatively high intergroup biological distances between the series situated on the Illinois River and series from Mississippi River sites. None of the results clearly suggests biological differentiation corresponding to river distance.

For face measurements, intersite distance by land was a somewhat better predictor of biological distance than intersite distance by river. The results from the alternative data sets are generally consistent with this interpretation, particularly when one considers the relatively small biological distances between Ledders–Schild and Ledders–Koster and the more substantial biological separation of Yokem from the other series. The results for the vault, mandible, and combination data sets are also like those from face measurements in that geographical distance is more closely reflected by biological distances among the female series than among male series. It is noteworthy, however, that for Schild and Koster males, the large biological distance based on face measurements is not reflected in the distances computed from the alternative measurement subsets. In this respect, the alternate data sets for male series give better support to the third model of intergroup relationships than does the face-measurement set.

Summary and Discussion

The univariate results indicate that the Schild Late Woodland male crania are smaller, on the whole, than the other male series. This tendency is most marked in the upper face breadth measurements. The female series are considerably more similar to one another than the male series. The Schild Late Woodland female crania are not smaller overall than crania in other female series.

Multivariate discriminant analyses based on four different data sets generally yielded consistent results. With a possible exception for Klunk females, the univariate and multivariate analyses did not suggest that differences in the incidence of cranial deformation or in the age profiles of the samples contributed significantly to the between-group variation.

For both male and female series, across all four data sets, the pattern of biological distances best supports a model of moderate intraregional heterogeneity, with intergroup biological distances corresponding more closely to intersite distance by land than to intersite distance by river. This pattern is similar to that found in Middle Woodland insofar as there is biological diversity within the region. It differs from the Middle Woodland pattern in that biological interactions were less river-oriented. These results are consistent with those of Buikstra (1977:76), who used nonmetric skeletal variants to estimate biological distances among these Late Woodland series. Her results also indicated that intersite land distances are more important than intersite river distances in explaining biological variability among these Late Woodland series.

For all data sets, the biological distance patterns among the female series generally approximate geographical distance among sites more closely than do the distance patterns for the male series. Except for distances involving the Klunk series, biological distances among the female series correspond very closely to intersite distance by land.

The biological distances among the female Late Woodland series are smaller, on the whole, than among the male series. The sex difference is not a consequence of differential cranial deformation. The Koster male and female series have artificially deformed crania, but the incidence of deformation by sex is approximately equal at Koster. The sex difference in the magnitude of intergroup distances suggests that the marriage system in Late Woodland times may have favored out-marriage of females, with exchange of males between groups occurring less frequently. This assumes, of course, that within-group variation is approximately equal in males and females. As there is some evidence that male crania are more variable metrically (within groups) than female crania in prehistoric midwestern skeletal series (Newman and Snow 1942:404; Smail 1964:73; Wilkinson 1971:33), this assumption probably errs in the conservative direction.

A marriage system favoring out-marriage of females would imply patrilocal residence, a pattern cited by a number of workers (Service 1962; Steward 1955) as the dominant type of residence among hunting and gathering societies. Lane and Sublett's (1972) study of nonmetric cranial variants in historic skeletal series from five Seneca cemeteries supports such an interpretation. Finding that male series were more heterogeneous between cemeteries than female series, Lane and Sublett concluded that residence was based on a male–male genetic relationship. Ethnohistorical data indicated that a patrilocal residence pattern did, in fact, predominate among these people, thus supporting the use of skeletal data to infer residence patterns.

The D^2 values between the Klunk female series and the other Late Woodland female series are relatively high for all four data sets. Inspection of the group means (Table 23) indicates that the morphological differences are primarily differences in shape rather than size. This in turn suggests that the differences are probably not explainable in terms of environmental factors. It is also unlikely that the effects of either cranial deformation or age can account for the distinctness of the Klunk female series, although age factors may be involved to some extent. Possibly the Klunk people were relatively isolated, biologically, from other Late Woodland groups in the region. Other possible explanations involve sampling error and/or the accidental inclusion of Middle Woodland material in the Klunk Late Woodland series.

Although the Klunk male series was too small to be included in the discriminant analysis as a group, the Klunk crania were classified (with relatively high inclusion probabilities) into the other Late Woodland male series in a manner which clearly reflected the geographical relationships of Klunk with other sites. These observations suggest that the Klunk male crania do not differ from the other male series to the extent that the Klunk females differ from other female series. This in turn suggests that sampling error or mixing of archeological components is preferable to biological isolation as an explanation for the morphological distinctness of the Klunk female series. More data than those presently available are necessary to clarify the relationships between Klunk and the other Late Woodland series in the region.

8

Late Woodland and Mississippian Biological Distances

This chapter presents the results of analyses directed toward the question of interactions among Late Woodland and later, Mississippian peoples in west–central Illinois. There is archeological evidence (see Chapter 2, pages 21–23) that the emergence of a Mississippian pattern in the west–central Illinois region was associated with major cultural and subsistence–settlement changes. Craniometric data are examined here for any evidence that the shift to Mississippian culture was associated with large-scale population movement into the region during the Late-Woodland–Mississippian interface period. Substantial morphological differences between Mississippian and Late Woodland cranial series would constitute evidence for such a movement of people into the region.

This chapter contains three sections. The first describes the results of univariate comparisons of cranial measurements among the study series. The second presents the results of multivariate discriminant analyses among Late Woodland and Mississippian series, and discusses their implications for alternate models of Late-Woodland–Mississippian interaction. The final section summarizes the findings regarding biological relationships among Late Woodland and Mississippian populations in the region.

Univariate Results

Males

As indicated by their *F* ratios, 13 of the 33 cranial measurements differ significantly ($p < .05$) among the male series (Table 33). The majority of the significant differences are for measures of facial morphology.

Like the other Late Woodland series, the two Mississippian series have generally larger cranial dimensions than the Schild Late Woodland series. For 7 of the 13 significant differences, Schild Late Woodland has the smallest mean measurements (see Table 23). These 7 measurements are internal biorbital breadth (IOB), subtense to IOB (SIOB), anterior interorbital breadth (AIB), minimum breadth of nasals (MN), breadth of ascending ramus (RL), inferior malar length (IML), maximum malar length (XML).

TABLE 33
One-way Analysis of Variance among Late Woodland and Mississippian Series

Variable	*F* ratio[a]	
	Male	Female
L	1.41	0.85
MF	1.76	1.57
FC	1.72	1.42
MFB	1.68	1.41
IOB	2.80*	3.76*
SIOB	2.23*	0.59
AIB	2.89*	1.83
LOBM	2.17	4.51*
LOH	1.23	2.21*
NH	2.73*	1.17
NB	1.73	0.71
DC	3.24*	2.12*
MN	2.66*	1.34
BNB	0.21	0.55
BA	1.29	0.86
RL	3.21*	2.36*
LM	0.42	0.29
G∠	0.86	1.69
ZZ	1.94	1.32
CyL	1.53	2.77*
IML	2.49*	2.75*
XML	2.40*	1.49
WMH	1.32	1.18
LCD	3.43*	0.25
BCD	4.92*	2.40*
ASB	0.96	0.20
FRS	4.38*	1.59
FRF	0.59	1.05
PAC	2.04	0.46
PAS	4.86*	1.96
OCC	0.73	1.32
MDB	1.19	3.60*
MLN	1.38	1.21

* $p < .05$.
[a] Males, $df = 5{,}132$; females $df = 6{,}178$.

There are other morphological differences between Late Woodland and Mississippian series. In particular, the Mississippian series generally tend to be larger than the Late Woodland series in face breadth measurements. Dacryal chord (DC) is an exception to this generalization; the Mississippian series have a smaller mean dacryal chord. Compared to Late Woodland crania, then, Mississippian crania tend to have broader faces and a smaller distance between orbits. They also have larger zygomatics and smaller occipital condyles.

Frontal and parietal subtense measurements (FRS, PAS) vary significantly among groups, primarily between Late Woodland and Mississippian series (especially Schild Mississippian). In the Schild Mississippian and, to a lesser extent, in the Yokem Mississippian series, the frontal subtense tends to be lower and the parietal subtense higher than in the Late Woodland series. The flatter forehead and more rounded parietals in the Schild male crania are likely a reflection of artificial frontal flattening and compensatory superior growth in the parietal area. This interpretation is supported by the fact that the Klunk crania (which were not included in the computation of the *F* ratios for males) also have a relatively low frontal subtense (FRS) and high parietal subtense (PAS). Like the Schild Mississippian crania, the Klunk crania have a relatively high incidence of artificial deformation in the frontal area. These findings are consistent with results reported in Chapter 5, which indicated that vault measurements are most affected by deformation.

Only two age-affected measurements (see Table 16) are included among measurements which varied significantly. They are minimum breadth of nasals (MN) and breadth of occipital condyle (BCD).

Examination of the group means (Table 23) and the age structures of the samples (Table 22) suggests that most of the intergroup variation in these two measurements cannot be attributed to age differences among samples. For reasons paralleling those given at the beginning of Chapter 7, the large contribution of the Schild Late Woodland group to intergroup variance in MN is unlikely to be due to age-related variation. MN is significantly smaller in old than in middle-aged adults. Hence, the relatively large Ledders MN appears not to be due to age factors, since old adults are not underrepresented in this series. The relatively large MN in Yokem Mississippian, however, may be attributable, in part, to a disproportionately low number of old adults. Since MN is included in the variable list for distance analysis, it may possibly introduce age-related effects into comparisons involving the Yokem Mississippian series.

Breadth of the occipital condyle (BCD) increases significantly from young to middle adulthood in the male study series. This measurement is smallest in the Yokem Mississippian series and largest in the Yokem Late Woodland series. Since there is a disproportionately high number of young adults in the Yokem Mississippian series and a disproportionately high number of middle adults in the Yokem Late Woodland group, some of the variation in BCD between these and other series can probably be attributed to age. It should be noted, however, that within-group variation in this measurement is relatively low, as indicated by the comparatively small standard deviations (Table 23). This tends to accentuate between-group differences. Thus age effects on BCD may not be as important in distinguishing Yokem from the other series as it first appears. Since BCD was not used in the multivariate distance analysis, it will not influence biological distance estimates among these series.

Females

Fewer of the cranial measurements vary significantly across the female series than across the male series. In females, 9 of the 33 measurements show statistically significant differences among series (Table 33). This suggests that the female series are, on the whole, more similar to one another morphologically than are the male series. This is despite two conditions. First, statistical significance can be obtained for less extreme differences in females because the female samples are generally larger than the male samples. Second, the most morphologically distinct series, Klunk, was included in the series used to compute F values for females but was not among the series used for the male F tests.

Five of the facial measurements—internal biorbital breadth (IOB), orbital breadth (LOBM), orbital height (LOH), dacryal chord (DC), and inferior malar length (IML)—vary significantly across groups. The Mississippian series generally have larger orbits (LOBM, LOH), greater face breadth in the orbital area (IOB), and larger zygomatics (IML) than the Late Woodland series, while the distance between the orbits (DC) is relatively small, especially in the Schild Mississippian series. These distinctions between female Late Woodland and Mississippian crania closely parallel the differences among males.

The four other significantly varying measurements are breadth of ascending ramus (RL), condylar length (CyL), breadth of occipital condyle (BCD), and mastoid breadth (MDB). For the two mandible measurements, RL and CyL, the differences appear to be due mainly to the larger size of these dimensions in the Mississippian series. On the other hand, intergroup differences in the means for BCD do not suggest a distinction between Late Woodland and Mississippian series, since both maximum and minimum mean values for this measurement are found in Late Woodland series. The significant intergroup difference in MDB may be due in large part to the relatively narrow mastoid breadth in the Schild Late Woodland series.

Age effects appear to be slightly greater in the female series than in the male series. Three measurements which differ significantly among female groups also vary significantly with age (see Table 17). All three—internal biorbital breadth (IOB), orbital breadth (LOBM), and mastoid breadth (MDB)—are significantly larger in old females than in middle-aged females. Both the Schild and Yokem Mississippian series have a greater proportion of old adults than any of the Late Woodland series (Table 22). It seems likely, therefore, that the larger means for IOB and LOBM in the Mississippian series are at least in part attributable to differences in age structures with respect to the Late Woodland series.

The effects of age variation are not as clear for mastoid breadth (MDB), the third variable which is both age-affected and significantly variable among series. Although mastoid breadth is smallest in the Schild Late Woodland female series, consideration of the age distribution for this series (discussed in Chapter 7) led to the conclusion that age effects can be discounted. The Schild Mississippian series, which has a relatively large MDB, has more old adults than middle-aged adults. It is possible, therefore, that the relatively large mastoid breadth in the Schild Mississippian crania is a reflection of the age structure of this series relative to the other series.

In summary, three of the measurements with statistically significant *F* ratios are age-affected in the female study series. Age effects are likely to affect biological distance estimates between Late Woodland and Mississippian series.

Multivariate Distance Results Based on Face Measurements

Two alternative models were evaluated according to their ability to explain the pattern of biological distances among Late Woodland and Mississippian cranial series. These models are—

1. The pattern of biological distances among Late Woodland and Mississippian series can be best explained in terms of a large influx

of people into the region at the Late-Woodland–Mississippian interface. Mississippian series are clearly distinguishable morphologically from Late Woodland series.

2. The pattern of biological distances indicates biological continuity, on a regional level, from Late Woodland through Mississippian times, with between-group morphological differences explainable in terms of factors other than a migration of Mississippians into the region.

Males

Discriminant analyses were carried out for six male series: the same Late Woodland series investigated in the preceding chapter, plus the Schild Mississippian and Yokem Mississippian series. As before, eight male Klunk Late Woodland crania were entered into the analysis as unclassified cases, to be classified with reference to the other series following the derivation of the discriminant functions. These analyses were based on the subset of 14 face measurements. Reasons for giving precedence to this measurement subset were discussed in the preceding chapter.

The possible effects on the biological distance pattern of artificial cranial deformation and age differences among series are evaluated first.

DEFORMATION EFFECTS

The incidence of frontal flattening in the Schild Mississippian series (sexes combined) is significantly higher than in any of the other series, according to statistical tests reported in Table 12. These tests also showed that the Schild Mississippian series has a significantly higher incidence of bifrontal flattening than the Schild Late Woodland series. Frontal and bifrontal flattening are both more frequent among males than among females in the Schild Mississippian series (Table 11). There is evidence, however, that cranial deformation among the Schild Mississippian males has not significantly altered the face measurements used in the discriminant analysis. Correlations between an individual's degree of cranial deformation and his distance from the group centroid derived from face measurements are not statistically significant for the Schild male series (Table 14).

The Koster and Klunk series (sexes combined) contain a significantly higher incidence of bifrontal deformation than the Schild Late Woodland, Yokem Late Woodland, or Yokem Mississippian series. However, for reasons discussed in Chapter 7, estimates involving the Koster series are not expected to be significantly distorted. Deformation in the Klunk series crania cannot bias the discriminant functions because they were not used to derive the functions for the male series.

In summation, there is no evidence to suggest that differences in the incidence of artificial cranial deformation between male series has served to significantly bias biological distance estimates, based on face measurements, among the study series. Generally, a relatively small proportion of these series is deformed. Among those crania which are deformed, the deformation is not severe. Finally, associations between deformation and D^2 were not statistically significant.

AGE EFFECTS

The standardized discriminant function coefficients (Table 34) resulting from analysis of Late Woodland and Mississippian male series indicate the relative importance of each of the 14 face measurements in distinguishing among the male series. The group centroids (Table 35) indicate distances among the group means on each discriminant function.

As noted in the preceding chapter (see page 150), 2 of the 14 face measurements—orbital height (LOH) and minimum breadth of nasals (MN)—vary significantly among adult age categories in the male study series. Neither of the two age-affected variables is weighted heavily in the first three discriminant functions, which together explain 85% of the between-group variation. Although MN is assigned the second highest weight in the fourth discriminant function, and LOH is the

TABLE 34

Standardized Discriminant Function Coefficients Resulting from Analysis of Face Measurements, Late Woodland and Mississippian Male Series

	Discriminant function				
Variable	I	II	III	IV	V
MFB	.64216	−.88930	−.69348	−.32554	−.61775
IOB	−.67981	.15241	−.21203	.41943	.07854
SIOB	−.01391	−.58003	.28497	−.35783	.20146
AIB	.46138	−.93611	.22942	−.09786	.01704
LOBM	−.05708	−.40275	.10190	.06037	−.32352
LOH	.29646	−.11085	−.01324	−.02145	.65027
NH	.30665	.21785	−.87615	−.13993	−.16154
NB	.34942	−.00542	.28680	−.27485	.54725
DC	.35674	.99196	−.14591	.65037	−.21117
MN	−.12454	−.33672	.00754	.53065	−.04022
BNB	−.47920	.88323	.26055	.08988	.18359
IML	−.28208	−.51278	−.43116	.03159	.00808
XML	−.37597	.83752	.15885	−.11972	.51745
WMH	−.08030	.08717	.11978	.33562	.42805

TABLE 35
Centroids of Late Woodland and Mississippian Male Groups in Reduced Space, Analysis Based on Face Measurements

Series	Discriminant function				
	I	II	III	IV	V
Koster LW	.60172	−.44787	.47658	−.09278	.16443
Schild LW	.44959	1.22513	.22297	−.63346	−.33032
Yokem LW	.40495	.66258	−.76183	.04344	.43530
Ledders LW	.21464	.57023	.29586	.83690	−.17464
Schild Miss	−.78374	−.09741	−.00066	−.04893	.00294
Yokem Miss	.61770	−.77928	−.71121	.00753	−.35125

most heavily weighted variable in the fifth function, these functions account for relatively little (10.2% and 4.8%, respectively) of the between-group variation. Since the variables which best discriminate among groups in the most important functions are not age-affected, it is unlikely that the discriminant analysis results are biased by age effects.

BIOLOGICAL DISTANCE

Based on the discriminant scores for each case, 47.8% of all males were classified into the group to which they actually belonged (Table 36). The proportion of correct classifications is lower than when only Late Woodland series were dealt with. In that analysis, 67% of the cases were correctly classified.

When the Ledders crania were incorrectly classified, they tended to be misclassified into other Late Woodland series. Incorrectly classified

TABLE 36
Group Membership Predictions Based on Analysis of Face Measurements, Late Woodland and Mississippian Male Series

Actual group	Predicted membership						
	Koster LW	Schild LW	Yokem LW	Ledders LW	Schild Miss	Yokem Miss	N
Koster LW	*14*	3	4	3	3	4	31
Schild LW	0	*8*	0	1	1	1	11
Yokem LW	1	3	*4*	2	1	3	14
Ledders LW	2	1	2	*7*	1	1	14
Schild Miss	6	6	4	4	*24*	9	53
Yokem Miss	2	0	2	1	1	*9*	15
Klunk LW	0	0	1	2	3	2	8

Note: Frequencies in italics are correct classifications.

crania from the other Late Woodland series, however, were misclassified into Mississippian groups as frequently as into Late Woodland series. Conversely, Mississippian crania were frequently misclassified into Late Woodland series. Although nearly half of the misclassified Schild Mississipian crania were classified as Yokem Mississippian, only 1 of 6 misclassified Yokem Mississippian crania was classified as Schild Mississippian. In general, then, the classification results do not suggest a clear morphological separation between Mississippian and Late Woodland series.

Table 37 presents Mahalanobis D^2 values of biological distance among the six male study series. The pattern of biological distances among the Late Woodland series closely parallels the pattern resulting from comparison of the Late Woodland series alone (Figure 12). This is expected since the only difference in the two analyses is that data from the Mississippian series are now admitted into the pooled sample covariance matrix. As evidenced by the statistically significant ($p < .05$) difference between the Schild and Yokem Mississippian series, intergroup heterogeneity was apparently maintained through the Mississippian period in west–central Illinois.

Seven of the 15 intergroup distances in Table 37 are statistically significant ($p < .05$). Five of the seven significant intergroup distances are between Mississippian and Late Woodland series. The Schild Mississippian series is significantly distant from all of the Late Woodland series except Ledders. These findings would seem to support the migration model. However, the Schild Mississippian sample is much larger than the other samples, and the significant differences are, at least in part, a reflection of this larger sample size. Support for the migration model is weakened further when the remainder of the results are considered.

On the whole, distances between Late Woodland and Mississippian

TABLE 37

Mahalanobis Distances (D^2) Based on Face Measurements, Late Woodland and Mississippian Male Series

	Koster LW	Schild LW	Yokem LW	Ledders LW	Schild Miss
Schild LW	3.42*				
Yokem LW	2.90*	2.35			
Ledders LW	2.20	2.81	3.13		
Schild Miss	2.30*	3.77*	2.78*	2.35	
Yokem Miss	1.80	5.33*	2.78	3.80	3.06*

* $p < .05$.

series are not larger than distances between pairs of Late Woodland series. In addition, the distances between Schild Mississippian and the Late Woodland series are generally smaller than the distance between the two Mississippian series, Schild and Yokem. Moreover, the distances between Yokem Mississippian and the Late Woodland series are, with the exception of the Schild-Late-Woodland–Yokem-Mississippian distance, not statistically significant. Clearly, Mississippian facial morphology is not markedly different from Late Woodland facial morphology. On the whole, the matrix of biological distances among the male series (Table 37) does not suggest that the Mississippian series represent immigrants to the region.

It was concluded in the preceding chapter that geographical distance among sites is related to biological distance among series. Since there are both Late Woodland and Mississippian series from the Schild and Yokem sites, Late-Woodland–Mississippian biological distance can be examined with the geographical factor controlled. Figure 16 displays the biological distance relationships among the four Schild and Yokem male series. The vertical dimension in this figure mainly reflects separation in time and culture, while the horizontal dimension reflects primarily spatial separation.

If the Mississippian series do, in fact, represent immigrants to the region, it would seem likely that the Mississippians at the Schild and Yokem sites came from the same place, since the Mississippian components at the two sites are very similar culturally, and both show close

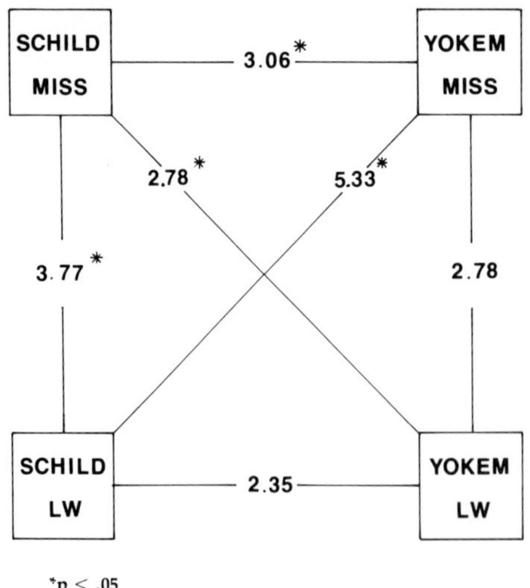

FIGURE 16. Biological distances (D^2) based on face measurements, Schild and Yokem male series.

cultural ties with Chaokia to the south. We would expect, therefore, that the distance between Mississippian series from the Schild and Yokem sites would be lower than within-site distances between the newly arrived Mississippians and the Late Woodland people who lived there previously. The results do not reflect this pattern, however. The Yokem Mississippian crania are more similar morphologically to earlier Late Woodland crania from the same site (the biodistance is relatively small and insignificant) than to Mississippian crania from the Schild site (the biodistance is larger and statistically significant). This result suggests biological continuity from the Late Woodland through the Mississippian periods at Yokem. Furthermore, the large distance between Mississippian components is not readily accounted for by the large geographic separation, since Schild Mississippians are more similar biologically to the Late Woodland series at Yokem than to Yokem Mississippians.

Late-Woodland–Mississippian relationships at the Schild site warrant closer examination in the context of a local continuity model, since the biological distance between the Schild Late Woodland and Schild Mississippian groups is one of the largest distances obtained.

If, in fact, local evolution from Late Woodland to Mississippian occurred among the Schild people, Late Woodland people should be more similar to early Mississippians than to late Schild Mississippians. In order to test this proposition, the Mississippian series from the Schild site was divided into two temporal subgroups corresponding to the Knoll A and Knoll B portions of the cemetery. Associated artifacts suggest that Knoll A is earlier than Knoll B (Perino 1971a). Discriminant analyses were carried out for Late Woodland, Knoll A, and Knoll B cranial subgroups from the Schild site. The sample sizes were 11, 21, and 32 for the Late Woodland, Knoll A, and Knoll B samples, respectively.

Mahalanobis sample distances (D^2) among the three Schild subgroups are given in Table 38. The Late Woodland series is more distinct from the later Mississippian series, Knoll B, than it is from the earlier Mis-

TABLE 38
Mahalanobis Distances (D^2) Based on Face Measurements, Schild Site Males

	Late Woodland	Early Miss (Knoll A)
Early Miss (Knoll A)	4.59	—
Late Miss (Knoll B)	5.71*	2.27

* $p < .05$.

sissippian series, Knoll A. The distance between the Late Woodland and Knoll B series is statistically significant, while the difference between Late Woodland and Knoll A is not. Although this distance pattern is not incompatible with a model involving the movement of a small number of individuals into the region during the latter phases of Mississippian occupation at the Schild site, it does not indicate the clear biological discontinuity between Late Woodland and early Mississippian expected if these early Mississippians represent a large-scale immigration into the region. In general, the biodistance relationships at the Schild site best support the *in situ* development model.

The pattern of within-group variability through time was also examined in the Schild male series. Figure 17 shows the relative positions of the three subgroups from the Schild site when the first discriminant function is plotted along the *x* axis and the second discriminant function

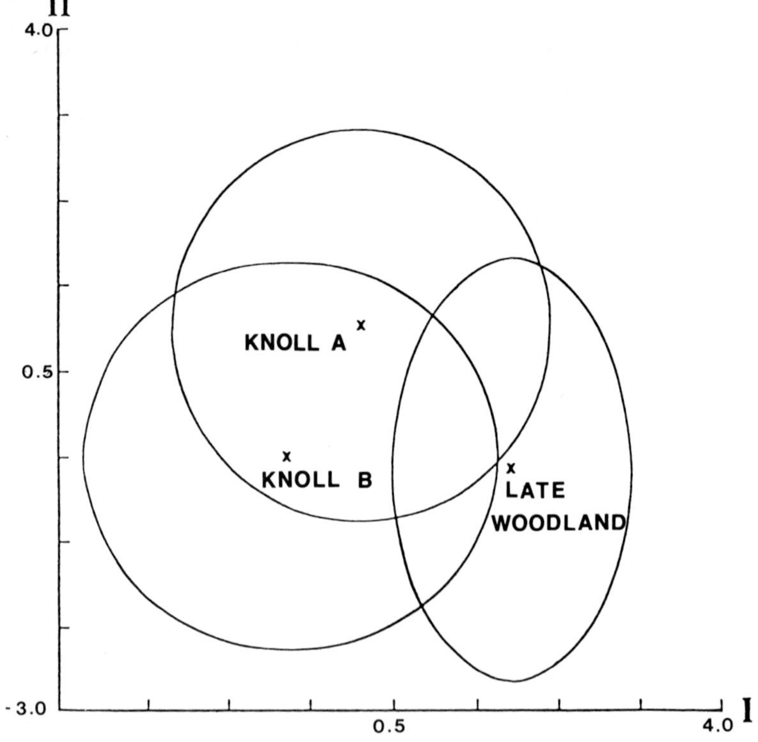

FIGURE 17. Plot of discriminant functions I and II based on face measurements, Schild male series.

is plotted along the *y* axis. The first function explains 65.5% of the total between-group variation, and the second function explains the remaining 34.5%. The ellipses enclose approximately 95% (two standard deviations) of the dispersion about the group centroids.

Within-group variation in cranial morphology increases considerably from Late Woodland to Knoll A, as shown in Figure 17, but increases very slightly from Knoll A to Knoll B. Although the small size of the Schild Late Woodland sample dictates caution in substantive interpretation of these results, a possible explanation for the increase in variability in early Mississippian can be suggested.

Archeological data indicate a trend in the Late-Woodland–Mississippian transitional period toward decreased localization, increased population numbers, and concentration of people adjacent to the arable river floodplains. It is possible that the increase in biological variation from Late Woodland to Mississippian at the Schild sites reflects this breakdown in localization and consequent enlargement of the effective gene pool in Mississippian times. In any case, the invasion of a Mississippian population is not necessary to explain the mosaic of Late-Woodland–Mississippian biological relationships. Both the network of intergroup biological distances and the pattern of intragroup variability can be more easily explained by changes in the structure of biosocial interactions along with ecological reorientations among the region's population. On the whole, then, the evidence from male cranial morphology points to the intraregional development of a Mississippian way of life among indigenous Late Woodland populations.

Females

Discriminant analyses, based on the set of 14 face measurements, were carried out among the same female Late Woodland series investigated in the previous chapter and among the Mississippian series from the Schild and Yokem sites.

DEFORMATION EFFECTS

As reported in Chapter 5, frontal deformation in the Schild Mississippian female series is significantly associated with the distance (D^2) of individual cases from the group centroid. Also, occipital deformation in Koster females is significantly associated with D^2. It is possible, therefore, that the biological distances calculated between these two series and the other cranial series are biased to some extent by deformation effects.

AGE EFFECTS

Analyses (Table 17) have shown that five of the female face measurements used in the distance analysis vary significantly between adult age classes. Four of these dimensions—internal biorbital breadth (IOB), orbital breadth (LOBM), nasal height (NH), and breadth of nasal bridge (BNB)—are significantly larger in old adult females than in middle-aged females. The remaining measurement, nasal breadth (NB), is significantly larger in middle-aged adults than in young adults.

The standardized coefficients associated with each variable in the discriminant functions (Table 39) reflect the importance of each measurement for discriminating among groups. The first discriminant function explains 39.4% of the total between-group variance, the second function explains 27.4%, the third 14.5%, the fourth 9.8%, the fifth 6.1% and the sixth 2.8%. The first three functions, which together explain 81.3% of the between-group variation, are clearly the most important functions for discriminating among the female series. The search for age effects is therefore confined to the first three discriminant functions.

As indicated by the group centroids (Table 40), the first discriminant function serves primarily to distinguish Late Woodland series from Mississippian series. With the exception of internal biorbital breadth (IOB), the age-affected variables are not heavily weighted in this function. Internal biorbital breadth, however, is the second most heavily

TABLE 39

Standardized Discriminant Function Coefficients Resulting from Analysis of Face Measurements, Late Woodland and Mississippian Female Series

	Discriminant function					
Variable	I	II	III	IV	V	VI
MFB	.09291	.18242	−.43755	−.63845	−.20885	−.76815
IOB	−.58173	−.74406	−.36352	.09536	.04488	.32919
SIOB	.35230	.33279	.04820	.16930	−.01188	−.41670
AIB	−.31052	.98624	−.58322	.52717	−.73227	.19456
LOBM	−.36996	.71785	.64389	−.21877	.35973	−.23825
LOH	−.14795	.35626	−.31267	−.65208	.03465	.21370
NH	−.04279	.11008	.10124	.52705	.03115	.17164
NB	.35345	.37826	.43974	−.34217	−.25078	.28196
DC	.65810	−.59621	.08420	−.23457	.76621	−.34809
MN	−.17081	−.29234	−.30554	−.14753	.74461	.20064
BNB	−.12679	−.62103	−.05770	.40239	−.24680	.06745
IML	−.00739	−.29401	.25242	−.20736	−.65492	−.62635
XML	−.26757	−.20955	−.07346	.46014	.28416	.34534
WMH	.29985	−.24865	.25527	−.45462	−.39813	.67002

TABLE 40
Centroids of Female Late Woodland and Mississippian Groups in Reduced Space, Analysis Based on Face Measurements

Series	Discriminant function					
	I	II	III	IV	V	VI
Koster LW	−.07503	.22839	.19882	.42655	−.13832	.15385
Klunk LW	.73912	−1.07036	.64015	.19598	.38570	−.11931
Schild LW	.79069	.97352	.15364	−.09982	.01343	−.22542
Yokem LW	.74666	−.48714	−.37512	−.14948	−.32127	.03319
Ledders LW	.40774	.31228	−.54136	−.14194	.57497	.30747
Schild Miss	−.51474	−.03475	.17963	−.29043	−.01935	.01764
Yokem Miss	−.62378	−.13331	−.50432	.28754	.09217	−.21720

weighted variable in the equation. The group means (Table 23) indicate that both of the Mississippian female series have a considerably larger IOB than the Late Woodland female series. The Mississippian series also have a higher proportion of old adult females than the Late Woodland series (Table 22). Since IOB increases with age, it is possible that the larger IOB in the Mississippian crania is due, at least in part, to the relatively high frequency of old adults in the two Mississippian series.

Three of the age-affected measurements—orbital breadth (LOBM), internal biorbital breadth (IOB), and breadth of nasal bridge (BNB)—are among the four most heavily weighted variables in the second discriminant function. This function serves primarily to separate the Klunk and Schild Late Woodland series from one another and from the other female series. The Klunk means for LOBM, IOB, and BNB tend to be lower than the corresponding means in the other series, and this difference is greatest with respect to the two Mississippian series. Since Klunk has a relatively small ratio of old to middle-aged adults (Table 22) and since measurements are significantly larger in old females (Table 23), it is likely that some of the variation between Klunk and the other series (especially the Mississippian series) is attributable to age effects.

In the Schild Late Woodland series the mean value for BNB is neither markedly higher nor lower than in the other study series, but the means for LOBM and IOB tend to be lower. Since the ratio of old to middle-aged adults in the Schild Late Woodland series is higher than in any of the other series, the relatively low mean values for LOBM and IOB cannot be attributed to the Schild age distribution. There is no evidence, therefore, that age effects can account for the distinction of the Schild Late Woodland series by the second discriminant function.

The third discriminant function serves primarily to distinguish Klunk from the two Mississippian series and from the Ledders series (Table 40). Note that two of the age-affected measurements, orbital breadth (LOBM) and nasal breadth (NB), are among the most heavily weighted variables in this function. In Chapter 7 (see page 157), it was concluded that age effects on LOBM do not seriously bias comparisons of Klunk with other Late Woodland series. On the other hand, the mean LOBM in the Yokem Mississippian series is approximately 1 mm larger than in the Klunk series. Since the ratio of old to middle-aged adults in the Yokem Mississippian series is considerably higher than in the Klunk series, it is possible that the Klunk–Yokem Mississippian distance is, to some extent, a reflection of age differences.

Since the Klunk series does not deviate markedly from the Ledders, Yokem Late Woodland, or Yokem Mississippian series in mean NB (Table 23) or in the critical ratio of middle-aged to young adults (Table 22), it is unlikely that variation in NB between Klunk and these three groups can be attributed to age effects.

In summary, the multivariate results, like the univariate results discussed earlier in this chapter, show that age effects are greater in the female series than in the male series. The distances most affected appear to be those between Late Woodland and Mississippian female series. Comparisons between Klunk and the two Mississippian series are probably most subject to age effects.

BIOLOGICAL DISTANCE

Table 41 summarizes the group membership predictions, based on discriminant analysis of face measurements, for the female Late Woodland

TABLE 41

Group Membership Predictions Based on Face Measurements, Late Woodland and Mississippian Female Series

	Predicted membership							
Actual group	Koster LW	Klunk LW	Schild LW	Yokem LW	Ledders LW	Schild Miss	Yokem Miss	*N*
Koster LW	*9*	4	6	3	3	4	6	35
Klunk LW	1	*7*	1	1	0	1	1	12
Schild LW	2	1	*8*	2	4	2	0	19
Yokem LW	1	4	2	*9*	3	3	3	25
Ledders LW	0	1	2	1	*4*	2	2	12
Schild Miss	6	6	4	6	4	*22*	10	58
Yokem Miss	3	3	0	3	2	3	*10*	24

Note: Frequencies in italics are correct classifications.

and Mississippian crania. Of the total number of individuals, 37.3% were assigned to the series to which they actually belong. The proportion of correct female classifications is lower than for males, among whom 47.8%, or nearly half, of the cases were assigned to the correct group. Thus, female series overlap in their facial morphology more than the male series.

Previously, when only Late Woodland series were included in the analysis, 50.5% of the cases were correctly classified (Table 32). The lower proportion of correct classifications with Mississippian crania included suggests that the Mississippian crania share considerable morphological variation with crania from the Late Woodland series. This conclusion is further supported by the observation that misclassified Late Woodland crania tend to be assigned to Mississippian series as frequently as they are assigned to other Late Woodland series, and vice versa.

Mahalanobis distances (D^2) among the seven female study series are given in Table 42. Ten, or nearly half, of the 21 D^2 values are statistically significant. The Klunk series accounts for a disproportionately large number (40%) of the statistically significant D^2 values. In Chapter 7 it was noted that Klunk is the most distinct Late Woodland series. The present results indicate that Klunk is distinct from Mississippian series as well. Possible reasons for the separation of Klunk, discussed in the previous chapter, are comparative biological isolation, environmental effects, accidental mixing of archeological components, and sampling error. Although other explanations cannot be eliminated given the available data, it appears that environmental effects are at least partially responsible for the distinctiveness of Klunk females. As concluded previously, both deformation and age effects probably account for some

TABLE 42
Mahalanobis Distances (D^2) Based on Face Measurements, Late Woodland and Mississippian Female Series

	Koster LW	Klunk LW	Schild LW	Yokem LW	Ledders LW	Schild Miss
Klunk LW	2.95*					
Schild LW	1.75	4.66*				
Yokem LW	1.90*	2.01	2.60*			
Ledders LW	1.64	3.75	1.67	1.66		
Schild Miss	0.81	3.42*	2.82*	2.22*	1.95	
Yokem Miss	1.14	4.15*	3.82*	2.44*	1.96	0.89

* $p < .05$.

of this separation. Age effects are likely more important in comparing Klunk with the Mississippian series than in comparing it with the other Late Woodland series.

Turning now to the alternative models of migration versus *in situ* Mississippian development, the data in Table 42 appear to lend some support to the first model. The majority of the significant distances are between Late Woodland and Mississippian series. The two Mississippian series are significantly distant from three of the five Late Woodland series, while the distance between the Mississippian series themselves is very low.

There are, however, a number of inconsistencies between the migration model and the biological distance results. First, the D^2 values between Mississippian and Late Woodland series are not, on the whole, of the magnitude expected if the Mississippian series represent immigrants. Late-Woodland–Mississippian distances are not *markedly* larger than Late-Woodland–Late-Woodland distances. In fact, the mean Late-Woodland–Mississippian D^2 (2.47) is virtually identical to the mean Late-Woodland–Late-Woodland D^2 (2.46). Second, both the multivariate and the univariate analyses reported in this chapter found that differences in the age structures of Late Woodland and Mississippian series have contributed to between-group variation. There is evidence as well for deformation effects in comparisons involving the Schild Mississippian female series. It is probable, therefore, that distances between Late Woodland and Mississippian series are partially a reflection of environmental, as opposed to epigenetic, variation between these series. Finally, the distinctness of Late Woodland from Mississippian series is not entirely consistent. Two Late Woodland series, Koster and Ledders, are not significantly different from either Mississippian series. In fact, Koster is more similar to the Mississippian series then to any Late Woodland series. In general, then, the results lend greater support to the *in situ* development model than to the migration model.

In the preceding chapter it was concluded that biological distances among the female Late Woodland series (excluding Klunk) are closely associated with intersite distance by land. The two series that are farthest apart geographically, Schild Late Woodland and Yokem Late Woodland, are also most distinct biologically. Since the Schild and Yokem sites contain both Late Woodland and Mississippian series, it is possible to compare biological distances between these sites in both the Late Woodland and Mississippian periods (Figure 18). All of the intersite distances in Figure 18 are statistically significant except D^2 between Schild and Yokem Mississippian.

The distance between Mississippian series is very small compared

Multivariate Distance Results Based on Face Measurements

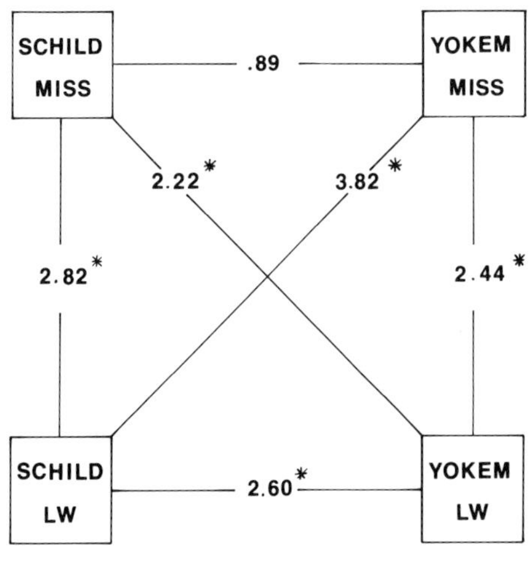

FIGURE 18. Biological distances (D^2) based on face measurements, Schild and Yokem female series.

to the distance between Late Woodland series at Schild and Yokem. Although the small Mississippian distance would support a migration model, the remaining results, as discussed above, do not generally support this model. In relation to the alternative model of intraregional Mississippian development, the small Schild–Yokem Mississippian distance suggests that the comparatively large geographical distance between the Schild and Yokem sites did not limit biological exchange among females. Since the corresponding distance between male series was relatively large, the discrepancy between the male and female patterns also suggests that out-marriage of females may have prevailed in the Mississippian period as well as in the Late Woodland period.

The remaining distances in Figure 18 support the model of intraregional biological continuity from Late Woodland to Mississippian times. Distances between Late Woodland and Mississippian series, although enhanced somewhat by age effects, are not markedly greater than the distance between the two Late Woodland series.

Although the distance between the female Schild Mississippian and Late Woodland series is not as great as that for males, it is larger than the female distances for Yokem Late-Woodland–Mississippian or for Schild–Yokem Late Woodland. When the Schild Mississippian series is divided into early (Knoll A, $N = 32$) and late (Knoll B, $N = 26$) subseries and compared to the Schild Late Woodland series ($N = 19$), Mahalanobis D^2 values among the three groups (Table 43) indicate that the Late Woodland series is more similar to the earlier Mississippians than to the later Mississippians. As was the case for males, the later Knoll B subgroup evidently accounts for the greater part of the distance

TABLE 43
Mahalanobis Distances (D^2) Based on Face Measurements, Schild Site Females

	Late Woodland	Early Miss (Knoll A)
Early Miss (Knoll A)	3.91*	—
Late Miss (Knoll B)	6.56*	1.29

* $p < .05$.

between the Late Woodland and the combined Mississippian female series. This correspondence of temporal and biological patterns supports a model of local development at the Schild site, although the pattern does not rule out the possibility that a small number of immigrants to the region are included in the Mississippian series.

Within-group variability was also compared for the three Schild female subgroups. Figure 19 shows the relative positions of the three

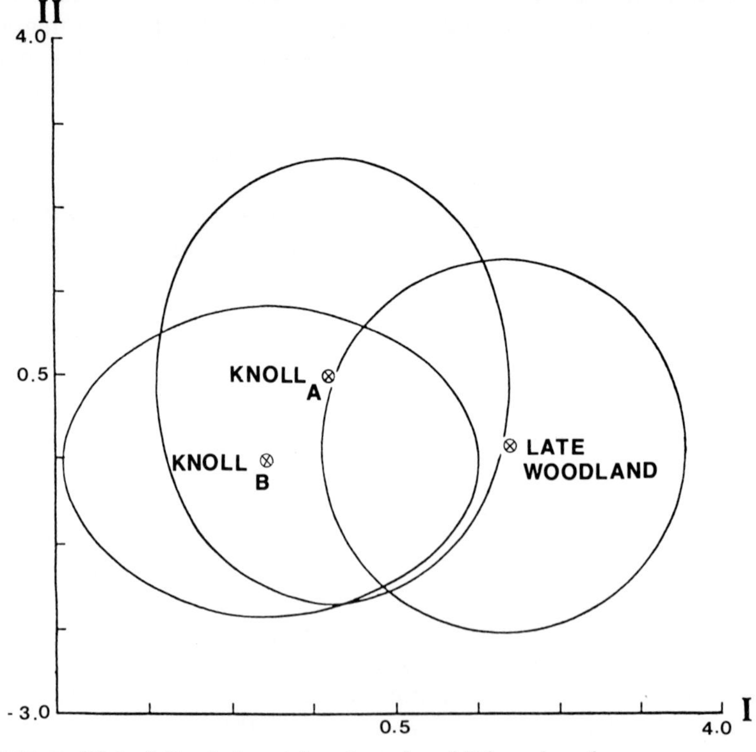

FIGURE 19. Plot of discriminant functions I and II based on face measurements, Schild female series.

subgroups with the first discriminant function plotted along the x axis and the second function plotted along the y axis. The first function explains 85.4% of the total between-group variation, and the second explains the remaining 14.6%. The ellipses enclose approximately 95% of the dispersion about the group centroids.

The ellipses indicate that within-group variation remained approximately constant from Late Woodland through late Mississippian (Knoll B). This contrasts with the results for males, for whom within-group dispersion in the two Mississippian subseries exceeded that of the Late Woodland series. Results for females are compatible with the suggestion on page 179 that the male increase in variability reflects enlargement of the gene pool in Mississippian times. Assuming that emergence of the Mississippian pattern involved the nucleation of the area's population, the Mississippian female sample would not necessarily be expected to show increased variation, since females were apparently being exchanged among local communities in Late Woodland times. On the other hand, increased variation in males would be expected, since Late Woodland males apparently tended to move from group to group less frequently than females.

Results from Alternative Data Sets

To supplement findings based on face measurements, analyses of Late Woodland and Mississippian cranial series were also carried out for the three alternative data sets consisting of vault measurements, mandible measurements, and a combination of vault, face, and mandible measurements. Since there are both Late Woodland and Mississippian series from the Schild and Yokem sites, biodistances among these four series provide a convenient representation of Late-Woodland–Mississippian relationships within the region. Figure 20 for males and Figure 21 for females show Mahalanobis D^2 values between these series.

The results obtained from the three alternative data sets are quite similar to those obtained from face measurements. There is no marked separation of Late Woodland and Mississippian series, such as one would expect if the Mississippians were recent immigrants to the area. The distance between Late Woodland and Mississippian series from the Yokem site is small relative to the other distances. This result is quite consistent in both sexes, across all data sets, suggesting biological continuity at Yokem.

For the alternative data sets, distances between the two Mississippian series tend to be less than distances between and two Late Woodland

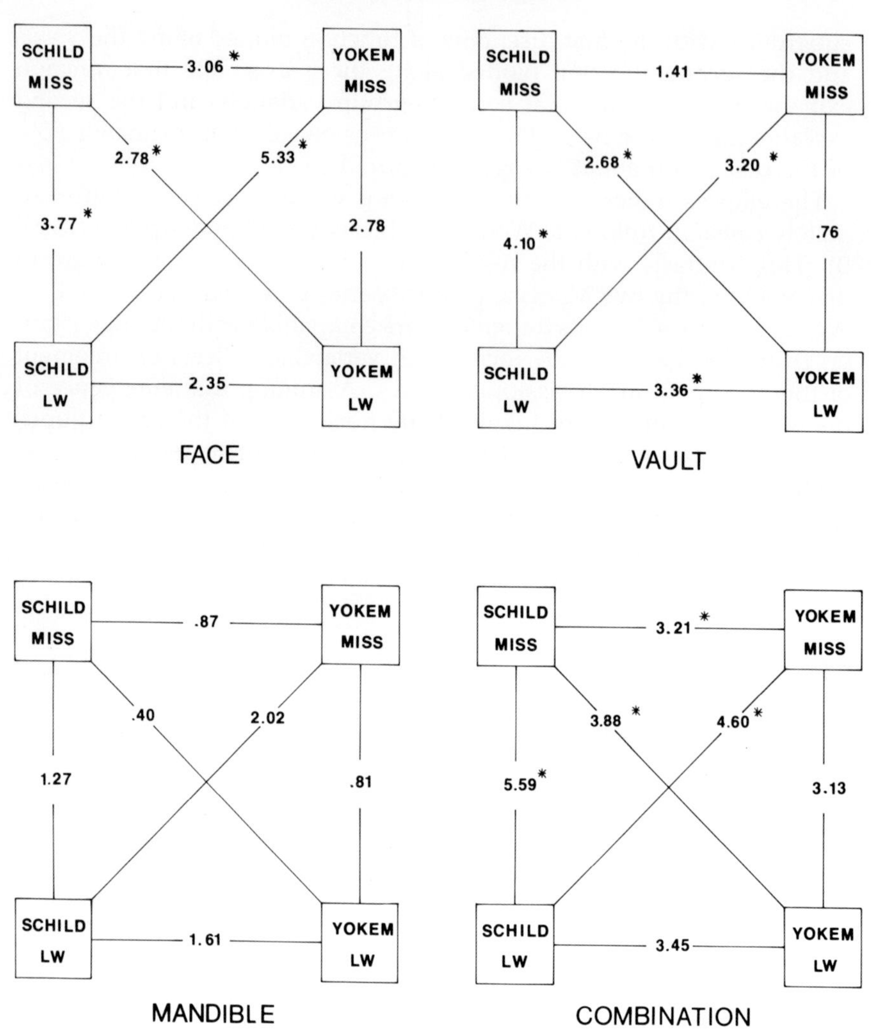

FIGURE 20. Biological distances (D^2) based on face, vault, mandible, and combination data sets, Schild and Yokem male series.

series. In contrast, for the data set of face measurements, the Schild–Yokem distance for Mississippian males is relatively larger. For the female series, however, all four data sets give consistent results.

Distances among female series are smaller, on the whole, than distances among male series. In this regard, the alternate data sets yield results consistent with those obtained from face measurements.

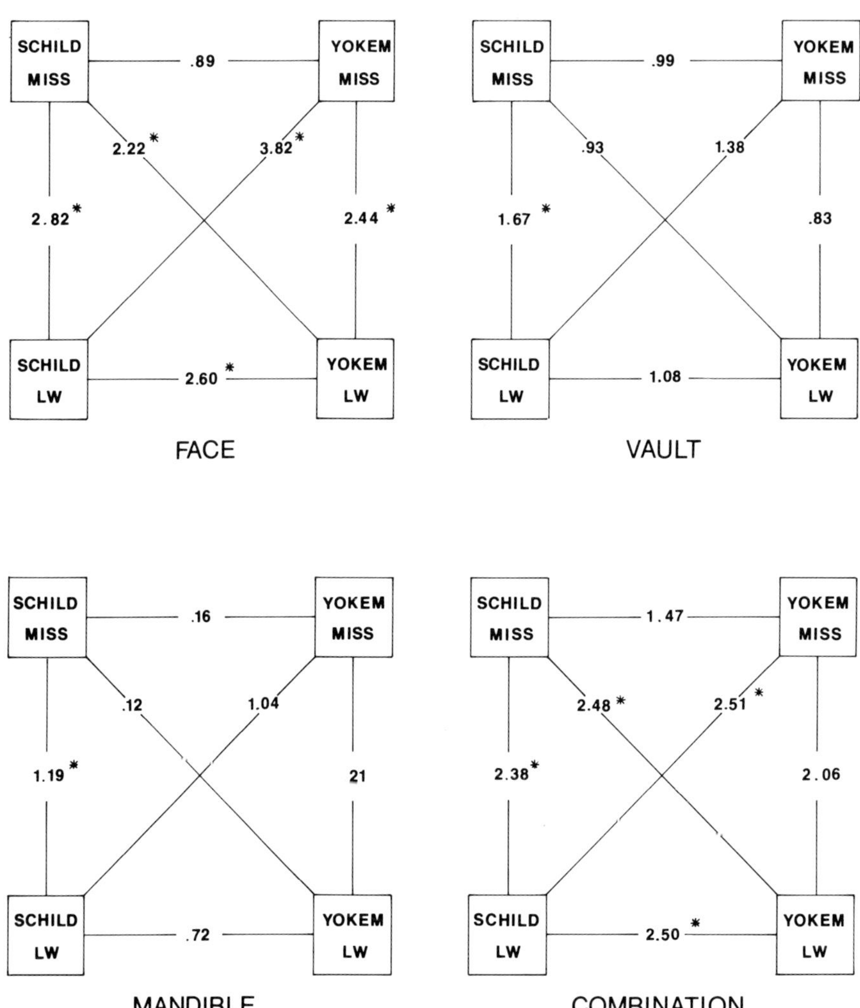

*p < .05.

FIGURE 21. Biological distances (D^2) based on face, vault, mandible, and combination data sets, Schild and Yokem female series.

The four measurement subsets are also consistent in that the biological distances between the Schild Mississippian series and the Schild and Yokem Late Woodland series are relatively large. Distances based on vault and combination data sets are especially large between male series, perhaps in part because of Mississippian cranial deformation.

When the Schild Mississippian crania are divided into earlier (Knoll

A) and later (Knoll B) subseries and compared to the Schild Late Woodland series (Table 44), a temporal sequence is seen which parallels the results based on face measurements. For both sexes, the Late Woodland series is more distinct from the later Mississippian series than from the earlier Mississippian series. This is true for all data sets, with one exception: when male distances are derived from vault measurements. Then, Schild Late Woodland males are slightly more distant from Knoll A than from Knoll B. Again, cranial deformation in the Mississippian series may have distorted the distances based on vault measurements. On the whole, these results, like those based on face measurements, do not indicate the clear biological discontinuity expected between Late Woodland and Mississippian series if the Mississippians were recent immigrants to the region.

Congruence of Distance Results

Tables 37, 42, and 45 give the Mahalanobis distances based on all four craniometric subsets and all Late Woodland and Mississippian series. Spearman's rank-order coefficients of correlation (r_s) were used to measure the strength of the association between D^2 values obtained from the four subsets of craniometric data. The SPSS subprogram NONPAR CORR (Nie *et al.* 1975) was used to perform the computations. The correlation results are presented in Table 46.

The correlations show that the various data sets tend to result in

TABLE 44

Mahalanobis Distances (D^2) Based on Alternative Measurement Subsets, Schild Site[a]

	Late Woodland	Early Miss (Knoll A)	Late Miss (Knoll B)
Vault variable subset			
Late Woodland	—	2.44*	2.84*
Early Mississippian (Knoll A)	5.32*	—	0.80
Late Mississippian (Knoll B)	4.04*	1.43	—
Mandible variable subset			
Late Woodland	—	0.99	1.86*
Early Mississippian (Knoll A)	0.67	—	0.27
Late Mississippian (Knoll B)	2.22*	1.33*	—
Combination variable subset			
Late Woodland	—	2.94*	4.54*
Early Mississippian (Knoll A)	5.92*	—	1.28
Late Mississippian (Knoll B)	9.22*	3.72*	—

* $p < .05$.

[a] D^2 values above the diagonals are between female series; D^2 values below the diagonals are between male series.

TABLE 45
Mahalanobis Distances (D^2) Based on Alternative Measurement Subsets, Late Woodland and Mississippian Series[a]

	Koster LW	Klunk LW	Schild LW	Yokem LW	Ledders LW	Schild Miss	Yokem Miss
Vault subset							
Koster LW	—	1.12	0.57	0.45	0.69	0.70	0.85
Klunk LW	—	—	1.53	1.13	2.66	2.25*	2.96*
Schild LW	2.00	—	—	1.08	1.06	1.67*	1.38
Yokem LW	0.59	—	3.36*	—	1.23	0.93	0.83
Ledders LW	0.88	—	2.16	1.02	—	0.98	0.86
Schild Miss	1.79*	—	4.10*	2.68*	1.97*	—	0.99
Yokem Miss	0.47	—	3.20*	0.76	0.96	1.41	—
Mandible subset							
Koster LW	—	0.42	0.34	0.25	0.53	0.51	0.63
Klunk LW	—	—	0.74	0.35	0.86	0.52	0.48
Schild LW	0.45	—	—	0.72	0.11	1.19*	1.04
Yokem LW	0.78	—	1.61	—	0.90	0.12	0.21
Ledders LW	0.45	—	1.10	1.39	—	1.22	1.03
Schild Miss	0.54	—	1.27	0.40	0.88	—	0.16
Yokem Miss	0.79	—	2.02	0.81	0.93	0.87	—
Combination subset							
Koster LW	—	2.55	1.33	1.68	1.28	1.10	1.37
Klunk LW	—	—	4.04*	3.60*	5.29*	3.36*	5.37*
Schild LW	2.54	—	—	2.50*	0.79	2.38*	2.51*
Yokem LW	1.84	—	3.45	—	1.71	2.48*	2.06
Ledders LW	1.04	—	2.60	3.27	—	2.39	1.54
Schild Miss	2.90*	—	5.59*	3.88*	2.92*	—	1.47
Yokem Miss	2.37	—	4.60*	3.13	2.00	3.21*	—

*$p < .05$.
[a]D^2 values above the diagonal are between female series; D^2 values below the diagonal are between male series. The Klunk male series was too small to be included in the discriminant analyses.

similar patterns of biological distance. All of the correlations are positive, ranging from 0.22 to 0.89. Half are statistically significant at the .05 level. For the male series, the smallest correlations involve the vault measurement subset and, to a lesser extent, the combination measurement subset, which includes vault measurements. This result is not surprising, since vault measurements are more susceptible to distortion by artificial cranial deformation than are face or mandible measurements (see Chapter 5).

Among the female series, the three lowest and nonsignificant correlations occur between distances derived from mandible measurements and distances derived from the other three subsets. In other words, the pattern of biological distances based on mandible measurements does not agree strongly with the highly intercorrelated biological distances resulting from analyses of the other three data sets. Analyses

TABLE 46
Correlations between D^2 Values Derived from Different Craniometric Subsets[a]

	Spearman's rank-order coefficients of correlation, r_s			
	Face	Vault	Mandible	Combination
Face	—	.7567*	.3065	.8892*
Vault	.3435	—	.3657	.7713*
Mandible	.4494*	.4039	—	.2222
Combination	.3363	.7321*	.5076*	—

* $p < .05$.
[a] Correlations above the diagonal are between female series ($N = 21$); correlations below the diagonal are between male series ($N = 15$).

reported in Chapter 6 indicated that dental loss is a significant factor in age trends, especially in measurements of structures associated with masticatory functions. Also, the incidence of dental loss was considerably higher in females than in males, especially in the largest series, Schild Mississippian. Therefore, among females, the discrepant results for biological distances derived from mandible measurements and those derived from the other data sets may be attributable, at least in part, to the confounding effects of dental loss on mandible measurements.

Summary and Discussion

Univariate *F* tests were carried out to determine which of 33 measurements varied most between groups. A major source of differences among the male series was the small size of the Schild Late Woodland crania. In addition, a number of morphological differences were evident between Late Woodland and Mississippian series.

Some of the differences are probably environmental in origin. The flatter frontals and more rounded parietals likely reflect the relatively high incidence of artificial frontal flattening in the Schild Mississippian male series. Very few age-affected measurements vary significantly among the male series. Age differences among series probably account for part of the between-group variation in two measurements, minimum breadth of nasals and breadth of the occipital condyle.

Univariate comparisons among the female series closely parallel the results for the male series, although fewer of the measurements vary significantly across female groups. Unlike the males, female intergroup differences due to artificial cranial deformation are not demonstrated. The differences in parietal and frontal morphology noted above for males are not evident in the female series, among whom the incidence of frontal deformation is relatively low.

Differences in the age structures of the various samples probably account for more variation in the female series than in the male series, in particular, for the relatively greater internal biorbital breadth and orbital breadth of the Mississippian female series. Mastoid breadth may also have age-related variation.

Distance analyses were carried out separately for the face, vault, mandible, and combination measurement sets. Results from the face measurements, which probably are the most reliable, were presented in detail.

The discriminant functions derived from face measurements were studied for evidence of age effects that might bias biological distance computations. Age effects were inferred for female distances but not for male distances, most seriously in comparisons of the Late Woodland series (especially Klunk) with the Mississippian series.

Two alternative models were evaluated according to their ability to explain the Late-Woodland–Mississippian patterns of biological distance. The first model proposes the movement of a large number of people into the lower Illinois Valley region in the Late-Woodland–Mississippian interface period. The second model proposes *in situ* development of a Mississippian way of life, accompanied by little, if any, movement of people into the region.

The biodistance results for both males and females give greater support to the second model. The discriminant analyses, using all four measurmement sets, point to a considerable morphological overlap among Late Woodland and Mississippian series. Distances between Late Woodland and Mississippian groups are not as great as expected if the Mississippians were immigrants to the region. In several instances, the two Mississippian series were more similar to Late Woodland series than to one another.

The biological distance between the Late Woodland and Mississippian series from the Schild site is relatively large, especially for males. For males, the primary difference between Schild Late Woodland and Mississippian crania appears to be that the Late Woodland crania are smaller overall. The difference between the Late Woodland and Mississippian Schild female series is not a matter of overall cranial size. Rather, the female biodistance is probably due in part to differences in the age structures of the two series.

When the Schild Mississippian series is divided into early and late subseries, biological distances clearly reflect a temporal sequence. For both males and females, the Schild Late Woodland series is more similar to the earlier Mississippian than to the later Mississippian subseries. This finding supports the model of local development from Late Woodland through Mississippian at the Schild site. Buikstra (1975:13) carried out a similar analysis of the three Schild samples using nonmetric traits. Her results, which corresponded closely with those of the present study, led her to conclude that "the major cultural change here, whatever it is, is *not* associated with an initial alteration in either population composition or breeding patterns. The appropriate behavioral model should emphasize a delayed biological response to changing patterns of social interaction."

The Klunk female series is quite distinct from the other Late Woodland series and from the Mississippian series, partly because of deformation and age effects. Biological isolation of the Klunk community, sampling error, and accidental mixing of archeological components are additional possible explanations for the differences.

Disregarding the Klunk series, which was not included in male group comparisons, the D^2 estimates among the female series are smaller, on the whole, than the corresponding D^2 estimates among the male series. This result suggests that a Late Woodland pattern of out-marriage of females continued in the Mississippian period.

Within-group variation in cranial morphology was examined at the Schild site by plotting the 95% limits of variation on the discriminant functions. For males, variation increases from Late Woodland to early Mississippian, then increases only very slightly from early to late Mississippian. For females, within-group variation remains approximately equal through time. The greater variation among Mississippian males may reflect the trend indicated by archeological data toward a breakdown in localization, with concentration of people adjacent to the fertile floodplains in the Late-Woodland–Mississippian transitional period.

Finally, the results obtained from the four measurement sets were compared. Correlations among D^2 values derived from face, vault, mandible, and combined data sets are moderately high, indicating that the different data sets tend to result in similar patterns of biological distance. This finding supports Sokal and Sneath's (1963:85) hypothesis of nonspecificity (cited in Chapter 1).

The distance results obtained from vault measurements in male series and from mandible measurements in female series are not highly correlated with the other sets of D^2 values, at least in part because of environmental effects. The vault data for males were subject to the effects of artificial cranial deformation. Female mandible measurements may reflect the confounding effects of dental loss.

In summary, the biological distance results support a model of biological continuity within the region from Late Woodland through Mississippian times, with very limited immigration, if any, accompanying the transition to a Mississippian way of life. These findings are consistent with those of Buikstra (1975), who carried out biological distance analyses, based on nonmetric skeletal variants, among these same skeletal series.

The skeletal evidence is, in turn, consistent with archeological evidence for Late-Woodland–Mississippian relationships in west–central Illinois and in the central Illinois Valley as well. In the lower Illinois Valley region, Perino's (1971a:141, 1971b:184) study of material cultural remains led him to the conclusion that Mississippian sites in the region do not represent major population movement from Cahokia. Rather, he suggested that Mississippian manifestations resulted from the acculturation of local Late Woodland people, a process which could have been initiated by a small number of Mississippian newcomers. Similarly, Harn (1975:427) views the Mississippian period in the central Illinois Valley as a predominantly local development, with very limited Cahokian immigration.

9

Summary and Discussion

Summary

Craniometric data were used to examine patterns of biological microvariability among Late Woodland and Mississippian groups who inhabited the west–central Illinois region from approximately A.D. 600 to A.D. 1300. Male and female series from five Late Woodland sites (Koster, Klunk, Schild, Yokem, and Ledders) and two Mississippian sites (Schild and Yokem) were studied. Multivariate discriminant analysis was selected as the statistical approach most appropriate to the available data and to the questions dealt with in this research.

Results related to five defined research goals are summarized below. The first two goals are concerned with problems in the prehistory of west–central Illinois, while the remaining three goals are concerned with methodological problems.

Biosocial Interaction among Late Woodland Communities of West–Central Illinois

The results of multivariate discriminant analyses based on four craniometric data sets are generally consistent with one another. Although the results indicate that the regional Late Woodland population was not morphologically homogeneous, intergroup biological differences are generally not marked.

Biological distances among the Late Woodland cranial series were examined in relation to three alternative models for intergroup relationships. For both male and female series, across all four data sets, the pattern of biological distances best supports a model of intraregional heterogeneity in Late Woodland times, with intergroup biological distances corresponding more closely to intersite distance by land than to intersite distance by river. This pattern is similar to that found in Middle Woodland insofar as there is biological diversity within the region. It differs from the Middle Woodland pattern in that biological interactions appear to have been less river-oriented. In general, the biological distance pattern among the female series approximates geographical distance among sites more closely than does the distance pattern for the male series.

Neither multivariate nor univariate analyses yielded evidence that differences in the incidence of cranial deformation or in the age profiles of the samples contribute significantly to the between-group variation. The Klunk female series represents a possible exception to this generalization. The D^2 values between the Klunk female series and the other Late Woodland series are relatively high, indicating comparatively little morphological overlap between Klunk and the other female Late Woodland series. The reasons for this distinction are unclear. Possible explanations include relative isolation, sampling error, age effects, and accidental mixing of skeletal material from different archeological components at the time of excavation. Although the Klunk male crania were too few to be included in the discriminant analyses as a group, there are indications that they do not differ from the other male series to the extent that the Klunk females differ from other female series.

The biological distances among female Late Woodland series are smaller, on the whole, than distances among the male series. In other words, Late Woodland female groups share more of the total range of morphological variation than Late Woodland male groups. This sex difference in intergroup variability suggests that the Late Woodland marriage system may have favored out-marriage of females, with exchange of males between groups occurring less frequently. Such a marriage system suggests a patrilocal residence pattern.

Biological Dimensions of the Late-Woodland–Mississippian Transition in West–Central Illinois

Two alternative models to explain the patterns of biological distance among Late Woodland and Mississippian cranial series were evaluated. The first model proposes the movement of a large number of people into the region in the Late-Woodland–Mississippian interface period, while the second model emphasizes *in situ* development of a Mississippian way of life among the region's resident populations, accompanied by very little, if any, movement of people into the region.

Summary

The biodistance results for both males and females best support the second model. The discriminant analyses point to considerable morphological overlap among Late Woodland and Mississippian series. Distances between Late Woodland and Mississippian groups are not as great as expected if the Mississippian series represent immigrants to the region. Furthermore, the two Mississippian series are in several instances more similar to Late Woodland series than to one another. Finally, differences in the age structures of Late Woodland and Mississippian female series probably bias some Late-Woodland–Mississippian biological distances. As a result, these distances probably reflect environmental, as well as epigenetic, differences between Late Woodland and Mississippian samples. There is no evidence that male biodistances are biased by age effects.

Although the results as a whole do not support the migration model, the distances between the Late Woodland and Mississippian series from the Schild site are relatively large, especially for males. When the Schild Mississippian series was divided into early and late subseries and compared to the Schild Late Woodland series, the pattern of biological distances clearly reflected the temporal sequence of the three subgroups. For both males and females, the Schild Late Woodland series is more similar to the early Mississippian subseries than to the later Mississippian subseries. This correspondence of temporal and biological patterning lends further support to the model of local development from Late Woodland through Mississippian.

Patterns of within-group variation were also examined at the Schild site. Within-group variation in male cranial morphology increases from Late Woodland to early Mississippian, then increases very slightly from early to late Mississippian. For females, within-group variation remains approximately constant. The increased variation in males may reflect the trend indicated by archeological data toward decreased localization and concentration of people adjacent to the fertile floodplains in the Late-Woodland–Mississippian transitional period.

In general, the female study series are more similar than the male study series. This suggests that, as in the preceding Late Woodland period, out-marriage of females was the prevailing Mississippian marriage pattern.

In conclusion, the results of this research support the second model of biological continuity within the west–central Illinois region from Late Woodland through Mississippian times, with very little, if any, immigration accompanying the transition to a Mississippian way of life. This conclusion agrees with that of Buikstra (1975) and others (Harn 1975; Perino 1971a, 1971b).

Artificial Cranial Deformation and Biodistance

Four kinds of cranial flattening (frontal, bifrontal, occipital, and lambdoid) were scored according to four rank scales of deformation severity. The scales were developed independently, using the Schild Mississippian crania.

On the whole, the degree of cranial deformation in the study series is mild as compared to series from areas such as South America, the Northwest Coast, or the American Southwest. The Schild Mississippian series has a significantly higher incidence of frontal flattening than the other study series. The highest incidences of bifrontal flattening occur in the Schild Mississippian, Klunk, and Koster series. Occipital flattening occurs with relatively low frequency in all of the study series, with no statistically significant between-group differences. It is most frequent in the Schild Mississippian, Koster Late Woodland, and Yokem Mississippian series. Lambdoid flattening is common in all series, and probably represents largely natural morphology.

Sex differences in the incidence of all four forms of deformation are not statistically significant, except for Schild Mississippian. There the frequencies of frontal and occipital flattening are significantly higher in males.

The susceptibility of each of four data sets (face, vault, mandible, and combined morphology measurement subsets) to deformation effects was examined by measuring the association between degree of cranial deformation and distance (D^2) of cases from the group centroids derived from the different data sets. The association is strongest when vault measurements are used to compute D^2 and weakest when face and mandible measurements are used. In other words, the presence of deformed individuals in cranial samples appears more likely to distort biological distances based on vault measurements than distances derived from face measurements. These findings are consistent with previous research which suggests that the cranial vault is most susceptible and the facial skeleton least susceptible to the effects of artificial cranial deformation. These analyses led to the decision to give most weight to results of biological distance analyses based on the subset of face measurements.

Adult Age Changes and Biological Distance

Few age changes in the study series are statistically significant for either sex. However, both significant and nonsignificant trends correspond fairly well to trends noted by previous investigators of adult cranial growth. Age trends in the female study series correspond more closely to the trends found in previous research than do trends in the male study series. In females, overall cranial size tends to increase with age.

Partial correlation analysis yielded results suggesting that some of the age changes, especially those associated with areas affected by alveolar bone loss, represent the effects of increased loss of teeth with age. These findings underscore the necessity for considering the dental status of the sample before attributing age changes in adulthood to appositional bone growth. Not all of the age changes in the study series can be explained by dental loss, however. This finding, together with the fact that age trends in the study series are fairly consistent with the findings of previous research, supports the assertion that the human craniofacial complex continues to grow in adult life.

The primary purpose of this analysis was to provide a basis for estimating the effects of developmental variation on patterns of biological distance among the study series. Accordingly, the relationship between age and each of the cranial measurements used to compute biological distance estimates was examined. Approximately 25% of the total variable list is age-affected in one or both sexes. In general, however, the proportion of variation explained by age is small, averaging about 7% for the variables which were significantly associated with age.

Age effects on distance estimates will be most serious when the age structures of the samples are dissimilar. Kolmogorov-Smirnov tests for differences in age distributions between cranial samples indicated statistically nonsignificant differences in all of the female sample comparisons and in most of the male comparisons.

Finally, the discriminant function weights assigned to individual measurements in the discriminant analyses were examined for evidence of age effects. These weights indicate the importance of each measurement in distinguishing between or among particular groups. This information, together with the associations between particular measurements and age and the variation in age structures, was used to estimate the degree to which particular biological distance estimates are biased by age effects. Evidence for age effects was found in several instances, more commonly among female series than among male series. There was also evidence that differences in age structures were a source of some of the morphological variation between Late Woodland and Mississippian series, especially in females.

Congruence between Alternative Data Sets

Biological distance analyses were carried out using four data sets—face measurements, vault measurements, mandible measurements, and a combination of the preceding measurements. Spearman's rank-order coefficients of correlation between D^2 values obtained from the four sets were moderately high, indicating that they tend to yield similar patterns of biological distance. In this respect, the results of this study support Sokal and Sneath's (1963) hypothesis of nonspecificity.

The distance results obtained from vault measurements in male series and from mandible measurements in female series are not highly correlated with the other sets of D^2 values, partly as a consequence of environmental effects. In males the vault data set is affected by artificial deformation of the cranial vault. In females, on the other hand, the discrepancy between biological distances derived from mandible measurements and those derived from the other data sets may reflect the confounding effects of dental loss on mandible measurements.

Buikstra (1975, 1977) carried out a parallel biological distance study, based on nonmetric skeletal variants, of the series which were examined in the present investigation. Buikstra's findings agree very closely with the models of Late Woodland and Mississippian change and continuity which were supported by my research. This consistency contributes to the strength of the conclusions. It also contributes additional support to Sokal and Sneath's hypothesis of nonspecificity, inasmuch as two different sets of biological data have led to the same conclusions.

Discussion

Research Methods and Strategies

In addition to its substantive contributions, this study has attempted to demonstrate the value of certain approaches to bioanthropological and archeological research problems.

First, consider the methodological response to cranial deformation, which has long posed problems for craniometrically based distance studies. Ideally, one would like to have a very large sample, half of which is deformed and half of which is underformed, with assurance that the deformed and undeformed subsamples were drawn from the same gene pool, that age structures were similar in the two groups, and that the two subsamples had been subjected to comparable environmental circumstances. One could then compare the undeformed to the deformed subsample and discover the effects of deformation on the cranium; the morphology of the two subsamples could then be equalized through a regression-based correction procedure. Unfortunately, the likelihood of at once obtaining such a large American Indian skeletal series containing both deformed and undeformed subgroups and assuring that both subgroups were equally representative is extremely small. Probably such a data pool could be obtained only in an experimental program using nonhuman primates. Given these limitations, the procedures followed here represent a realistic and practical means of dealing with the deformation problem.

The deformation scoring procedure of this study was developed as a compromise between the need for detailed deformation data and the observational limits of the phenomena themselves. The scoring system is applicable to most other midwestern Mississippian cranial series and, with the Schild Mississippian series as a reference, can be used by future investigators. With this system as a model, similar deformation scoring systems can be developed using other reference series.

The matter of ultimate concern here was the effects of deformation on the biological distance estimates. The analyses devoted to measuring the association between D^2 and deformation severity for various craniometric data sets provides support for the frequently stated, but often untested, assertions that face measurements are least susceptible to the effects of artificial cranial deformation. These analyses also illustrate a means of testing for deformation effects on alternative data sets. As bioanthropologists continue to adopt and develop more sophisticated statistical procedures and computer software, this approach can be further refined.

Age changes in adult cranial morphology have been investigated in living populations for many years. To my knowledge, however, age changes have not previously been examined in detail in relation to distance studies of American Indian skeletal series. My results demonstrate that differences in the age structures of samples being compared *do* need to be taken into account in morphology-based studies of biological distance.

It is important to point out that, although factors such as age effects and cranial deformation certainly pose serious analytical problems for craniometric studies, these problems are not insurmountable. The present study shows, I believe, that craniometric data *can* be used with satisfactory results despite these problems. A large body of research points to the value of cranial morphology as an epigenetic measure. Craniometrics ought not to be hastily discarded in favor of data bases which—while showing much promise in overcoming some of the problems inherent in metrical data—are not as thoroughly tested in a research context as cranial measurements. In any case, testing hypotheses on multiple data sets can only strengthen research findings.

This study is predicated on and, I hope, illustrates the value of using data from several subdisciplines of anthropology to study extinct biocultural systems. In particular, this research joins several other bioanthropological studies undertaken within the west–central Illinois research program in illustrating the value for the archeologist of using human biological data to generate and to test models of human behavior. Although the logic of studying the actual bodily remains of extinct people for clues to their behavior in life may be obvious, in practice, skeletal data have not been employed to their full potential.

Finally, it should be noted that this work was conducted within the context of an intensive, multidisciplinary, *regional* research program which unites the efforts of bioarcheology, the archeology of cultural remains, and prehistoric ecology. The strategy of long-term research in west–central Illinois is

> founded on the premise that intensive regional investigations are an important means of probing more deeply into processes of prehistoric culture change [and biological change]—that the accumulation of archeological knowledge about a region leads not to an attenuation in the returns of further research but rather to an expansion in the capacity for recognizing and solving processual problems [Asch 1976:70].

The regional perspective is particularly appropriate to the study of complex systems and to the investigation of slow process in biobehavioral systems, an area of research that is the unique domain of archeology.

Directions for Future Research

1. My results suggest that the degree of biosocial intercourse among Late Woodland communities was related to the geographical distance among these communities. Since only two Mississippian series were studied, it was not possible to determine to what extent such spatial factors continued to be important in Mississippian times. In other words, it was not possible to examine a *pattern* of Mississippian biological distances. As more Mississippian skeletal series are recovered from the region, the pattern of biological relationships among Mississippian communities should be examined and compared to the preceding Late Woodland pattern.
2. All of the cranial series examined in this study come from west–central Illinois. This posed difficulties for deciding how large a biological distance should be before genetic isolation is inferred. It would be desirable, therefore, to compare the series studied

here with Late Woodland and Mississippian series from outside the region. Skeletal series from the Cahokia and Dickson areas would be particularly appropriate for this purpose.

3. This study supports a particular model of changing interactions among west–central Illinois communities from Late Woodland through Mississippian times. A logical extension would be to test this model in other areas of the Midwest, ideally, in areas adjacent to the study region such as the Cahokia and Dickson areas as well as in more remote localities such as Aztalan and Kincaid. Such investigations would provide insights into the process of Mississippian development in general, as well as into the degree and nature of variations in particular regional circumstances.
4. The Late Woodland male crania from the Schild site are smaller, overall, than the Koster Late Woodland and Schild Mississippian male crania. At the same time, the biological distances between these series and the Schild Late Woodland male series are quite large compared to the rest of the biological distances among the study series. Since size, more than shape, is likely to vary with environmental factors such as nutritional level and disease stress (Eveleth and Tanner 1976:243; Newman 1975:234; Stini 1974:29; Tanner 1977:341), these size differences may reflect largely environmental differences between groups rather than intergroup genetic differences. There is considerable evidence from living populations that deprivation of protein and/or calories in early life can result in reduced mean adult body size (Eveleth and Tanner 1976:241; Tanner 1977:341; Weiner 1977:419; Newman 1975:232; Stini 1974:20, 1975:69). Males typically undergo a greater reduction in size than females, the latter being less easily thrown off their growth curves by environmental factors (Tanner 1977:343; Stini 1974:30, 1975:69). Future research could be directed at determining if the Schild Late Woodland male series is smaller than other series in body size as well as cranial size. If so, then it could be hypothesized that the smaller size of the Schild males stems from unfavorable environmental circumstances. This hypothesis could then be tested using other kinds of data such as archeological evidence for dietary practices at the Schild and Koster sites and chemical composition of human bone (cf. Szpunar and Lambert 1977).
5. My research indicates that a particular pattern of biological relationships existed among west–central Illinois Late Woodland communities and, further, that these biological relationships were regulated by social factors. Microstyle analysis of Late Woodland

ceramics from habitation sites should be carried out to test the model of biosocial relations suggested here. The productivity of integrating microstyle ceramic analysis with biodistance analysis has been demonstrated previously by the coordinated research of Buikstra (1975) and Houart (1975) on Middle Woodland data. The relationship of Klunk to the other Late Woodland sites in the region would be of particular interest in such a ceramic analysis, as its position biologically is unclear at the conclusion of the present study.

6. The research problems toward which craniomtric data were directed in this study were also approached with the use of nonmetric data by Buikstra (1975). That our results pointed to similar conclusions establishes them more firmly than on the basis of either study alone. Nevertheless, these studies should be replicated using additional data sets. To the extent that new results support those of Buikstra and myself, this support will add an extra measure of confidence to our conclusions. To the extent that new results do not agree, the areas of discrepancy may be useful for discovering differences in the capacity of various data sets to measure epigenetic relationships or for learning why one data set may be preferable to another, both within the framework of the present research problems and within the more general context of bioanthropological methodology.

APPENDIX

Master Data File

Tables 47 and 48 record data concerning individual crania—provenience, burial number, sex, age, deformation, and the 33 variables employed in the discriminant analyses. All of the 507 measurable crania are listed in the tables, of which 331 were sufficiently complete to be included in the discriminant analyses. Coding for Tables 47 and 48 is explained below.

Analytical status

D = used in discriminant analyses
— = not used in discriminant analyses

Age

Y = young adult, 20–34.9 years
M = middle adult, 35–49.9 years
O = old adult, 50+ years

Deformation score

0 = no flattening
1 to 4 = increasing degrees of flattening
— = not scored due to incompleteness of cranium

Frontal, bifrontal, and occipital flattening are scored on a scale of 0 to 3, lambdoid flattening on a scale of 0 to 4. See Figures 4–7 for reference crania to illustrate deformation scoring.

Cranial measurements

— = not measurable; cranium too incomplete for multiple regression estimate
italics = estimated by multiple regression

Measurements are recorded in millimeters except for gonial angle (GZ), which is in degrees.

TABLE 47 *Male*

Case	Bur. no.	Mound/ knoll	Analytical status	Age	Deformation score: Frontal	Bifrontal	Occipital	Lambdoid	Measurement: L	MF	FC	MFB	IOB	SIOB	AIB	LOBM	LOH	NH	NB	DC
Schild Mississippian:																				
1	48	A	D	M	2	3	0	4	172	86	113	94	94	17	17	42	34	48	24	18
2	52	A	D	Y	3	0	0	1	188	96	113	105	103	18	20	43	32	54	25	21
3	58a	A	D	O	0	0	0	2	171	86	105	93	94	17	19	41	32	48	28	22
4	117	A	D	Y	0	0	0	0	189	94	120	87	97	22	21	42	33	53	24	20
5	136	A	D	O	2	0	0	1	182	96	109	102	98	20	18	42	32	53	25	19
6	137	A	D	M	0	0	0	3	184	91	105	99	101	18	21	43	36	54	26	22
7	154	A	D	Y	1	1	0	0	192	99	123	103	105	25	22	46	36	51	26	21
8	160	A	D	O	0	0	0	1	174	88	110	104	94	16	18	42	32	50	26	17
9	58b	A	D	O	0	0	0	0	168	92	112	89	94	20	18	42	33	51	22	16
10	67h	A	—	O	—	—	—	—	—	94	111	—	—	*19*	—	—	—	—	—	—
11	101	A	—	Y	—	—	—	—	*177*	86	102	98	95	19	*18*	*42*	—	—	*26*	*20*
12	122a	A	D	Y	0	0	0	1	184	92	108	101	*98*	*18*	18	43	35	51	25	20
13	70	A	D	M	0	2	0	0	*182*	95	118	97	102	23	18	46	36	55	24	19
14	83a	A	D	M	3	0	2	4	171	93	105	99	98	17	20	41	35	53	23	19
15	84	A	D	Y	2	0	3	4	164	92	115	94	99	18	19	42	35	50	25	20
16	127	A	D	O	1	0	0	1	173	91	113	100	97	15	20	41	28	47	26	20
17	149	A	D	Y	0	0	1	2	170	96	111	98	98	18	21	40	34	52	25	20
18	153	A	D	Y	0	0	0	0	186	92	116	97	97	20	19	41	36	54	22	20
19	156	A	D	Y	2	0	1	4	181	96	118	107	105	19	17	47	36	56	26	19
20	163	A	D	Y	2	0	1	4	176	91	104	100	97	19	19	41	34	51	*26*	24
21	159	A	D	Y	2	1	1	1	170	88	109	105	96	17	18	42	32	53	24	17
22	41a	A	—	Y	—	—	—	—	—	93	119	—	100	20	—	*43*	—	—	—	—
23	45	A	—	O	—	—	0	2	—	—	—	*99*	—	—	—	—	—	—	*26*	—
24	50a	A	—	Y	0	0	1	4	188	96	118	*100*	102	17	*20*	*44*	—	—	*26*	*21*
25	50b	A	—	M	—	—	—	—	—	—	—	95	—	—	—	—	—	—	*25*	—
26	42	A	D	M	1	3	2	4	*181*	85	*109*	101	100	*18*	18	44	38	51	25	20
27	63	A	D	Y	0	0	0	0	181	*94*	116	94	98	*19*	21	40	33	51	25	24
28	185	B	D	Y	2	0	0	3	187	92	112	101	101	19	23	42	35	52	28	24
29	193	B	D	Y	1	0	0	2	170	89	111	105	94	16	17	42	34	51	24	18
30	194	B	D	Y	0	0	1	2	179	95	118	97	99	18	18	45	36	52	26	17
31	204	B	D	O	0	2	0	2	178	93	109	98	96	17	16	43	34	50	25	16
32	212	B	D	Y	1	0	0	3	184	104	125	108	105	22	25	46	36	58	29	26
33	244	B	D	Y	0	0	0	3	178	107	112	98	101	23	23	44	34	54	26	24
34	248	B	D	Y	0	0	0	1	182	96	115	89	96	21	19	43	35	53	22	17
35	250	B	D	M	2	0	0	1	185	93	111	103	100	21	17	44	34	53	23	17
36	251	B	D	Y	1	0	1	2	172	97	108	98	97	17	18	41	34	53	27	19
37	255	B	D	M	0	3	0	0	182	100	110	103	109	19	18	48	34	53	28	21
38	262c	B	D	M	1	0	0	3	183	90	113	98	101	20	19	44	35	51	24	20
39	265	B	D	O	0	0	0	0	182	97	117	101	103	20	19	44	35	54	27	21
40	270	B	D	Y	0	2	0	2	182	98	113	98	101	18	20	43	34	57	25	23
41	192a	B	D	O	0	2	0	1	174	94	110	103	96	18	16	42	34	53	26	17
42	207	B	D	O	—	—	1	3	183	100	113	97	102	21	20	45	33	54	27	20
43	221	B	D	Y	0	0	0	2	175	87	103	96	*98*	*20*	20	43	35	52	25	20
44	256	B	—	O	—	—	—	—	*178*	90	*109*	97	102	—	*19*	*44*	—	—	27	*21*
45	261b	B	D	M	0	0	0	1	184	98	116	104	103	20	21	45	35	54	26	21
46	229	B	D	M	—	—	—	—	*180*	97	111	112	103	19	20	44	33	53	28	23
47	273	B	D	Y	—	—	—	—	*179*	103	*116*	95	101	*21*	18	47	35	52	25	*19*
48	303	B	D	Y	—	—	—	—	*180*	100	110	102	107	*19*	*20*	45	34	53	24	*21*
49	235	B	D	Y	1	0	0	3	172	96	111	98	100	21	21	44	37	51	27	22
50	241	B	D	O	1	0	0	0	170	88	112	103	94	17	19	40	35	53	27	21

Case	MN	BNB	BA	RL	LM	GL	ZZ	CYL	IML	XML	WMH	LCD	BCD	ASB	FRS	FRF	PAC	PAS	OCC	MDB	MLN
	Measurement																				
Schild Mississippian (cont.):																					
1	7	49	102	33	97	117	42	18	31	54	22	24	15	102	20	54	117	28	86	34	44
2	10	65	102	37	112	111	47	23	34	56	28	27	13	106	17	52	119	28	97	40	56
3	8	52	99	34	98	122	44	21	37	57	20	25	15	108	20	45	107	24	98	35	45
4	8	54	92	31	111	131	46	19	34	51	23	28	15	104	25	48	123	26	103	36	50
5	9	65	116	37	117	124	50	23	32	52	28	28	13	104	18	48	106	23	104	37	41
6	9	64	105	31	104	121	44	21	36	54	23	25	15	110	20	53	111	23	101	34	40
7	8	66	103	35	112	123	49	21	36	54	25	28	14	107	24	56	111	21	107	35	50
8	8	65	85	34	101	112	46	22	30	52	25	25	14	104	22	49	108	25	97	33	53
9	8	50	102	34	104	120	46	22	35	55	24	29	14	100	22	47	104	23	95	34	50
10	—	—	—	—	—	—	—	—	—	—	—	—	—	—	21	54	—	—	—	35	43
11	*9*	58	102	36	101	121	47	21	34	53	22	30	14	—	17	49	*108*	*25*	—	34	45
12	10	60	121	32	*103*	108	46	*21*	32	53	23	28	13	110	22	48	118	26	102	32	51
13	7	64	106	29	104	123	42	20	35	54	24	28	12	106	21	53	106	22	*104*	35	47
14	7	54	102	30	104	120	46	20	30	53	22	25	14	106	18	45	113	32	*92*	30	42
15	7	50	106	31	103	117	49	21	37	59	24	20	13	113	20	57	100	27	97	32	44
16	10	63	114	36	95	110	45	19	33	53	23	26	13	105	22	51	112	27	98	38	48
17	11	62	113	35	110	130	44	21	32	49	21	26	16	108	23	49	110	28	89	38	48
18	*9*	61	99	32	112	123	46	20	37	56	21	26	15	108	25	48	116	25	*98*	34	51
19	6	66	115	36	110	121	47	22	34	57	25	26	17	113	22	53	109	25	105	36	52
20	*9*	50	100	35	100	105	47	22	35	57	25	23	13	98	17	49	109	30	101	33	45
21	11	62	96	32	102	112	49	22	*32*	*51*	28	24	11	107	17	54	111	24	98	34	52
22	—	—	—	34	—	125	—	17	—	—	—	—	—	—	*24*	*53*	—	—	—	34	46
23	—	*60*	—	—	*111*	—	46	*22*	—	—	27	—	—	—	—	—	112	20	*103*	32	48
24	*10*	*61*	*109*	36	104	118	45	21	*35*	*56*	*24*	*25*	—	114	21	60	117	29	*97*	30	49
25	—	*59*	103	35	104	114	50	20	—	—	*23*	—	—	—	—	—	—	—	—	—	—
26	8	60	102	33	102	111	46	22	31	50	25	23	14	107	*21*	*52*	*109*	*22*	108	33	45
27	10	58	102	32	109	124	46	21	29	49	24	28	16	108	23	48	105	22	102	30	56
28	12	64	100	33	112	114	47	22	36	56	24	25	14	107	19	55	102	21	107	35	43
29	8	55	97	35	106	119	45	21	30	55	26	27	16	107	22	47	105	25	93	32	46
30	8	61	109	32	109	122	51	20	34	52	24	24	14	105	26	54	116	29	97	34	54
31	8	65	100	34	103	117	43	18	29	49	22	23	12	108	22	54	101	20	106	35	44
32	12	68	110	38	111	111	49	24	36	55	26	23	12	111	23	57	114	27	96	38	45
33	13	61	101	32	104	126	45	*21*	33	53	20	24	14	104	23	58	111	27	101	36	51
34	10	50	99	35	108	127	44	17	36	58	22	26	13	104	22	51	112	28	102	32	44
35	8	58	114	35	108	104	45	21	32	54	27	29	12	110	21	47	112	26	98	35	48
36	7	54	115	37	110	130	49	20	35	57	22	26	15	101	22	47	104	25	93	35	44
37	11	62	120	32	109	124	50	*21*	39	59	24	25	13	103	23	45	115	26	104	35	42
38	11	54	103	36	116	125	48	21	39	61	25	28	15	105	21	59	107	25	99	30	38
39	10	62	106	32	107	115	44	21	33	53	20	24	13	110	25	52	111	25	101	34	48
40	9	56	104	38	114	117	44	23	40	61	26	25	14	111	21	55	118	30	93	39	50
41	7	59	105	36	106	116	44	23	35	56	25	24	13	104	22	50	111	25	94	40	46
42	7	57	*106*	*36*	*107*	*117*	*46*	*21*	39	60	24	27	14	102	*21*	*51*	111	25	92	31	47
43	8	59	106	40	*106*	*114*	46	*21*	38	56	23	28	14	*107*	19	46	105	24	100	34	48
44	—	63	—	36	105	114	49	22	33	53	23	26	14	—	—	—	—	*25*	—	34	52
45	11	62	110	36	112	121	45	*21*	36	57	24	30	14	111	24	56	119	27	102	35	48
46	10	63	113	40	111	116	48	22	37	58	25	28	16	*107*	25	45	*114*	*26*	*101*	32	48
47	10	61	110	33	105	125	43	20	32	49	21	24	13	*107*	*24*	*50*	*111*	*23*	*101*	36	46
48	*9*	62	106	32	102	116	44	17	32	50	23	25	11	107	24	47	*111*	*23*	*104*	29	45
49	9	67	101	31	103	125	40	20	32	49	22	23	15	102	21	53	99	22	100	30	43
50	7	66	101	36	*106*	117	47	21	36	51	24	*26*	*14*	98	21	55	97	20	107	33	42

TABLE 47 (cont.)

Case	Bur. no.	Mound/ knoll	Analytical status	Age	Deformation score				Measurement											
					Frontal	Bifrontal	Occipital	Lambdoid	L	MF	FC	MFB	IOB	SIOB	AIB	LOBM	LOH	NH	NB	DC
Schild Mississippian (cont.):																				
51	298a	B	D	M	0	0	0	1	174	84	107	94	91	17	16	42	36	56	23	16
52	165	B	D	M	1	0	0	3	180	92	112	102	100	20	17	45	34	52	26	18
53	197	B	D	M	2	3	0	3	180	94	114	96	98	20	23	42	35	54	26	22
54	211a	B	D	O	2	0	0	2	183	92	106	110	104	20	20	45	32	50	27	22
55	279	B	D	O	2	0	0	2	184	90	111	106	100	16	20	44	29	58	26	20
56	226a	B	D	Y	—	—	—	0	184	99	120	101	99	18	20	45	34	57	25	20
57	245a	B	D	O	0	0	0	3	192	96	115	103	101	22	*20*	*43*	*35*	55	26	*21*
58	267	B	D	M	2	3	0	0	185	95	110	102	99	17	18	45	36	53	24	18
59	290	B	D	M	0	0	0	2	195	90	111	94	94	20	21	42	33	54	27	22
60	296	B	D	Y	2	0	0	0	187	95	119	96	100	20	19	43	35	57	24	22
Schild Late Woodland:																				
61	18a	9	—	O	0	0	0	0	—	87	111	*102*	102	17	—	*44*	—	—	—	—
62	24	9	—	O	—	—	—	—	—	—	—	*100*	—	—	—	—	—	—	*26*	—
63	25	9	—	M	0	0	—	—	*179*	94	108	*99*	96	21	*20*	*42*	—	—	*26*	*21*
64	28	9	D	M	0	2	0	3	192	*99*	120	101	101	22	19	45	33	56	25	22
65	36	9	D	Y	0	0	0	1	175	90	117	98	93	15	16	41	32	50	23	17
66	31	2	—	Y	—	—	—	—	*184*	*95*	*115*	106	*100*	*18*	20	43	34	*52*	*27*	22
67	1	3	D	M	0	0	0	2	177	92	115	95	94	18	19	42	34	50	26	21
68	4a	3	—	O	—	—	—	—	—	—	—	—	—	—	—	—	—	—	—	—
69	6	3	D	Y	0	0	0	2	194	90	112	100	92	14	*20*	*41*	—	—	28	*22*
70	7a	3	—	M	—	—	—	—	—	—	—	—	—	—	—	—	—	—	—	—
71	20	3	—	M	0	0	—	—	—	—	—	*98*	—	*18*	19	—	—	—	*26*	23
72	22	3	—	Y	—	—	—	—	—	—	—	—	—	—	—	—	—	—	—	—
73	25	3	—	M	—	—	—	—	—	—	—	—	—	—	—	—	—	—	—	—
74	27	3	—	Y	—	—	—	—	—	*96*	*114*	100	*101*	—	*20*	45	—	—	25	*21*
75	5a	6	—	O	0	0	—	—	*185*	100	119	99	103	19	*22*	*44*	37	56	28	24
76	5b	6	—	O	0	0	0	0	*184*	88	107	*94*	89	15	—	*40*	—	—	—	—
77	SCa	6	D	O	0	0	0	3	180	91	115	99	97	16	18	41	36	52	25	18
78	SCb	6	—	O	0	1	0	2	189	94	113	*101*	*99*	*19*	*20*	*43*	—	—	*26*	21
79	6	1	—	M	—	—	0	1	*183*	96	*116*	104	104	19	*20*	*44*	—	—	25	*21*
80	7	1	—	M	—	—	—	—	*184*	*94*	123	*100*	99	*21*	*20*	*43*	—	—	26	*21*
81	23	1	D	O	0	0	0	0	187	89	120	99	93	17	19	40	34	55	24	20
82	62	1	D	O	0	0	0	1	180	92	108	101	95	19	18	43	31	55	27	20
83	16	3	—	M	—	—	—	—	*192*	98	117	109	100	25	25	45	37	57	31	28
84	17	1	D	M	0	0	0	4	188	84	118	98	95	16	16	41	36	53	25	18
85	34	1	—	O	0	0	0	2	—	—	—	—	—	—	—	—	—	—	—	—
86	17a	2	—	M	0	—	0	0	188	—	115	101	—	*19*	*20*	—	—	—	*26*	*21*
87	53a	1	—	Y	—	—	—	—	—	—	—	—	—	—	—	—	—	—	—	—
88	67	1	—	O	—	—	—	—	—	—	—	—	—	—	—	—	—	—	—	—
89	73	1	—	M	—	—	—	—	—	—	—	—	—	—	—	—	—	—	—	—
90	7b	2	—	M	—	—	—	—	—	—	—	98	—	—	—	—	—	—	23	—
91	11	2	D	Y	—	—	—	—	*182*	86	*112*	97	96	16	16	43	36	55	26	20
92	15	2	—	Y	—	—	0	1	*183*	90	*113*	102	90	16	20	*39*	36	54	26	21
93	20	2	—	Y	—	—	—	—	—	90	117	98	*96*	*18*	*19*	—	—	—	*26*	*20*
94	25c	2	—	M	—	—	—	—	—	—	—	—	—	—	—	—	—	—	—	—
95	15	9	—	M	0	0	0	2	190	—	116	*99*	—	—	—	—	—	—	*26*	—
96	38	9	—	Y	—	—	—	—	*184*	*96*	*115*	*102*	102	*20*	*22*	42	34	53	30	25
97	34	9	D	M	0	0	0	0	168	92	105	104	97	16	18	41	35	48	28	22
98	4b	1	—	Y	—	—	—	—	—	—	—	—	—	—	—	—	—	—	—	—
99	51	1	—	M	0	0	0	2	188	94	110	—	96	20	*20*	*42*	—	—	27	*22*
100	52	1	—	M	—	—	—	—	*187*	*94*	121	103	*99*	*19*	*19*	43	35	51	24	*20*

										Measurement											
Case	MN	BNB	BA	RL	LM	GL	ZZ	CYL	IML	XML	WMH	LCD	BCD	ASB	FRS	FRF	PAC	PAS	OCC	MDB	MLN
Schild Mississippian (cont.):																					
51	7	60	102	35	114	120	45	20	32	55	22	27	14	103	20	52	105	23	99	31	54
52	8	62	113	37	103	127	48	21	39	62	24	29	13	105	21	53	103	26	107	34	49
53	10	63	87	34	98	*113*	43	21	35	54	25	24	13	101	23	57	108	22	96	29	45
54	8	62	118	34	107	120	48	21	30	54	24	28	14	108	17	53	112	26	98	35	48
55	8	63	110	36	113	116	46	24	36	55	26	29	12	111	21	49	111	27	102	34	43
56	8	66	106	38	116	119	50	25	39	58	28	*27*	*14*	118	24	54	113	20	104	35	43
57	*10*	65	105	38	*107*	117	47	23	*36*	*55*	24	27	15	104	20	52	118	26	103	32	50
58	8	72	102	39	105	115	44	22	35	50	26	24	13	108	20	48	111	25	100	40	56
59	9	59	*109*	34	105	116	43	23	39	58	22	27	14	109	22	47	124	26	104	29	39
60	7	58	108	34	112	113	47	22	36	55	28	28	12	111	23	52	116	26	109	34	37
Schild Late Woodland:																					
61	—	—	—	30	—	*123*	—	19	35	52	24	—	—	—	23	48	*112*	—	—	28	43
62	—	*61*	—	35	*107*	*120*	47	19	—	—	*24*	—	—	—	—	—	—	—	—	—	—
63	*10*	*60*	*103*	—	*108*	—	47	*21*	—	—	*24*	*26*	—	—	19	55	110	24	*99*	*33*	*46*
64	8	57	92	32	*113*	125	44	23	32	54	24	*28*	*14*	*107*	25	51	109	20	103	33	45
65	7	54	99	29	107	122	41	16	34	55	22	28	14	103	27	53	117	30	97	29	45
66	9	*61*	105	35	105	109	47	19	37	58	26	*27*	—	—	*23*	*52*	*113*	*25*	*100*	29	36
67	8	57	104	29	*108*	*124*	45	*20*	33	54	19	28	16	100	24	52	106	21	96	32	41
68	—	—	—	—	—	—	—	19	—	—	—	—	—	—	—	—	—	—	—	28	43
69	*9*	60	*99*	34	*107*	119	49	*21*	31	50	23	*26*	15	*107*	21	51	98	19	100	30	39
70	—	—	—	—	*109*	—	—	—	—	—	—	27	16	—	—	—	—	—	—	26	41
71	10	*60*	103	35	—	123	44	*21*	37	56	23	—	—	—	—	—	—	—	—	29	47
72	—	—	—	—	—	—	—	—	—	—	—	—	—	—	—	—	—	—	—	31	40
73	—	—	—	*34*	—	*119*	—	22	34	*54*	—	—	15	—	—	—	—	—	—	35	43
74	—	*60*	111	34	*110*	*118*	50	*23*	33	54	29	—	—	—	—	—	—	—	—	45	42
75	*10*	59	*110*	*36*	*110*	*119*	*46*	*22*	39	60	24	*27*	—	118	25	47	*115*	*25*	*103*	44	47
76	—	—	—	*32*	—	*120*	—	*21*	31	46	22	—	—	—	21	47	117	23	*96*	32	45
77	7	61	100	34	102	119	42	22	33	54	25	28	14	98	26	48	107	21	99	34	45
78	*9*	*61*	119	31	*110*	*124*	48	*20*	*33*	*52*	20	*26*	—	111	21	59	129	27	*98*	36	47
79	*9*	63	103	32	115	124	54	20	34	54	28	27	17	—	*23*	—	*111*	*23*	—	34	54
80	*9*	*61*	94	33	114	120	47	21	32	57	31	26	15	—	21	57	*109*	*23*	105	39	54
81	8	59	111	32	96	114	45	22	29	52	27	29	14	117	25	52	102	20	114	30	45
82	8	67	106	33	108	127	51	17	31	50	23	27	16	100	20	45	106	22	93	37	47
83	13	70	*99*	*35*	*114*	*121*	49	23	31	51	29	*28*	—	—	*20*	*53*	*108*	*21*	*103*	31	48
84	7	58	106	32	104	116	46	20	30	49	21	30	15	112	24	54	115	22	104	28	46
85	—	—	—	—	—	—	—	—	—	—	—	—	—	110	—	—	118	25	97	32	42
86	10	*61*	*105*	*33*	—	*120*	*47*	*21*	31	56	24	—	—	111	*23*	*52*	*110*	—	—	32	44
87	—	—	—	*34*	—	*117*	—	24	33	46	24	—	—	—	—	—	—	—	—	30	53
88	—	—	—	35	—	133	—	—	—	—	—	—	—	—	—	—	—	—	—	*33*	44
89	—	—	—	*32*	—	*121*	—	*20*	32	43	19	—	—	—	—	—	—	—	—	29	45
90	—	60	—	*34*	*106*	*118*	*46*	*21*	34	56	24	—	—	—	—	—	—	*25*	—	30	42
91	5	63	125	34	111	114	48	20	35	51	24	33	15	*107*	*21*	*51*	*111*	*22*	*100*	29	37
92	8	57	104	31	*110*	123	47	21	—	*50*	22	*27*	—	106	*22*	*51*	—	—	97	29	45
93	*8*	62	*104*	32	*110*	124	45	20	32	57	23	*27*	—	—	24	50	*111*	—	—	31	45
94	—	—	—	*33*	—	—	—	—	30	47	—	—	—	—	—	—	—	—	—	33	44
95	—	*60*	99	32	110	120	45	*23*	28	*49*	30	28	14	106	21	46	104	20	108	37	50
96	12	64	112	35	*112*	129	*47*	22	32	51	25	*27*	—	—	*23*	*50*	*110*	*23*	*102*	32	51
97	10	59	95	31	112	124	45	20	28	52	24	23	14	106	24	50	101	21	99	35	45
98	—	—	—	30	*106*	119	—	20	—	—	—	—	—	—	—	—	—	—	—	—	—
99	*10*	*60*	*104*	32	*105*	118	—	20	*33*	*52*	—	*26*	—	107	*21*	*50*	109	21	96	29	37
100	*8*	60	*103*	—	*110*	—	*47*	*21*	—	—	25	*27*	—	—	*24*	*54*	107	19	*104*	36	49

Case	Bur. no.	Mound/ knoll	Analytical status	Age	Deformation score: Frontal	Bifrontal	Occipital	Lambdoid	Measurement: L	MF	FC	MFB	IOB	SIOB	AIB	LOBM	LOH	NH	NB	DC
Schild Late Woodland (cont.):																				
101	12a	3	—	Y	0	0	0	0	192	*92*	111	102	*96*	*20*	*20*	41	36	54	26	*21*
102	11	4	—	M	—	—	—	—	—	—	—	*99*	—	—	—	—	—	—	*26*	—
103	16d	2	—	Y	—	—	—	—	—	—	106	100	—	—	—	—	—	—	*26*	—
104	60b	1	D	O	0	0	0	2	179	92	110	94	96	20	22	41	35	52	27	24
Koster Late Woodland:																				
105	4	1	—	M	—	—	—	—	—	—	—	90	—	—	—	—	—	—	26	—
106	9	1	D	M	0	0	0	2	*192*	98	118	102	104	26	22	47	33	57	26	24
107	28	1	—	M	—	—	0	3	—	—	—	—	—	—	—	—	—	—	—	—
108	7	2	—	M	—	—	—	—	—	—	—	—	—	—	—	—	—	—	—	—
109	30	2	—	M	—	—	—	—	—	—	—	*104*	—	—	—	—	—	—	*26*	—
110	31a	2	—	O	—	—	—	2	—	—	—	106	—	—	—	—	—	—	*27*	—
111	31b	2	D	O	0	0	0	4	188	87	109	100	97	19	21	41	35	53	27	21
112	1	3	—	Y	0	0	0	—	*182*	—	110	84	—	—	—	—	*35*	56	*24*	—
113	14	3	—	Y	—	—	—	—	*181*	95	*115*	101	92	*18*	20	42	32	52	26	24
114	1a	4	D	M	0	1	0	4	189	95	120	106	*103*	*20*	22	44	36	60	32	21
115	1b	4	D	Y	0	3	0	3	175	94	110	98	96	22	20	40	36	53	25	21
116	18	4	D	Y	0	1	0	0	175	89	115	100	99	18	20	43	35	54	26	20
117	24	4	D	M	0	0	3	4	164	101	120	103	*102*	*20*	22	44	36	51	26	*23*
118	25a	4	D	M	0	1	0	0	174	92	108	88	94	18	*20*	*41*	34	52	26	*21*
119	25b	4	—	M	0	1	0	3	171	92	108	—	98	16	—	*43*	—	—	—	—
120	25d	4	—	M	0	0	0	3	187	97	113	*99*	100	19	*20*	*43*	—	—	*26*	*21*
121	27a	4	D	M	0	0	0	3	188	96	111	*102*	101	25	*20*	*43*	—	—	*26*	*22*
122	3	5	D	M	0	0	0	4	185	90	116	93	94	18	19	41	34	49	24	17
123	17	5	D	M	0	2	0	1	185	95	116	100	95	19	19	39	33	49	26	21
124	41	5	D	Y	0	0	0	1	181	97	114	93	97	20	22	41	35	51	24	23
125	48	5	D	M	—	—	0	2	*186*	*91*	116	95	*93*	*17*	18	40	35	52	24	19
126	50b	5	D	M	—	—	1	1	190	91	114	97	97	22	19	44	34	52	27	18
127	57	5	—	O	0	0	0	2	*178*	94	114	102	93	20	*20*	43	32	47	*26*	*21*
128	4	6	D	Y	0	0	0	0	178	93	113	95	96	20	22	42	39	53	25	22
129	10a	6	—	Y	0	0	0	2	*186*	96	117	*101*	97	20	*20*	*42*	—	—	*26*	*21*
130	14	6	—	Y	—	—	—	—	*181*	*94*	*114*	92	*99*	—	*20*	43	—	—	26	*21*
131	—a	6	D	Y	0	0	0	3	177	89	106	101	96	15	18	43	33	49	26	20
132	8	7	—	M	0	2	0	—	*183*	91	113	104	102	15	*18*	45	38	55	*26*	*20*
133	10a	7	D	M	3	3	0	0	187	96	112	99	101	19	19	44	39	56	27	18
134	23	7	D	M	0	3	0	1	180	90	114	104	96	18	20	43	35	50	26	22
135	7	8	D	Y	0	0	0	3	177	95	111	108	95	16	17	41	34	53	26	17
136	2	Kn1	—	O	—	—	—	—	*182*	95	115	100	*99*	*19*	*20*	*43*	—	—	*26*	*21*
137	1	Kn4	—	Y	0	0	0	1	182	98	110	102	*99*	*19*	20	43	36	54	24	*21*
138	8	Kn4	—	O	—	—	—	—	*182*	*94*	111	99	*99*	18	*20*	43	*34*	52	26	*21*
139	—a	Kn4	D	M	0	0	0	4	172	100	115	102	98	18	20	42	34	50	26	21
140	5	Kn5	D	Y	0	1	0	3	185	93	111	98	101	23	25	42	36	53	26	26
141	6a	Kn5	D	Y	1	0	0	1	179	98	114	101	98	20	19	42	36	56	26	22
142	6b	Kn5	D	Y	0	0	0	0	180	94	112	97	97	20	17	43	34	49	25	21
143	6e	Kn5	D	M	0	0	0	0	188	92	116	98	95	20	18	42	33	51	27	20
144	6	Kn7	D	Y	0	0	0	1	184	100	117	99	100	20	24	42	34	51	26	24
145	1	Kn8	D	M	0	0	0	3	191	93	118	109	94	*18*	20	44	33	49	30	*23*
146	5a	Kn8	D	Y	0	0	1	4	179	89	111	105	97	18	22	40	36	50	26	23
147	8	Kn8	D	Y	0	0	0	0	190	98	119	102	101	20	22	42	32	56	27	22
148	1	Ridge	D	O	2	0	0	1	188	94	115	101	100	17	22	42	34	51	28	24
149	3	Ridge	D	Y	0	0	—	—	*180*	93	109	93	92	19	18	43	34	52	24	20
150	9	7	—	O	0	0	—	—	—	98	115	*101*	101	*19*	*20*	*43*	—	—	24	*21*

	Measurement																				
Case	MN	BNB	BA	RL	LM	GL	ZZ	CYL	IML	XML	WMH	LCD	BCD	ASB	FRS	FRF	PAC	PAS	OCC	MDB	MLN
Schild Late Woodland (cont.):																					
101	*10*	60	*101*	34	*106*	114	48	*22*	30	53	25	*27*	—	—	18	50	100	17	113	34	46
102	—	*60*	—	—	—	—	46	—	—	—	*24*	—	—	—	—	—	—	—	—	31	44
103	—	66	—	*31*	—	*121*	*47*	*21*	28	49	22	—	—	—	*20*	*49*	*107*	—	—	32	49
104	6	64	100	32	107	119	47	21	35	50	21	28	14	110	20	48	100	22	112	35	48
Koster Late Woodland:																					
105	—	58	—	*33*	—	*120*	*44*	*21*	34	53	22	—	—	—	—	—	—	—	99	36	54
106	9	63	105	34	117	120	47	21	33	55	23	*27*	*14*	105	22	54	116	20	113	34	49
107	—	—	—	—	—	—	—	—	—	—	—	—	—	115	—	—	114	25	*99*	32	50
108	—	—	—	—	—	—	—	—	—	—	—	—	—	—	—	—	—	—	—	30	*45*
109	—	*62*	116	37	110	117	51	24	—	—	*24*	—	—	—	—	—	—	—	—	—	—
110	—	72	—	*34*	—	*120*	*48*	*20*	36	*55*	21	—	—	115	—	—	111	23	94	36	58
111	8	61	106	29	112	131	47	21	35	52	22	30	16	110	22	52	102	20	111	32	35
112	—	56	103	34	*108*	115	44	*21*	*34*	—	*21*	*27*	—	—	21	53	112	23	*101*	35	51
113	10	53	*105*	33	*112*	122	*47*	23	34	57	26	*26*	—	—	*23*	*51*	*111*	*25*	*97*	32	48
114	13	63	98	36	*110*	124	47	*23*	36	58	28	23	13	112	27	58	103	24	98	36	40
115	11	60	*107*	33	*104*	120	*46*	19	34	53	20	26	14	111	22	47	116	26	102	32	45
116	10	60	115	34	104	111	45	21	34	53	24	*27*	12	108	23	51	114	25	96	36	38
117	*10*	62	100	33	111	129	47	22	28	50	24	25	16	115	26	57	100	24	91	34	42
118	10	51	90	31	103	125	43	20	31	53	24	*26*	*14*	100	22	55	104	23	95	30	42
119	—	—	—	32	—	127	—	21	*32*	—	—	—	—	103	23	44	106	21	*103*	28	42
120	*9*	*60*	98	32	120	121	44	23	*34*	*53*	*24*	28	17	105	24	52	122	29	99	30	45
121	*9*	63	107	32	103	116	48	23	*33*	*53*	23	27	15	114	22	48	115	22	100	34	50
122	6	60	94	32	96	106	45	18	31	50	22	*26*	*14*	*107*	22	51	114	24	*98*	35	51
123	9	50	100	35	*111*	122	46	19	32	55	25	27	16	*107*	24	56	112	24	*98*	35	51
124	9	64	102	32	121	144	45	*20*	30	47	20	28	15	108	26	52	115	26	91	38	40
125	10	53	105	28	102	126	43	19	30	52	22	26	15	101	*24*	*52*	117	22	100	31	47
126	8	64	110	32	*108*	126	47	20	39	55	24	*27*	*14*	*107*	*22*	*52*	113	22	101	31	53
127	*9*	62	—	36	*105*	122	*47*	*20*	—	*52*	22	24	14	—	20	50	—	—	—	34	47
128	9	62	*103*	33	105	123	44	*21*	34	49	22	26	15	107	23	48	115	25	96	35	48
129	*9*	*64*	*104*	31	101	113	50	23	33	51	25	*26*	—	107	23	52	112	22	102	34	55
130	—	65	—	35	*106*	118	43	*20*	—	*53*	20	—	—	—	—	—	—	—	—	*32*	—
131	6	60	96	32	109	122	47	22	29	49	22	25	15	104	22	50	109	25	92	32	49
132	7	52	*106*	35	*109*	124	*48*	21	33	60	25	*28*	14	—	20	56	*109*	*24*	*103*	33	41
133	8	51	108	35	*109*	*119*	49	*22*	34	55	24	*27*	*14*	110	20	48	114	23	107	33	52
134	11	54	104	35	105	127	43	20	34	58	25	29	15	105	25	52	115	25	89	34	45
135	11	62	104	33	108	126	46	22	31	52	23	26	15	109	24	50	105	24	93	28	47
136	*9*	60	*106*	36	*107*	113	*47*	24	36	54	24	*27*	—	—	*23*	*52*	*112*	*24*	—	35	55
137	*9*	66	*102*	*33*	*107*	*119*	*47*	*22*	29	46	25	*27*	—	—	24	53	113	20	*104*	*35*	*48*
138	*9*	60	115	31	*114*	131	47	21	30	52	19	*27*	—	—	*23*	*51*	*110*	*23*	*100*	34	45
139	9	58	110	32	99	109	47	21	36	55	22	28	14	104	23	52	105	22	*102*	35	45
140	13	60	98	33	110	118	45	22	33	54	24	25	15	107	20	54	117	24	102	37	52
141	8	59	96	32	99	108	50	22	28	53	27	27	15	110	21	44	96	18	111	33	55
142	7	63	107	34	110	121	46	23	30	48	21	24	15	109	23	50	115	23	93	32	49
143	8	62	*106*	*32*	*109*	*122*	*46*	*20*	32	51	21	25	16	108	26	56	119	28	96	29	46
144	11	58	*110*	37	101	109	47	22	39	58	25	*26*	*14*	115	23	50	116	28	100	32	52
145	*9*	68	110	35	114	125	49	19	28	45	20	27	16	107	26	48	114	22	103	33	45
146	7	66	107	37	116	119	47	22	37	55	24	26	15	98	25	45	113	27	90	33	42
147	11	62	111	37	*112*	128	48	19	37	57	25	28	14	115	24	51	115	24	105	39	53
148	8	57	111	*34*	112	119	50	23	35	55	24	*26*	*14*	113	23	52	113	24	110	39	50
149	12	56	*103*	30	*110*	*124*	43	*21*	32	50	23	25	14	102	22	46	*110*	*23*	101	27	43
150	9	*61*	115	35	112	123	47	22	—	*55*	*24*	*26*	—	—	*23*	*52*	—	—	—	35	49

Case	Bur. no.	Mound/ knoll	Analytical status	Age	Deformation score: Frontal	Bifrontal	Occipital	Lambdoid	Measurement: L	MF	FC	MFB	IOB	SIOB	AIB	LOBM	LOH	NH	NB	DC
Koster Late Woodland (cont.):																				
151	1	5	D	M	0	0	0	2	184	98	115	102	98	16	20	45	34	54	26	20
152	2	8	D	M	0	0	0	0	184	98	115	96	99	20	22	42	39	56	27	22
Yokem Mississippian:																				
153	17	1	—	Y	—	—	—	—	*183*	—	—	99	—	*20*	*22*	—	*35*	55	27	*22*
154	30	1	D	Y	0	0	—	—	*181*	94	110	102	94	19	21	40	33	50	27	22
155	43	1	D	M	0	0	0	0	186	97	106	100	104	19	23	42	35	54	25	24
156	52	1	D	O	0	0	0	1	182	96	110	101	100	18	19	43	36	54	27	20
157	67	1	—	M	—	—	—	—	*178*	96	116	*101*	105	14	20	*44*	—	—	24	21
158	1	1	D	Y	0	0	0	3	183	92	114	100	96	17	*19*	42	33	56	25	*20*
159	7	1	D	M	0	0	0	2	187	106	116	105	103	20	22	44	35	54	27	21
160	34	1	D	Y	0	0	0	1	181	98	118	100	101	20	19	46	33	51	26	*21*
161	36	1	D	O	0	0	0	1	*184*	89	116	104	93	25	21	44	36	57	27	*22*
162	56	1	D	Y	0	0	0	2	183	97	113	106	105	19	24	42	35	54	28	23
163	64	1	D	O	0	0	0	0	186	101	118	111	104	19	21	42	33	53	26	21
164	6	2	D	M	0	0	0	0	177	94	118	106	96	15	18	42	33	54	26	20
165	13	2	D	Y	—	—	0	0	*180*	98	115	103	102	*20*	20	46	34	57	27	22
166	16	2	D	Y	0	0	0	0	185	93	114	102	98	20	19	43	36	55	26	19
167	92	3	D	Y	2	3	1	2	177	94	113	110	103	20	20	44	36	56	28	22
168	97	3	D	Y	0	0	0	0	178	—	105	97	—	*19*	*20*	—	—	—	22	*21*
169	103	3	D	Y	0	0	0	1	*183*	88	114	100	95	18	*19*	43	36	56	25	*20*
170	116	3	—	Y	—	—	—	—	—	—	—	96	—	—	—	—	—	—	*25*	—
171	21	1	—	Y	0	0	1	—	179	94	110	102	99	14	21	40	34	52	26	*22*
Yokem Late Woodland:																				
172	14	3	—	M	—	—	—	—	*184*	94	112	94	98	20	21	43	36	53	24	22
173	16	3	D	M	0	0	—	—	*183*	90	121	98	96	21	22	39	36	52	28	*23*
174	20d	3	—	O	0	0	1	2	176	—	114	100	—	*19*	*20*	—	*34*	50	26	*21*
175	21	3	D	M	0	0	0	4	183	98	116	106	109	18	*20*	*46*	—	—	*27*	*21*
176	22a	3	—	Y	—	—	—	—	*184*	*94*	*114*	102	*99*	—	*20*	43	34	53	*26*	*21*
177	24c	3	—	O	0	0	0	4	189	102	112	—	—	*19*	—	—	—	—	—	—
178	24d	3	—	O	0	0	—	—	*178*	93	*111*	94	97	18	20	41	34	51	26	20
179	29	3	—	O	0	1	0	0	*186*	—	119	—	—	*19*	*21*	—	—	—	—	*22*
180	44	3	—	M	—	—	—	—	*180*	95	*113*	104	97	16	20	42	32	50	24	21
181	45	3	—	M	—	—	—	—	—	—	—	102	—	—	—	—	—	—	*26*	—
182	46	3	—	Y	—	—	—	—	—	—	—	102	—	—	—	—	—	—	27	—
183	49	3	D	Y	0	2	0	0	182	92	114	109	100	18	18	44	35	55	27	20
184	50a	3	—	O	—	—	—	—	*179*	94	*113*	88	97	*18*	*19*	42	*34*	51	25	*20*
185	79	3	D	M	0	0	0	0	190	92	118	88	93	21	20	43	34	59	25	21
186	80	3	—	M	—	—	—	—	*186*	*94*	118	94	*99*	*19*	*20*	43	*36*	59	24	*21*
187	85	3	—	O	0	0	0	4	180	83	111	110	100	17	*18*	*43*	—	—	*27*	*20*
188	—a	3	D	M	0	0	0	1	*189*	90	119	96	96	14	18	41	36	52	23	*19*
189	—b	3	—	O	—	—	—	—	—	—	—	98	—	—	—	—	—	—	25	—
190	6	4	D	M	0	0	0	2	169	94	114	95	93	19	16	41	37	54	27	22
191	9	4	D	O	0	0	0	2	177	92	115	99	97	19	18	43	36	55	26	22
192	10a	4	—	Y	0	0	—	1	*183*	94	112	*97*	96	16	*20*	*42*	—	—	*25*	*21*
193	18c	4	—	Y	0	3	—	—	*179*	95	111	102	98	19	*19*	41	38	53	22	*19*
194	32	4	D	Y	0	0	—	3	*174*	95	105	108	99	20	20	43	34	53	23	21
195	4a	5	D	M	1	0	0	1	184	98	108	103	101	18	23	42	34	54	25	23
196	15a	5	D	M	0	0	0	2	180	96	112	104	98	13	18	43	36	56	29	21
197	17	5	—	M	0	0	—	—	*181*	94	111	*101*	99	16	21	*42*	—	—	*26*	23
198	20	5	D	O	0	0	0	0	190	96	119	99	103	20	21	44	32	56	30	22

Case	MN	BNB	BA	RL	LM	GL	ZZ	CYL	IML	XML	WMH	LCD	BCD	ASB	FRS	FRF	PAC	PAS	OCC	MDB	MLN
										Measurement											
Koster Late Woodland (cont.):																					
151	8	62	114	35	106	108	52	23	33	55	25	27	14	112	25	52	108	23	98	34	48
152	10	63	100	31	109	117	46	20	31	49	22	23	15	107	25	54	119	25	98	34	40
Yokem Mississippian:																					
153	12	62	105	34	107	118	46	23	35	55	22	27	—	—	—	52	—	24	—	32	49
154	10	64	109	33	104	124	43	22	34	52	20	26	13	107	24	48	112	24	97	33	43
155	10	63	114	35	106	121	46	25	33	52	22	24	15	110	22	48	119	24	96	33	44
156	8	57	110	39	110	116	51	23	40	60	23	27	12	103	21	56	116	23	105	32	42
157	9	59	105	34	108	112	43	19	34	53	17	27	17	—	27	52	114	25	—	32	47
158	8	60	105	33	107	119	47	22	31	46	25	27	14	107	25	49	117	27	92	34	53
159	10	64	104	37	99	103	50	22	34	56	25	24	13	108	26	51	114	24	97	41	54
160	10	58	99	39	112	118	47	20	36	54	24	28	13	101	23	56	116	25	93	33	47
161	10	64	107	31	111	126	46	20	36	59	22	27	14	107	22	52	112	25	100	33	46
162	12	64	111	34	116	133	46	22	34	54	25	28	13	105	22	52	112	24	103	34	49
163	8	63	106	35	112	110	53	21	35	57	26	28	14	112	27	49	112	25	114	33	51
164	7	60	113	34	106	122	48	22	32	51	28	26	13	108	23	54	108	23	108	44	53
165	10	53	103	34	104	111	49	23	30	55	25	26	14	114	22	52	108	23	98	34	50
166	11	61	97	35	106	109	49	23	29	50	23	26	13	109	22	49	111	22	103	29	41
167	10	64	107	33	117	120	54	23	32	55	26	31	14	114	19	56	105	25	105	35	52
168	9	52	107	34	—	109	46	20	34	54	23	24	13	110	19	50	98	16	110	32	38
169	9	62	88	34	104	119	45	20	31	47	22	27	14	107	24	46	111	21	101	32	46
170	—	59	—	32	107	126	44	19	—	—	23	—	—	—	—	—	—	—	—	—	—
171	7	56	100	31	108	122	47	21	28	47	22	27	—	—	24	46	117	24	100	32	47
Yokem Late Woodland:																					
172	7	56	95	34	109	122	43	21	33	56	22	27	—	—	22	51	110	24	100	32	43
173	10	62	103	34	109	128	49	18	32	51	24	29	15	110	22	56	110	23	99	34	50
174	9	60	—	35	104	116	49	21	35	—	25	27	—	116	23	53	116	27	107	30	45
175	9	66	115	38	103	114	50	20	33	56	26	27	14	118	25	56	122	29	103	40	54
176	—	58	106	32	104	112	49	22	32	57	22	27	14	—	—	52	—	24	101	36	51
177	—	—	—	—	—	—	—	—	—	—	—	—	—	107	26	51	116	23	101	31	50
178	8	61	—	—	105	—	45	21	—	—	24	25	—	—	22	—	—	—	—	30	48
179	11	—	—	—	—	—	—	22	—	—	26	—	—	—	22	49	106	19	104	43	44
180	7	59	106	34	106	120	50	19	35	57	24	26	13	—	23	51	112	25	98	33	44
181	—	62	123	38	115	122	50	21	42	60	24	—	15	—	—	—	—	26	—	33	40
182	—	66	—	31	106	120	47	22	—	—	26	—	—	—	—	—	—	—	—	30	53
183	6	53	108	33	111	120	52	25	32	58	25	28	14	101	23	54	109	25	100	32	53
184	8	58	106	35	113	124	44	20	32	52	22	28	15	110	22	51	110	24	99	31	49
185	11	62	109	38	110	118	47	21	35	53	25	29	18	103	23	54	110	20	107	31	39
186	9	64	—	34	110	116	47	22	—	52	24	28	—	107	24	53	—	—	106	34	57
187	8	52	108	32	110	121	49	22	29	53	28	27	—	108	21	54	103	20	105	31	50
188	6	56	106	31	105	122	48	15	33	51	24	25	17	107	28	57	120	23	100	32	42
189	—	68	—	38	111	124	49	23	36	55	23	27	—	98	—	—	—	24	—	36	38
190	6	54	102	34	103	111	43	21	30	50	23	26	15	108	22	49	107	22	88	36	49
191	6	58	120	32	103	118	45	24	36	54	24	25	14	109	25	51	106	21	97	33	45
192	9	57	112	30	97	109	44	21	32	52	20	28	11	—	24	51	112	23	100	31	51
193	9	52	—	—	109	—	47	21	—	—	23	26	—	—	19	57	—	—	—	34	42
194	9	65	110	36	107	120	47	20	34	53	24	28	14	107	20	52	106	25	99	34	45
195	10	61	101	37	108	111	44	22	38	56	25	30	15	108	19	43	118	24	99	30	51
196	11	62	114	33	107	121	44	22	35	55	24	28	15	115	27	50	114	23	99	33	44
197	8	61	—	—	105	—	48	21	—	—	22	26	—	—	21	48	—	—	—	26	40
198	8	59	108	40	124	119	49	21	38	58	28	28	14	109	23	52	113	21	105	37	53

Case	Bur. no.	Mound/ knoll	Analytical status	Age	Deformation score: Frontal	Bifrontal	Occipital	Lambdoid	Measurement: L	MF	FC	MFB	IOB	SIOB	AIB	LOBM	LOH	NH	NB	DC
Yokem Late Woodland (cont.):																				
199	39	5	D	M	0	0	0	3	183	93	116	98	95	16	18	42	35	54	28	20
200	2	8	D	M	0	0	0	1	190	*97*	124	108	*101*	*18*	22	42	*35*	53	26	22
201	10b	4	D	Y	0	0	0	0	186	100	119	104	102	19	21	43	36	57	26	23
Klunk Late Woodland:																				
202	13	8	D	O	0	0	0	0	178	98	116	95	100	20	21	43	32	52	24	22
203	15	8	D	M	0	3	0	3	178	83	110	98	94	14	18	42	32	52	24	21
204	32	8	D	O	0	0	0	1	176	93	113	100	102	20	17	46	38	53	23	18
205	1	10	D	M	1	2	0	3	174	79	107	100	95	18	16	41	32	50	25	19
206	1	14	D	M	0	1	0	1	179	89	108	96	98	16	18	43	33	53	25	20
207	4	14	D	M	0	0	0	2	185	99	115	103	100	19	20	42	35	56	24	23
208	7	14	D	O	0	1	0	1	180	93	114	99	98	21	18	43	38	58	28	20
209	12	14	—	Y	—	—	—	—	—	—	—	99	—	—	—	—	—	—	26	—
210	18	14	—	O	0	0	0	2	183	93	112	98	97	17	19	*42*	—	—	*25*	*20*
211	21	14	—	M	0	0	—	—	—	90	111	99	94	16	18	*41*	—	—	*25*	*20*
212	?	14	D	M	1	2	1	2	178	92	107	99	99	20	21	43	35	57	24	21
Ledders Late Woodland:[a]																				
213	98	1	—	Y					*180*	*91*	*112*	95	*95*	—	*19*	40	—	—	24	*20*
214	34	2	D	O					176	95	110	92	94	19	17	43	35	58	23	18
215	38	1	—	Y					—	100	116	106	106	18	*21*	*45*	—	—	27	*23*
216	70	1	—	O					—	—	—	—	—	—	—	—	—	—	—	—
217	102	1	—	O					*179*	94	112	100	100	18	*21*	44	—	—	29	*23*
218	135	1	D	O					178	86	110	103	97	15	21	40	33	53	26	20
219	5	1	D	O					180	100	113	105	102	20	21	42	33	50	26	21
220	7	1	—	O					172	95	*113*	98	*99*	—	*20*	*43*	—	—	26	*21*
221	1	1	—	O					—	—	—	—	—	—	—	—	—	—	26	—
222	16	1	D	M					*181*	91	*115*	96	98	19	18	42	35	54	25	21
223	24	1	D	O					181	91	114	102	96	19	21	41	34	52	27	22
224	17	1	D	O					*184*	98	118	105	102	18	*20*	*44*	*34*	49	25	22
225	25	1	D	M					195	94	121	102	99	18	*21*	*43*	*34*	49	26	*22*
226	49	1	—	Y					183	*97*	*114*	110	103	*20*	*20*	*44*	—	—	26	*22*
227	56	1	D	M					182	102	114	98	100	*18*	18	42	34	52	25	21
228	54	1	D	O					*185*	103	*117*	100	105	18	22	45	35	53	28	28
229	81	1	D	M					193	95	114	95	95	24	23	43	34	53	26	24
230	91	1	D	M					*182*	94	115	102	102	18	23	40	*34*	52	27	*24*
231	96	1	D	O					185	*96*	115	104	*101*	*20*	22	43	35	55	26	22
232	12	2	D	Y					*180*	92	*114*	91	94	17	18	42	35	56	28	21
233	143	1	D	M					184	88	111	104	100	10	19	45	34	45	27	26

[a]Deformation in the Ledders cranial series is effectively absent, and crania were not scored individually. Hence, the Ledders data file does not discriminate between *lack of deformation* (0) and *unscorable due to incompleteness of cranium* (—).

										Measurement											
Case	MN	BNB	BA	RL	LM	G*L*	ZZ	CYL	IML	XML	WMH	LCD	BCD	ASB	FRS	FRF	PAC	PAS	OCC	MDB	MLN
Yokem Late Woodland (cont.)																					
199	10	60	108	29	108	126	44	18	34	54	19	24	*14*	108	23	54	112	22	103	29	45
200	10	70	105	34	107	122	50	21	32	54	27	*27*	15	100	*25*	*55*	122	27	103	35	52
201	9	60	112	36	109	111	47	26	38	60	25	28	14	114	26	54	119	26	97	38	54
Klunk Late Woodland:																					
202	7	61	106	29	113	130	43	19	36	54	22	27	18	104	27	54	108	23	111	38	48
203	9	58	*106*	37	112	117	47	*21*	34	55	24	26	16	106	21	53	120	27	94	34	49
204	8	59	99	30	111	121	47	21	31	54	23	25	15	105	22	53	112	26	98	36	46
205	8	59	101	31	108	126	51	20	35	54	26	24	15	105	19	53	108	22	92	32	47
206	8	55	98	37	104	114	44	20	32	51	25	27	14	110	20	47	102	18	101	32	42
207	11	58	88	31	102	111	48	22	30	52	26	28	14	*107*	22	53	109	22	109	31	45
208	10	66	111	31	120	132	52	20	35	50	24	29	12	110	21	54	111	24	101	36	52
209	—	64	—	37	104	110	46	22	—	—	*24*	32	13	—	—	—	—	—	—	35	*47*
210	*9*	*60*	113	33	114	132	44	21	*33*	*53*	*23*	25	15	113	20	48	110	27	105	34	46
211	10	*60*	—	34	*109*	*119*	49	*21*	—	*52*	*24*	26	11	—	20	53	—	—	—	28	43
212	12	57	102	38	111	109	47	24	34	55	27	25	12	99	16	51	113	28	101	38	49
Ledders Late Woodland:																					
213	—	56	—	32	*107*	117	*45*	20	34	51	21	24	14	104	—	—	—	*23*	88	30	41
214	6	52	96	31	107	125	44	21	28	51	20	27	15	100	26	48	108	23	101	33	45
215	*10*	61	*110*	36	—	119	*48*	19	32	54	25	23	15	106	22	59	*110*	—	—	33	35
216	—	—	—	39	—	*116*	—	*22*	33	55	27	—	—	—	—	—	—	—	—	35	55
217	*10*	*60*	*107*	31	*110*	*124*	44	*20*	*32*	*53*	20	*27*	—	—	22	49	106	*22*	*101*	29	39
218	9	60	108	34	109	126	49	23	31	50	24	28	12	101	22	47	108	23	101	32	45
219	11	62	111	36	116	117	48	25	38	57	26	31	13	122	21	50	113	24	100	37	45
220	—	64	102	32	*103*	126	*46*	*21*	34	50	22	26	13	104	—	—	112	23	97	33	45
221		—	—	—	—	—	—	—	—	—	—	28	16	104	—	—	107	19	*104*	38	*49*
222	9	57	103	35	106	116	44	21	30	52	24	28	13	106	*22*	*51*	*109*	*23*	*101*	34	44
223	8	57	91	34	112	118	47	18	36	57	23	30	16	109	21	57	116	26	94	35	44
224	9	66	*103*	34	*108*	120	*48*	20	31	52	26	27	15	*107*	21	47	102	17	*108*	34	49
225	11	62	*104*	32	116	120	*47*	23	33	56	25	*26*	*14*	*107*	23	58	115	24	*100*	30	47
226	*10*	62	*107*	33	108	124	*49*	21	*32*	*54*	19	*27*	—	—	20	50	107	22	*104*	24	41
227	9	66	105	30	109	118	45	24	27	50	24	26	16	103	22	49	100	16	111	33	42
228	11	64	108	32	106	120	51	21	36	52	23	*27*	*14*	*107*	*24*	*51*	*113*	*23*	*102*	37	48
229	13	62	95	34	101	112	40	25	34	55	24	28	13	*107*	21	50	117	23	*99*	31	46
230	11	*64*	100	37	102	112	46	20	33	50	24	*27*	*14*	*107*	21	55	105	*21*	*105*	33	48
231	9	66	99	35	103	113	48	23	36	56	25	26	13	106	23	51	112	25	101	32	51
232	8	58	*108*	32	114	120	48	*21*	35	47	22	24	14	*107*	*22*	*50*	*112*	*22*	*100*	29	38
233	*9*	62	108	34	110	119	48	*20*	33	52	27	30	15	111	25	50	111	22	*103*	32	47

Case	Bur. no.	Mound/ knoll	Analytical status	Age	Deformation score: Frontal	Bifrontal	Occipital	Lambdoid	Measurement: L	MF	FC	MFB	IOB	SIOB	AIB	LOBM	LOH	NH	NB	DC
Schild Mississippian:																				
1	56	A	D	O	0	0	0	3	180	93	110	100	96	18	16	44	37	50	25	17
2	62	A	D	Y	0	0	0	3	179	88	106	91	91	16	16	41	38	53	24	18
3	74	A	D	M	0	0	0	1	172	87	107	97	95	18	18	42	32	52	27	18
4	76	A	D	M	0	0	0	0	172	87	107	99	98	16	19	43	35	52	28	20
5	90	A	D	O	0	0	0	1	179	92	115	101	97	18	18	45	34	52	23	19
6	96a	A	D	Y	1	2	0	3	168	92	103	96	96	20	22	40	32	52	24	22
7	103	A	D	M	1	3	0	0	180	102	118	103	100	18	19	43	36	51	28	22
8	107a	A	D	O	0	0	0	3	170	84	102	93	93	13	18	40	35	49	24	19
9	111	A	D	Y	0	1	0	3	169	88	110	101	91	16	17	41	36	52	27	17
10	157	A	D	Y	0	0	0	1	169	84	107	89	93	14	16	41	33	45	24	20
11	158	A	D	O	0	0	0	4	180	94	112	95	99	19	20	43	34	51	25	22
12	132d	A	D	M	0	0	0	3	169	86	109	91	89	15	15	41	34	49	27	17
13	59	A	D	O	0	1	0	4	176	96	105	92	97	17	21	43	34	48	26	20
14	49	A	D	M	1	1	0	0	170	96	104	98	98	17	22	42	36	49	26	24
15	53a	A	D	O	1	0	0	2	177	93	113	100	100	21	21	43	38	54	25	20
16	94	A	D	O	0	0	0	0	173	90	112	95	95	16	16	43	36	53	25	18
17	69a	A	D	Y	0	0	0	3	183	94	108	92	91	19	20	38	34	46	25	20
18	142	A	D	O	1	0	0	0	175	86	107	101	98	15	18	45	36	68	28	18
19	66a	A	D	Y	—	—	—	—	*178*	103	117	95	102	16	22	42	35	47	24	25
20	132a	A	D	M	0	0	0	1	180	91	117	96	95	17	19	42	30	48	28	20
21	72	A	D	O	0	0	0	3	159	88	102	90	94	17	20	41	33	49	27	22
22	77d	A	D	M	3	0	1	0	171	82	102	96	96	*16*	18	45	34	47	24	20
23	82	A	D	M	1	0	0	3	176	91	113	100	97	14	20	41	35	55	27	20
24	83b	A	D	Y	0	0	0	3	167	84	103	94	89	15	19	38	32	49	23	20
25	85	A	D	Y	—	—	—	—	*176*	98	112	102	100	18	20	46	38	48	25	21
26	91	A	—	O	0	0	0	1	175	87	108	*94*	94	*17*	*19*	*41*	—	—	*26*	*20*
27	109	A	—	Y	—	—	—	—	*167*	82	101	95	87	14	17	40	32	44	22	19
28	110	A	D	M	0	0	0	2	173	90	109	*96*	95	18	*19*	*41*	36	*51*	*26*	*20*
29	122b	A	—	Y	—	—	—	—	—	—	—	—	—	—	—	—	—	—	—	—
30	138	A	D	Y	1	0	0	3	167	89	107	94	98	16	20	42	39	49	26	22
31	65	A	D	Y	0	0	0	1	178	95	112	97	95	19	20	41	36	54	25	19
32	43	A	—	Y	—	—	—	—	*179*	95	*111*	—	105	24	22	*45*	—	—	*27*	22
33	44b	A	—	Y	—	—	0	2	*171*	—	—	—	—	—	—	—	—	—	—	—
34	46	A	—	Y	0	2	—	—	*172*	92	115	103	100	15	*20*	*43*	*34*	*51*	24	*20*
35	47a	A	D	M	1	0	0	1	175	94	107	95	96	17	16	43	36	50	26	19
36	55b	A	D	Y	0	0	0	2	175	94	106	104	99	16	23	40	35	55	30	24
37	155	A	D	O	0	0	0	4	180	90	110	101	98	19	20	43	32	53	27	20
38	162	A	D	Y	—	—	—	—	180	88	109	93	95	17	18	40	35	46	24	18
39	186	B	D	O	2	0	0	3	167	85	105	98	96	17	19	43	36	53	26	21
40	187a	B	D	M	—	—	0	0	174	89	109	96	102	19	20	44	34	50	29	22
41	201	B	D	Y	0	0	0	2	177	92	106	99	98	18	19	42	34	49	25	19
42	217	B	D	Y	0	0	0	2	159	85	108	99	93	17	15	40	34	50	24	17
43	230	B	D	Y	0	0	0	2	185	92	112	97	97	16	19	42	32	51	21	19
44	231	B	D	Y	0	0	1	3	155	87	105	98	91	13	17	40	32	47	23	18
45	239a	B	D	Y	0	0	0	4	177	100	109	101	101	21	24	42	34	52	28	26
46	263	B	D	M	0	0	0	2	169	90	102	101	94	15	18	41	32	50	24	17
47	269	B	D	O	0	0	0	4	172	92	110	101	93	17	19	40	34	49	25	18
48	285	B	D	O	1	0	2	4	162	89	109	93	94	16	17	42	30	50	25	19
49	295b	B	D	Y	1	0	0	1	172	90	108	91	95	13	18	40	36	50	25	20
50	236f	B	—	Y	—	—	—	—	171	87	105	—	96	17	*20*	*42*	—	—	*26*	*21*

Measurement

Case	MN	BNB	BA	RL	LM	GL	ZZ	CYL	IML	XML	WMH	LCD	BCD	ASB	FRS	FRF	PAC	PAS	OCC	MDB	MLN
Schild Mississippian:																					
1	8	64	98	33	109	121	44	21	32	47	18	26	18	109	22	50	106	20	108	34	52
2	9	54	95	32	103	124	45	20	30	51	22	28	14	105	21	46	112	25	106	30	41
3	10	60	92	33	109	123	44	19	31	52	22	24	13	106	22	46	107	24	99	30	44
4	9	56	89	32	118	129	48	22	32	53	20	23	15	100	22	48	112	27	97	27	39
5	8	60	101	34	107	122	46	22	32	52	24	26	13	107	22	48	108	23	102	35	39
6	9	57	96	37	97	107	43	22	32	55	24	29	11	104	19	50	103	26	92	34	51
7	12	65	105	36	112	122	48	23	38	54	25	23	15	104	22	49	112	24	103	35	43
8	9	52	96	33	108	123	49	16	33	50	18	25	12	100	21	45	109	27	98	31	44
9	9	60	86	30	106	120	43	18	30	51	22	24	13	99	21	47	106	24	99	30	44
10	6	57	94	27	92	115	42	20	28	45	20	21	12	105	22	44	96	20	104	29	44
11	10	60	97	35	104	124	47	20	38	55	22	28	16	100	26	50	114	27	97	33	43
12	8	57	89	29	95	114	45	17	29	49	20	23	12	113	22	52	99	18	106	32	44
13	12	60	95	31	98	121	45	16	34	54	22	27	14	103	22	48	112	23	97	33	42
14	9	68	91	34	100	117	45	20	32	45	21	20	14	109	19	50	101	21	98	28	44
15	10	58	105	33	101	124	46	20	32	52	27	24	14	101	22	53	110	27	95	35	40
16	9	61	94	29	103	123	44	20	28	44	21	26	15	101	22	50	109	25	98	32	40
17	11	57	91	36	106	133	48	18	34	51	23	22	14	101	27	47	118	26	89	24	34
18	7	59	96	30	105	136	45	19	28	49	23	25	15	103	20	52	105	23	99	28	40
19	10	65	102	31	98	123	44	18	30	47	22	27	16	106	26	60	110	23	118	36	46
20	10	58	96	32	104	120	44	20	33	51	25	22	13	107	24	48	109	24	109	31	45
21	12	59	90	33	98	108	45	18	29	48	21	22	12	108	18	50	93	20	88	27	43
22	10	53	97	32	105	124	45	19	33	51	21	25	18	105	13	47	108	22	104	34	45
23	8	56	96	36	116	128	46	20	32	49	24	27	14	103	21	48	114	28	100	34	45
24	8	48	94	31	96	123	45	19	30	54	23	20	15	104	20	43	108	28	91	29	32
25	10	65	96	35	105	122	46	17	30	47	22	28	14	104	24	47	108	23	98	32	41
26	9	58	92	32	—	121	41	18	31	50	20	23	13	107	20	49	111	23	101	29	41
27	9	63	87	32	100	122	43	18	—	46	19	24	—	—	22	44	—	—	98	26	32
28	9	59	97	37	104	116	45	19	31	54	21	26	15	105	19	52	104	23	99	30	38
29	—	—	—	—	—	—	—	—	—	—	—	26	13	—	—	—	—	—	—	—	—
30	12	57	102	33	101	123	44	20	33	50	22	25	14	104	18	46	112	26	94	27	42
31	9	55	86	35	110	122	46	19	34	55	25	24	15	107	23	49	99	17	104	34	45
32	9	65	95	30	—	126	48	19	—	51	—	24	16	114	23	—	—	—	—	30	45
33	—	—	95	—	—	—	—	—	—	—	—	25	15	105	—	—	103	21	101	29	45
34	9	62	99	34	105	126	45	19	31	51	23	25	—	—	19	52	105	23	—	32	43
35	6	52	95	28	101	128	41	20	28	52	21	25	14	112	19	47	106	21	97	30	46
36	10	59	108	33	108	128	47	18	32	53	25	25	15	103	22	48	103	20	105	30	40
37	8	64	104	35	112	124	45	18	30	51	22	27	15	113	22	52	111	25	99	35	47
38	7	56	88	29	104	126	45	20	33	50	21	23	17	104	22	47	111	25	93	27	39
39	11	62	96	35	110	115	44	20	32	49	23	20	16	99	17	51	107	20	89	32	46
40	9	56	98	35	107	118	46	24	40	58	22	28	15	106	20	47	110	27	102	33	48
41	9	59	99	37	100	117	45	18	34	53	24	25	16	102	21	47	108	25	104	29	48
42	10	55	95	33	106	127	46	20	29	49	22	21	15	100	22	44	95	21	91	35	42
43	9	49	85	32	100	106	46	18	34	58	24	24	14	103	22	45	113	25	93	34	47
44	7	58	97	35	101	115	47	20	31	50	23	18	12	98	22	47	100	25	93	29	37
45	11	68	103	32	104	133	45	19	33	49	21	29	13	96	25	51	107	25	97	30	46
46	9	51	97	38	108	114	45	20	35	55	27	24	16	107	19	47	109	24	100	29	35
47	9	52	101	31	101	122	40	16	27	51	20	25	14	104	24	52	112	28	97	28	32
48	6	57	99	33	105	120	49	22	32	52	22	24	12	112	19	54	97	21	104	31	43
49	8	60	100	28	108	136	44	18	34	51	18	27	13	102	20	54	108	24	103	32	45
50	10	59	96	36	—	120	42	22	34	52	—	25	—	—	20	45	108	24	99	35	45

Case	Bur. no.	Mound/ knoll	Analytical status	Age	Deformation score: Frontal	Bifrontal	Occipital	Lambdoid	Measurement: L	MF	FC	MFB	IOB	SIOB	AIB	LOBM	LOH	NH	NB	DC
Schild Mississippian (cont.):																				
51	266a	B	—	M	0	0	0	0	—	—	—	96	—	*18*	—	*42*	*35*	*50*	*27*	*21*
52	240a	B	—	O	—	—	—	—	*175*	97	113	—	98	15	*20*	*42*	—	—	*26*	*21*
53	219	B	—	M	0	0	0	2	167	87	107	90	90	18	19	39	34	*50*	*25*	22
54	249	B	D	O	0	2	0	2	177	88	103	99	100	19	17	44	34	51	25	20
55	191a	B	D	O	0	0	0	3	174	94	121	103	*97*	*17*	18	*42*	34	51	27	19
56	252	B	D	O	0	0	0	3	172	*89*	107	92	*93*	*16*	16	42	33	47	23	19
57	259	B	D	Y	0	0	0	1	169	*90*	100	92	*95*	*17*	21	40	34	48	25	21
58	222a	B	D	M	0	2	0	1	171	96	114	92	101	14	23	45	34	48	29	25
59	300	B	—	Y	—	—	—	—	—	—	—	—	—	*16*	16	—	*34*	*49*	*24*	*18*
60	306	B	—	O	0	0	0	4	181	95	114	96	97	16	*20*	*42*	—	—	*26*	*21*
61	257a	B	D	O	0	0	0	3	180	94	110	100	99	17	20	44	35	53	28	21
62	233	B	D	O	0	0	0	3	182	92	110	96	94	15	19	42	36	53	21	20
63	214	B	—	O	—	—	0	2	*179*	—	—	100	—	*16*	—	—	*34*	*50*	*25*	—
64	280	B	D	Y	0	0	0	1	166	88	110	94	90	15	19	39	34	50	27	18
65	172a	B	D	O	0	0	0	3	*183*	97	115	102	97	17	21	44	33	53	28	22
66	178	B	D	O	2	0	0	0	175	95	114	103	100	12	17	46	37	55	27	17
67	166	B	D	Y	0	0	0	4	182	99	121	102	95	18	20	40	33	52	25	20
68	175a	B	D	M	2	0	0	1	174	94	109	99	99	16	17	45	38	54	26	18
69	195	B	D	Y	0	0	0	1	170	90	106	95	96	13	18	42	35	53	24	23
70	308b	B	—	Y	—	—	—	—	*174*	91	111	98	93	15	*19*	*41*	*34*	*51*	*27*	*21*
71	305	B	D	Y	0	1	0	1	174	89	110	89	93	18	17	40	31	46	26	19
72	171	B	D	M	0	1	0	1	179	96	107	102	99	17	20	44	36	50	29	22
Schild Late Woodland:																				
73	13	9	D	O	0	0	0	1	184	85	112	93	94	20	18	42	35	52	24	20
74	17	9	D	Y	0	0	0	0	177	93	118	95	94	19	19	41	34	51	24	22
75	35	9	D	Y	0	0	—	—	*173*	85	108	94	91	20	*22*	37	33	50	29	*22*
76	7	9	D	Y	0	0	0	1	*188*	92	116	98	97	20	22	42	35	*52*	*27*	22
77	22	9	—	M	—	—	—	—	—	—	—	—	—	—	—	—	—	—	—	—
78	32	9	—	M	—	—	—	—	—	—	—	—	—	—	—	—	—	—	—	—
79	37a	9	D	Y	0	0	0	0	*176*	94	114	99	94	14	18	44	35	49	25	21
80	40	9	D	Y	0	0	0	1	182	83	109	94	89	19	16	41	34	50	26	*18*
81	9	3	D	O	0	0	0	1	171	86	105	88	90	18	17	41	36	52	24	19
82	13a	3	D	M	0	0	0	2	188	85	112	105	90	17	18	42	33	*50*	*26*	18
83	10	3	—	M	—	—	—	—	*171*	*89*	106	—	*94*	*16*	18	—	*34*	—	*25*	18
84	11	3	—	Y	—	—	—	—	*167*	86	102	96	90	13	*18*	*40*	*35*	*50*	25	*19*
85	17a	3	D	M	0	0	—	1	172	91	107	94	90	15	20	40	35	50	27	21
86	19	3	—	Y	—	—	—	—	*172*	91	110	—	91	13	*19*	*40*	—	—	*25*	—
87	21	3	D	Y	0	0	0	1	*176*	91	109	103	94	15	21	38	35	48	30	22
88	9c	4	—	Y	—	—	—	—	—	—	110	98	—	—	—	—	—	—	—	—
89	Scd	6	—	Y	—	—	—	—	*173*	83	*109*	—	91	16	*18*	*40*	*34*	—	24	—
90	24	3	—	Y	—	—	—	—	*170*	83	109	96	92	11	21	39	34	47	24	*22*
91	5	1	D	M	0	0	0	0	170	93	104	102	92	19	*18*	*40*	32	48	24	*20*
92	6b	1	—	M	—	—	—	—	—	—	—	—	—	—	—	—	—	—	—	—
93	10	1	—	O	0	0	—	—	*172*	93	108	92	95	16	19	42	35	55	25	20
94	11	1	D	O	0	0	—	—	*174*	*96*	109	99	103	*17*	19	45	33	50	31	*20*
95	13	1	D	O	0	0	0	4	176	92	110	92	93	20	21	39	35	52	28	21
96	16	1	—	Y	0	0	0	1	*176*	90	*108*	93	95	20	*18*	42	39	47	26	24
97	19	2	—	M	—	—	—	—	*174*	*90*	*109*	106	*95*	*18*	*20*	41	36	57	30	*22*
98	20a	1	—	Y	—	—	—	—	—	—	—	—	—	—	—	—	—	—	—	—
99	21	1	—	O	—	—	—	—	—	—	—	96	—	*17*	—	*42*	33	*50*	*26*	*20*
100	24	1	—	Y	0	0	0	3	*172*	—	108	—	—	—	—	—	—	—	—	—

	Measurement																				
Case	MN	BNB	BA	RL	LM	GL	ZZ	CYL	IML	XML	WMH	LCD	BCD	ASB	FRS	FRF	PAC	PAS	OCC	MDB	MLN
Schild Mississippian (cont.):																					
51	*9*	64	99	34	*105*	113	43	17	32	49	21	22	16	—	—	—	—	*23*	—	30	42
52	9	*61*	*95*	30	—	131	42	16	33	48	—	26	16	—	22	47	*110*	*24*	—	33	49
53	9	53	*97*	30	—	*126*	*44*	*18*	34	52	20	24	12	96	23	54	110	27	92	32	41
54	11	58	97	33	100	119	43	*20*	30	52	22	26	16	106	20	43	112	25	100	32	45
55	8	60	*101*	*31*	*103*	124	47	18	*31*	*50*	20	24	12	108	31	52	115	31	93	34	44
56	8	50	98	34	97	110	46	18	32	55	20	25	13	103	20	47	108	25	99	30	41
57	8	64	99	34	98	120	44	17	29	46	22	25	13	*104*	23	43	107	23	93	35	*45*
58	12	62	96	30	102	122	41	*19*	35	51	19	25	16	104	25	48	108	23	*98*	29	50
59	8	—	91	29	101	128	42	18	33	48	18	20	13	—	—	—	—	*24*	—	28	*41*
60	*9*	*60*	92	36	103	119	43	18	33	50	21	*24*	—	106	26	51	118	26	99	31	50
61	7	62	99	34	111	121	44	22	34	54	24	24	16	102	23	46	117	26	98	35	45
62	9	59	87	32	*103*	110	47	*18*	31	52	22	27	*14*	102	24	44	112	22	104	30	41
63	—	56	95	37	113	118	40	17	—	—	22	24	16	101	—	—	121	30	97	29	43
64	11	56	99	30	97	125	44	16	29	45	19	24	12	106	26	42	108	25	93	28	37
65	11	*60*	*101*	34	118	121	50	21	*32*	*51*	22	25	15	*104*	22	48	118	25	112	34	40
66	9	69	99	34	110	125	44	22	30	49	23	28	16	102	24	50	102	20	100	30	38
67	9	64	97	32	101	124	45	20	31	50	24	25	16	110	26	51	113	23	99	31	46
68	9	64	92	32	115	126	47	18	31	45	19	25	15	108	19	48	105	26	103	35	49
69	9	54	96	37	103	114	43	21	35	55	24	26	13	101	24	50	105	22	100	36	43
70	*9*	68	*97*	30	*103*	*126*	*45*	17	29	50	23	*25*	—	—	24	46	*107*	*22*	—	33	44
71	8	57	92	32	102	132	45	18	29	45	19	25	15	95	25	44	111	26	99	30	43
72	11	74	103	34	113	128	47	21	33	46	20	25	17	105	21	42	112	24	105	34	44
Schild Late Woodland:																					
73	7	55	91	31	101	116	41	20	*32*	*51*	19	*24*	*14*	112	25	47	116	25	97	28	44
74	8	57	96	30	107	125	45	18	*31*	*50*	24	25	13	106	25	52	105	24	94	27	50
75	13	57	90	27	106	125	44	17	30	48	22	*24*	*14*	94	22	46	102	*21*	*98*	27	35
76	10	62	*92*	31	*105*	130	43	18	32	50	24	*24*	*14*	*104*	23	52	116	22	*98*	22	37
77	—	—	*97*	—	—	—	47	—	—	—	—	*25*	—	—	—	—	—	—	—	31	41
78	—	—	*94*	28	—	*128*	—	—	—	—	—	*25*	—	—	—	—	—	—	—	27	44
79	8	63	90	32	*106*	123	45	19	32	48	22	*24*	13	*104*	24	48	112	24	102	33	45
80	8	56	*95*	30	*104*	126	45	18	28	48	18	26	16	103	23	46	104	21	100	30	47
81	6	62	*89*	26	*102*	125	41	*17*	*30*	*45*	18	24	13	*104*	21	45	102	21	*98*	25	35
82	9	61	*97*	32	*106*	128	50	21	*30*	*47*	22	*25*	16	*104*	22	44	112	21	*98*	30	41
83	10	—	88	30	*103*	124	44	21	32	44	—	26	14	—	19	47	*107*	*23*	—	29	48
84	8	54	97	30	100	125	47	*18*	30	45	21	25	—	—	22	41	*105*	*23*	—	25	44
85	8	62	*94*	32	*105*	130	*45*	17	25	41	18	*25*	*14*	104	20	49	101	20	104	26	33
86	—	*56*	*94*	35	—	126	—	*18*	—	*50*	—	*25*	—	—	23	48	—	—	—	27	47
87	7	61	*96*	34	*105*	128	*46*	18	*30*	*49*	22	24	15	*104*	23	46	107	20	94	30	35
88	—	—	*92*	—	—	—	—	—	—	—	21	*24*	—	—	*23*	—	—	—	—	25	40
89	—	*56*	*95*	28	*105*	112	*45*	17	—	*48*	—	*25*	—	—	22	51	—	—	—	*29*	*42*
90	10	58	*94*	32	*104*	*124*	*45*	*19*	30	49	22	*25*	—	—	*22*	—	*107*	*23*	—	27	43
91	*8*	64	90	32	100	127	47	18	27	47	21	28	15	103	24	45	104	22	92	27	40
92	—	—	*94*	—	—	—	—	—	—	—	—	*25*	—	—	—	—	—	—	—	28	37
93	9	64	88	33	109	127	46	18	32	*51*	22	*24*	—	—	*22*	—	*108*	*23*	—	29	36
94	*9*	63	99	29	105	127	44	20	30	48	22	*25*	13	*104*	26	46	*107*	*23*	*98*	29	37
95	8	59	107	31	101	131	45	16	30	48	21	21	16	106	25	48	115	25	96	29	45
96	8	50	*88*	31	*101*	124	40	20	*32*	*53*	20	*24*	—	—	24	43	104	20	—	25	45
97	10	62	*96*	35	—	*121*	*47*	*18*	32	*51*	28	27	14	—	*23*	—	*108*	*23*	—	31	49
98	—	—	*92*	—	—	—	—	—	—	—	—	*24*	—	—	—	—	—	—	—	25	42
99	*9*	59	—	33	*104*	127	44	*18*	30	51	23	—	—	—	—	—	—	*23*	—	—	—
100	—	—	*95*	—	—	—	—	—	—	—	—	*25*	—	103	25	47	110	26	—	29	42

Case	Bur. no.	Mound/ knoll	Analytical status	Age	Deformation score: Frontal	Bifrontal	Occipital	Lambdoid	Measurement: L	MF	FC	MFB	IOB	SIOB	AIB	LOBM	LOH	NH	NB	DC
Schild Late Woodland (cont.):																				
101	31j	1	D	O	0	0	0	2	*177*	*91*	105	99	96	19	22	42	35	55	29	23
102	38	1	—	O	—	—	—	—	*173*	*90*	*109*	106	94	*17*	17	40	*35*	53	25	17
103	40	1	—	M	—	—	—	—	—	—	—	—	—	—	—	—	—	—	—	—
104	46b	1	—	O	0	0	0	1	179	87	109	98	87	15	*18*	*39*	35	53	*25*	*20*
105	48	1	—	O	—	—	—	—	—	—	—	—	—	*16*	17	—	—	—	24	20
106	14a	1	—	O	0	0	1	0	183	94	126	93	99	16	21	42	36	55	26	*22*
107	37a	1	—	M	—	—	—	—	—	—	—	102	—	*18*	—	*42*	*35*	—	32	*23*
108	27a	2	—	M	—	—	—	—	—	—	114	—	—	—	—	—	—	—	—	—
109	34a	3	—	M	—	—	—	—	*179*	—	—	—	—	—	—	—	—	—	—	—
110	28	3	D	Y	—	—	—	—	*173*	93	*110*	99	92	15	19	39	32	48	27	20
111	8a	4	D	Y	0	0	0	0	*173*	87	110	95	92	15	*17*	43	31	49	25	*18*
112	1	5	D	Y	0	0	0	0	170	90	109	91	88	16	19	39	33	52	24	19
113	71	1	—	M	—	—	—	—	*173*	89	*108*	92	85	16	*16*	40	35	52	25	*18*
114	74	1	D	Y	0	0	0	2	174	91	107	96	93	16	18	40	35	48	25	20
115	28	1	D	Y	—	—	—	—	*179*	85	115	97	89	19	19	40	35	51	24	21
116	7a	2	—	O	0	0	0	0	—	—	—	—	—	—	—	—	—	—	—	—
117	18	2	—	M	—	—	—	—	*172*	83	104	94	90	19	18	39	*34*	49	25	*19*
118	47b	1	—	Y	—	—	—	—	—	—	—	94	—	*16*	—	—	*34*	*50*	23	—
119	30	2	—	M	—	—	—	—	—	—	—	—	—	—	—	—	—	—	—	—
120	65	1	—	M	—	—	—	—	*173*	89	*108*	—	93	*17*	*19*	*41*	—	—	*25*	—
121	16c	2	—	Y	—	—	—	—	*174*	91	*109*	97	95	*17*	*20*	*41*	*34*	—	27	—
122	16e	2	—	Y	—	—	—	—	—	—	—	99	—	*17*	—	*41*	—	—	*26*	*21*
123	1c	7	—	Y	—	—	—	—	—	—	—	—	—	—	—	—	—	—	—	—
Koster Late Woodland:																				
124	1	1	—	M	0	0	—	—	*172*	*87*	107	99	90	*16*	*19*	39	33	47	26	*21*
125	3	1	D	Y	0	0	—	—	*177*	88	113	96	91	16	19	39	34	49	27	20
126	14	1	D	Y	0	0	—	—	*174*	91	109	100	93	17	19	42	36	51	*26*	21
127	20	1	D	M	0	1	0	3	180	84	114	*99*	90	19	*18*	*40*	*35*	—	*25*	24
128	23a	1	D	Y	0	0	0	1	171	89	108	92	95	19	21	39	30	49	27	22
129	29	1	D	M	0	0	—	—	*178*	87	111	92	90	16	*17*	43	32	49	28	*18*
130	8	2	—	M	0	0	0	2	*173*	89	*108*	93	93	*17*	*20*	*41*	*34*	*51*	28	*21*
131	11	2	D	M	0	0	0	1	174	92	114	89	93	17	20	39	35	49	*25*	21
132	5	3	—	Y	—	—	—	—	*174*	89	109	—	94	18	*19*	*41*	—	—	*26*	20
133	7	3	—	Y	—	—	—	—	*173*	*90*	*109*	96	*94*	*16*	20	40	—	—	*25*	20
134	15	3	D	Y	0	0	—	—	*181*	95	117	101	100	21	18	43	35	57	25	12
135	2	4	D	Y	0	0	0	2	173	90	99	94	91	14	18	39	33	50	24	18
136	6	4	D	O	0	0	0	3	186	88	114	97	95	18	23	40	33	50	27	23
137	7	4	—	Y	0	0	0	2	181	—	111	—	—	—	—	—	—	—	—	—
138	8a	4	D	O	0	0	0	2	166	85	101	96	93	14	17	40	31	48	24	17
139	15	4	D	Y	—	—	0	1	*168*	*90*	106	96	*94*	*17*	19	41	35	52	24	18
140	16	4	D	M	0	1	0	4	175	86	112	95	94	14	*20*	38	34	52	27	*21*
141	20	4	—	M	0	0	—	—	*176*	98	109	93	100	20	*20*	43	37	52	26	—
142	21	4	D	O	0	0	0	4	169	87	103	100	96	14	22	42	29	47	28	22
143	22	4	D	O	0	0	0	2	177	81	110	94	93	16	21	41	33	50	24	22
144	25c	4	D	Y	0	0	0	2	167	84	98	85	92	15	*19*	*40*	*34*	*50*	26	*21*
145	25e	4	—	O	2	1	2	4	160	86	107	—	96	15	20	*42*	—	—	*26*	21
146	27b	4	—	Y	0	0	—	—	—	—	—	—	—	—	—	—	*35*	—	—	—
147	28	4	D	O	1	0	3	4	156	91	104	87	93	14	21	39	34	54	23	20
148	2	5	D	Y	0	0	0	1	175	88	109	91	90	15	16	40	33	53	23	16
149	4	5	D	Y	0	0	0	0	*171*	94	106	94	94	22	20	41	35	55	24	28
150	14	5	D	O	0	0	—	—	*172*	94	107	99	103	17	19	42	*35*	54	28	18

	Measurement																				
Case	MN	BNB	BA	RL	LM	GL	ZZ	CYL	IML	XML	WMH	LCD	BCD	ASB	FRS	FRF	PAC	PAS	OCC	MDB	MLN
Schild Late Woodland (cont.):																					
101	13	59	*97*	34	*105*	133	*45*	17	28	49	22	26	14	99	19	51	107	20	*98*	32	41
102	8	58	95	31	—	126	47	19	—	*50*	23	25	14	—	*22*	—	—	—	102	28	43
103	—	—	*94*	—	—	—	—	—	—	—	—	*25*	—	—	—	—	—	—	—	28	43
104	*9*	*54*	*95*	32	*104*	129	*45*	*18*	32	50	25	*25*	—	—	22	52	113	23	—	29	39
105	7	—	—	30	—	123	—	—	31	46	—	—	—	—	—	—	—	*23*	—	—	—
106	10	62	*99*	*33*	*109*	—	*45*	*19*	*34*	*51*	*21*	*25*	—	116	30	55	116	21	108	30	45
107	*10*	67	*98*	*33*	*108*	*127*	*46*	*19*	30	47	25	*25*	—	—	—	—	—	*23*	—	32	*43*
108	—	—	—	—	—	—	—	—	—	—	—	—	—	—	*24*	—	—	—	—	—	—
109	—	—	90	28	101	125	40	18	—	—	19	*24*	—	—	—	—	113	23	92	28	38
110	13	53	89	36	104	118	44	20	29	52	25	*24*	*14*	*104*	*22*	*48*	*107*	*22*	*98*	27	32
111	7	50	100	32	101	125	43	20	29	52	24	26	15	*104*	*22*	*48*	*107*	*22*	*98*	30	47
112	10	51	89	33	100	124	43	16	30	50	20	23	14	98	24	51	104	*22*	91	24	45
113	9	51	*95*	28	*105*	140	*44*	15	—	*47*	21	*25*	—	—	*23*	—	—	—	—	29	40
114	8	51	100	30	105	140	47	17	29	51	22	25	13	108	24	47	115	*26*	95	30	34
115	7	56	97	30	97	115	44	17	31	51	20	24	15	*104*	23	55	*110*	*23*	*98*	27	42
116	—	—	—	—	—	—	—	—	—	—	—	—	—	—	—	—	—	—	—	—	49
117	10	55	*96*	25	*104*	*131*	*45*	20	33	50	20	*24*	15	—	26	48	*107*	*24*	—	31	40
118	—	54	—	30	*105*	122	45	18	—	—	22	—	—	—	—	—	—	—	—	—	—
119	—	—	*94*	—	—	—	—	—	—	—	—	*25*	15	—	—	—	—	—	—	27	38
120	—	*57*	*94*	—	—	—	—	*18*	—	—	—	*25*	—	—	*22*	—	107	*23*	—	27	45
121	—	60	*96*	—	*101*	—	*45*	*18*	—	—	20	*25*	—	—	*23*	—	—	—	—	*30*	*42*
122	*9*	61	—	30	—	*126*	*45*	*19*	30	48	21	—	—	—	—	—	—	*23*	—	—	—
123	—	—	*97*	31	—	*125*	45	—	32	*51*	23	*25*	—	—	—	—	—	*23*	—	32	44
Koster Late Woodland:																					
124	9	61	*94*	*32*	*101*	*125*	*45*	18	32	46	22	*24*	—	—	21	44	*107*	*23*	—	29	43
125	6	55	104	30	100	123	44	16	24	44	19	*26*	14	*104*	25	53	113	*25*	94	28	40
126	10	63	*100*	34	—	120	51	18	34	52	21	*25*	*14*	*104*	22	47	*109*	*24*	*98*	32	43
127	9	*55*	100	31	118	133	47	18	30	50	26	26	15	*104*	22	54	100	22	93	28	40
128	10	60	104	32	101	129	43	19	34	50	20	*26*	13	102	22	47	101	21	*98*	36	43
129	9	57	*94*	30	104	130	42	17	30	50	22	26	11	*104*	23	49	114	24	*98*	29	40
130	*10*	62	*95*	31	*103*	*125*	45	*18*	*32*	*48*	24	*25*	—	98	*22*	—	106	22	—	28	47
131	9	*53*	94	29	101	123	44	16	35	52	*21*	23	13	102	24	53	106	22	109	27	39
132	—	*58*	*96*	—	—	—	—	*18*	—	—	—	*25*	—	—	27	48	—	—	—	*30*	*42*
133	9	54	*96*	34	—	*122*	47	*19*	31	50	25	24	14	104	*22*	—	*107*	*23*	—	29	34
134	10	60	116	32	107	111	42	21	33	56	26	*27*	*14*	*104*	22	55	*111*	*24*	*98*	36	49
135	9	55	100	29	108	123	46	21	30	47	21	25	14	99	19	42	112	25	105	31	42
136	10	57	91	31	112	132	47	20	34	52	25	*24*	*14*	105	21	50	106	19	*98*	32	37
137	11	—	*96*	—	—	—	—	—	—	—	—	30	15	102	24	48	112	22	—	31	43
138	8	56	87	34	103	121	42	19	27	47	23	23	13	95	22	44	103	20	99	27	43
139	10	56	90	32	104	114	43	20	30	52	22	25	14	*104*	*21*	*48*	*102*	22	96	28	38
140	*10*	62	*94*	30	*106*	140	*45*	18	*32*	*48*	20	26	13	113	24	49	112	23	101	25	42
141	—	57	*98*	33	*103*	*123*	*45*	*19*	—	*53*	21	*25*	—	—	*22*	—	—	—	—	35	50
142	8	59	91	35	102	123	45	21	33	53	21	21	13	111	22	48	114	*25*	95	33	36
143	9	57	98	30	107	134	45	16	28	45	20	25	14	102	21	49	106	21	91	26	40
144	*9*	52	90	36	99	113	43	18	*32*	*52*	*20*	22	15	102	20	36	105	23	89	29	42
145	8	*59*	94	31	95	115	42	19	—	*50*	—	24	13	104	17	59	105	24	96	31	40
146	—	—	107	—	*110*	128	50	18	—	—	—	*26*	—	—	—	—	—	—	—	30	48
147	*10*	52	87	32	98	122	41	19	36	53	20	*24*	*14*	106	17	47	98	22	88	27	32
148	8	47	104	33	103	126	45	15	30	55	23	24	14	107	27	47	108	23	97	31	46
149	12	59	87	33	98	116	43	17	31	50	24	20	13	*104*	23	45	98	20	*98*	29	44
150	8	59	100	34	104	126	46	20	35	55	24	24	14	*104*	21	50	*109*	*24*	*98*	35	50

TABLE 48 (cont.)

Case	Bur. no.	Mound/ knoll	Analytical status	Age	Deformation score: Frontal	Bifrontal	Occipital	Lambdoid	Measurement: L	MF	FC	MFB	IOB	SIOB	AIB	LOBM	LOH	NH	NB	DC
Koster Late Woodland (cont.):																				
151	16	5	D	Y	0	1	0	0	183	*91*	*111*	102	95	23	20	45	35	50	27	*21*
152	18	5	D	M	0	0	—	—	*176*	90	103	93	95	15	*19*	42	34	50	*24*	*20*
153	28	5	D	M	0	1	0	0	179	94	104	90	99	21	21	42	35	52	27	22
154	31	5	D	M	0	1	0	1	182	93	115	96	102	18	21	44	36	54	*27*	24
155	42	5	D	O	—	—	0	0	173	89	106	97	93	16	21	40	31	48	26	20
156	50a	5	—	O	—	—	—	—	—	—	—	—	—	—	—	—	—	—	—	—
157	51a	5	—	O	0	0	—	—	*172*	87	106	*95*	91	17	20	*40*	*34*	—	*25*	22
158	56	5	D	M	0	0	—	—	*177*	92	107	90	96	16	17	41	33	49	23	17
159	10c	6	D	M	0	0	2	4	175	88	110	94	92	16	20	39	34	*52*	29	21
160	1c	Kn1	—	Y	0	2	—	—	*176*	*91*	112	103	*96*	*17*	*20*	42	36	53	26	—
161	5	Kn1	—	O	0	0	—	—	*167*	98	108	*95*	98	16	*18*	*42*	—	—	*26*	*20*
162	11	Kn1	D	M	0	0	0	1	165	*91*	*110*	90	96	15	19	43	32	47	*26*	*20*
163	1	Kn2	—	Y	—	—	0	1	*175*	—	—	—	—	—	—	—	—	—	—	—
164	5a	Kn4	D	Y	0	1	0	2	169	88	104	91	92	17	16	40	37	50	23	20
165	6d	Kn5	D	Y	0	0	0	0	175	92	113	108	99	19	15	47	34	53	25	18
166	?	Kn6	D	M	0	2	—	—	161	87	103	96	92	*16*	*17*	40	32	46	24	17
167	4g	Kn7	D	Y	0	0	0	1	183	99	110	99	99	16	23	42	34	50	30	24
168	5	Kn7	D	M	0	0	0	0	174	93	107	102	97	20	20	43	36	55	26	21
169	6b	Kn8	D	M	0	0	0	3	170	89	104	100	92	16	18	40	35	49	25	19
170	26a	4	—	Y	0	1	—	—	*173*	85	109	—	94	16	*19*	*41*	—	—	*26*	—
171	4e	Kn7	D	M	0	0	0	3	174	91	110	88	98	15	20	41	34	*49*	*25*	23
172	4f	Kn7	D	O	0	0	1	2	166	91	110	*95*	93	19	*18*	43	—	—	*25*	*19*
Yokem Mississippian:																				
173	2	1	D	M	0	0	2	0	168	89	110	99	96	*17*	21	42	35	50	25	20
174	5	1	D	M	0	0	0	2	174	88	110	87	92	16	17	41	33	51	23	16
175	10	1	D	Y	0	0	0	3	172	95	114	99	96	19	21	42	33	53	24	22
176	14	1	D	Y	0	0	0	1	170	91	108	98	94	18	18	41	35	50	24	19
177	19	1	—	M	0	0	—	—	*178*	*87*	110	88	90	23	*18*	42	33	*49*	*25*	—
178	26	1	—	M	—	—	—	—	—	—	—	—	—	—	—	—	*34*	*51*	—	—
179	44	1	D	M	0	0	0	0	172	91	102	100	98	16	19	41	34	47	27	21
180	49	1	D	M	0	0	0	2	170	90	112	93	94	15	18	40	32	48	24	20
181	53	1	D	O	0	0	0	2	172	94	104	98	100	17	24	40	36	50	25	*24*
182	55	1	D	O	0	0	0	0	173	*92*	118	96	97	*18*	18	43	34	51	25	21
183	57	1	D	Y	1	0	0	4	178	98	113	103	101	18	23	42	35	*52*	*27*	23
184	63	1	D	Y	0	2	0	4	175	84	114	96	96	17	20	41	36	49	23	20
185	65	1	D	O	1	0	0	1	172	88	107	99	98	18	19	42	36	53	27	21
186	68	1	D	M	0	0	0	0	175	95	108	98	95	14	20	42	35	52	24	22
187	3	1	D	O	2	2	2	2	161	95	109	93	99	17	19	45	36	51	26	*20*
188	9	1	D	O	0	0	0	1	180	94	109	87	95	16	17	42	34	*50*	*25*	20
189	28	1	D	O	0	0	0	1	176	97	106	102	97	17	21	41	34	54	25	22
190	5	2	D	M	0	0	0	1	178	90	112	100	98	14	20	44	35	55	28	20
191	7	2	D	O	0	0	0	1	*175*	92	110	97	97	18	20	43	33	48	25	20
192	9a	2	D	Y	0	0	0	3	*177*	97	112	94	*91*	15	*18*	38	34	51	22	*19*
193	9b	2	D	M	0	0	0	1	173	95	113	95	95	17	20	40	33	46	25	19
194	10	2	—	Y	—	—	—	—	—	—	—	—	—	—	—	—	—	—	—	—
195	11	2	—	M	—	—	—	—	—	—	—	—	—	—	—	—	—	—	29	—
196	12	2	—	Y	—	—	—	—	—	95	*111*	—	*97*	—	—	—	—	—	—	—
197	17	2	—	Y	—	—	0	3	*174*	—	—	106	—	*18*	—	*42*	—	—	*27*	*21*
198	19	2	D	O	0	0	0	1	179	99	113	100	102	18	22	44	36	52	26	22
199	115	3	D	M	0	0	0	1	171	85	107	92	89	18	20	38	34	50	26	21

	Measurement																				
Case	MN	BNB	BA	RL	LM	GL	ZZ	CYL	IML	XML	WMH	LCD	BCD	ASB	FRS	FRF	PAC	PAS	OCC	MDB	MLN
Koster Late Woodland (cont.)																					
151	9	65	105	36	112	130	48	20	30	51	22	25	15	109	22	48	111	20	95	31	38
152	9	48	93	30	105	126	43	15	32	52	20	24	14	96	25	44	106	17	98	31	43
153	9	64	90	30	104	125	44	18	35	51	16	26	14	102	21	42	106	24	108	33	36
154	9	68	97	28	108	133	42	21	35	48	20	21	12	109	25	48	104	20	106	29	42
155	12	53	96	31	103	112	46	20	28	50	24	25	15	103	21	48	105	22	100	29	38
156	—	—	93	33	—	135	42	18	—	—	—	24	—	—	—	—	—	—	—	—	—
157	9	56	95	31	105	128	44	18	32	51	21	25	—	—	20	48	107	23	93	33	38
158	6	54	94	33	105	123	42	18	33	53	22	25	14	100	22	48	118	27	98	30	47
159	9	62	96	30	—	126	44	19	30	49	25	25	14	104	25	50	110	26	98	30	47
160	—	59	97	33	105	123	46	19	—	51	23	25	—	—	21	40	—	—	—	31	43
161	6	61	91	28	—	128	42	17	24	42	19	26	14	—	25	48	96	19	—	24	38
162	10	64	99	32	103	133	43	18	30	49	22	26	17	100	23	47	102	21	91	35	42
163	—	—	—	31	—	—	47	20	28	43	20	26	13	98	—	—	111	25	100	—	36
164	9	57	93	32	103	125	44	19	31	48	22	28	14	106	21	44	110	25	98	30	45
165	6	66	99	28	107	126	48	20	30	51	22	25	13	107	26	47	105	23	94	33	45
166	6	51	92	31	103	124	44	19	27	50	20	24	14	104	20	44	107	24	98	28	32
167	14	66	90	29	97	128	45	20	36	51	21	24	14	112	20	51	115	25	98	27	41
168	9	59	95	32	104	122	45	19	30	52	23	25	15	105	21	45	108	22	99	31	47
169	8	57	88	30	105	126	46	18	30	52	21	28	13	102	23	43	103	21	94	33	43
170	—	58	93	—	—	—	—	18	—	—	—	23	—	—	23	47	—	—	—	26	48
171	5	53	94	34	103	115	39	20	32	50	19	27	15	103	20	52	108	24	104	30	39
172	9	57	103	34	100	118	43	19	28	48	21	26	12	108	23	48	103	25	94	33	53
Yokem Mississippian:																					
173	10	62	97	32	100	122	44	21	28	46	25	25	13	101	21	47	106	24	107	32	43
174	8	52	104	33	116	128	48	19	34	52	18	25	12	102	24	53	105	20	101	27	38
175	10	60	99	32	110	142	44	18	32	48	22	25	14	102	24	54	105	24	101	28	41
176	10	53	98	34	108	119	45	20	31	54	20	25	14	106	21	44	106	21	100	28	38
177	—	56	97	30	107	125	43	17	—	48	20	25	—	—	19	49	—	—	—	29	41
178	—	—	96	37	105	119	47	—	31	50	22	25	—	—	—	—	—	23	—	28	42
179	9	56	98	30	100	122	47	20	32	52	21	28	15	104	21	44	108	20	98	30	43
180	8	50	95	35	102	113	47	19	33	52	21	25	14	100	23	48	119	30	92	28	46
181	12	67	95	30	102	127	46	19	29	44	19	25	14	106	21	53	112	21	100	29	40
182	10	66	86	30	101	123	41	18	31	48	22	27	14	103	26	51	100	20	98	32	46
183	12	60	94	36	106	114	47	20	36	58	24	29	15	108	20	53	111	25	102	32	47
184	9	54	102	35	101	119	47	20	33	56	22	26	14	109	24	54	108	22	102	31	41
185	10	66	100	30	109	125	48	20	36	49	23	27	14	99	17	45	108	24	98	37	46
186	9	56	95	32	109	125	46	18	33	54	20	25	15	104	23	47	110	22	98	29	40
187	9	60	101	31	104	132	44	19	32	51	21	27	12	104	20	48	100	25	90	31	36
188	10	56	95	32	105	121	42	20	36	51	20	26	13	112	24	47	107	19	107	27	48
189	11	54	99	34	107	127	48	21	32	55	22	28	13	104	21	51	102	18	105	32	48
190	9	62	96	30	103	131	40	18	30	50	21	23	14	107	24	52	114	25	97	26	41
191	7	70	90	31	105	130	43	17	31	43	21	24	16	102	24	47	104	20	98	30	50
192	8	56	92	35	105	116	46	19	30	50	22	19	15	104	23	48	107	20	93	28	41
193	10	57	93	32	106	119	46	20	30	50	20	18	13	101	28	53	110	25	99	30	46
194	—	—	98	40	—	125	46	23	37	52	23	25	—	—	—	—	—	25	—	34	47
195	—	—	96	35	—	121	—	17	—	—	21	25	—	—	—	—	—	—	—	30	35
196	—	—	106	32	106	120	47	19	—	—	—	26	—	108	23	—	—	—	—	33	43
197	10	64	98	37	105	116	50	22	33	50	21	25	13	106	—	—	109	24	99	31	43
198	12	64	97	36	106	124	47	20	31	51	22	23	12	104	24	49	107	23	97	31	46
199	11	56	99	29	97	127	44	19	30	50	19	25	13	106	24	50	101	21	91	27	38

Case	Bur. no.	Mound/ knoll	Analytical status	Age	Deformation score: Frontal	Bifrontal	Occipital	Lambdoid	Measurement: L	MF	FC	MFB	IOB	SIOB	AIB	LOBM	LOH	NH	NB	DC
Yokem Mississippian (cont.):																				
200	6	1	D	O	0	0	0	2	172	95	109	94	95	17	18	42	32	50	26	18
201	15	1	D	Y	0	0	0	4	177	88	110	103	99	19	21	42	34	50	27	23
202	104	3	D	M	0	0	0	2	177	95	110	95	100	20	23	41	36	53	25	23
Yokem Late Woodland:																				
203	2	3	—	Y	—	—	—	—	—	—	—	—	—	—	—	—	*34*	*50*	24	*20*
204	3	3	D	M	0	2	0	1	171	91	100	99	92	18	22	39	33	49	25	26
205	7	3	D	O	0	0	1	0	179	88	110	96	91	18	18	39	31	50	28	20
206	9	3	D	O	0	0	0	2	181	90	115	106	100	19	21	43	38	55	31	23
207	11	3	D	M	0	0	1	0	178	97	113	91	98	19	*20*	43	34	47	29	*21*
208	12a	3	D	Y	0	0	0	0	169	87	108	93	96	14	20	39	35	52	24	21
209	15	3	D	M	0	0	0	0	174	86	110	101	94	17	17	41	32	50	26	20
210	20c	3	—	Y	0	0	—	—	*174*	98	110	100	97	12	*21*	*42*	*35*	*51*	31	*23*
211	23a	3	D	M	0	0	0	3	184	91	115	92	94	*16*	*19*	41	35	50	24	*20*
212	23b	3	—	Y	0	0	—	—	*176*	93	113	98	96	16	20	42	34	48	26	21
213	24a	3	D	O	0	0	3	0	173	99	117	97	103	21	21	42	38	54	25	*22*
214	24e	3	—	O	0	0	—	—	*174*	92	110	100	93	16	*17*	42	33	53	24	17
215	36b	3	D	O	0	0	0	2	175	91	106	101	93	19	*20*	38	33	*50*	25	*21*
216	48	3	—	O	—	—	—	—	—	—	—	98	—	*18*	—	*42*	*34*	*51*	22	*19*
217	57	3	—	Y	0	0	0	2	*170*	—	107	—	—	—	—	—	—	—	—	—
218	84	3	—	M	—	—	—	—	*173*	—	114	97	—	—	—	*41*	*34*	*50*	—	18
219	106	3	D	M	0	0	0	1	172	94	113	101	94	17	21	39	34	52	28	23
220	107	3	D	M	0	0	0	2	183	*90*	114	92	*94*	*16*	20	40	34	51	26	21
221	1	4	D	M	0	0	0	0	164	83	101	96	92	15	18	40	33	51	25	22
222	7	4	D	Y	0	0	0	3	167	90	106	91	91	18	18	39	31	46	25	21
223	11	4	D	Y	0	0	0	1	170	90	102	95	92	16	18	40	34	49	25	21
224	14	4	D	Y	0	0	0	2	173	94	114	98	96	16	20	41	34	52	25	20
225	16	4	D	O	0	0	0	0	*175*	93	113	105	98	14	22	41	31	51	25	23
226	17	4	D	Y	0	0	0	0	165	89	106	101	98	20	20	41	36	50	25	21
227	18a	4	D	M	0	0	0	2	164	82	105	86	85	14	17	38	33	48	21	18
228	18b	4	—	M	0	0	—	—	*174*	89	110	94	93	17	20	38	34	52	25	21
229	31	4	D	Y	0	0	0	3	168	92	111	100	95	18	23	40	29	46	25	24
230	5	5	—	M	—	—	—	—	—	—	—	—	—	—	—	—	*35*	—	22	—
231	7	5	D	O	0	0	—	0	174	91	108	100	99	12	20	42	31	48	29	22
232	10	5	—	M	0	0	—	—	*177*	*92*	106	112	*97*	*17*	*18*	43	34	51	*27*	*20*
233	11	5	D	M	0	0	0	2	172	86	103	95	90	17	23	37	34	50	30	23
234	14	5	D	Y	0	0	0	1	167	94	108	93	91	17	19	38	38	50	26	*20*
235	15b	5	D	M	0	0	0	2	174	96	110	104	100	20	22	42	37	52	26	24
236	18	5	—	M	—	—	0	1	*177*	*94*	*110*	86	*100*	*16*	*20*	45	33	50	25	*20*
237	21	5	D	Y	0	0	0	0	171	*87*	105	88	*90*	*17*	19	38	30	42	24	19
238	25	5	—	O	0	0	—	—	*174*	91	104	94	95	23	18	42	33	48	26	19
239	50	5	—	O	0	0	—	—	*170*	90	105	93	*95*	*15*	22	*40*	*34*	51	23	*23*
240	59	5	—	Y	0	0	0	2	*177*	*94*	*110*	95	100	*18*	21	41	*35*	*50*	27	*22*
241	1	8	D	M	0	0	0	1	180	*90*	108	102	*93*	*18*	18	41	34	48	25	20
242	93	3	—	M	0	0	0	3	175	90	109	—	91	18	*19*	*40*	—	—	*25*	—
Klunk Late Woodland:																				
243	8	8	D	Y	0	0	0	3	175	87	106	94	92	16	19	40	34	52	28	21
244	9	8	D	Y	0	0	0	4	176	91	108	93	95	16	18	41	32	48	24	19
245	12	8	D	Y	0	0	0	0	172	99	104	94	100	19	20	42	32	51	25	22
246	14	8	D	O	0	0	0	1	175	87	107	98	94	13	18	40	33	46	25	21

									Measurement												
Case	MN	BNB	BA	RL	LM	G*L*	ZZ	CYL	IML	XML	WMH	LCD	BCD	ASB	FRS	FRF	PAC	PAS	OCC	MDB	MLN
Yokem Mississippian (cont.)																					
200	8	56	93	34	107	118	47	19	32	51	20	25	12	103	23	46	105	22	102	37	44
201	10	68	102	34	106	114	53	24	34	51	23	25	13	100	21	50	112	25	97	31	43
202	11	57	96	33	107	121	48	19	35	54	24	26	14	105	22	49	108	23	98	37	44
Yokem Late Woodland:																					
203	*9*	—	95	28	105	128	43	16	31	48	20	24	13	—	—	—	—	*23*	—	37	40
204	11	58	86	35	103	118	43	18	34	51	22	23	15	96	24	41	108	23	88	26	37
205	9	54	*93*	33	106	127	43	*18*	28	50	25	*24*	13	102	24	46	116	29	95	28	43
206	11	68	101	34	110	125	45	23	34	54	24	27	15	104	24	50	114	25	100	*32*	40
207	11	60	*96*	33	*103*	123	45	18	34	52	20	*25*	*14*	*104*	23	51	113	26	*98*	28	47
208	9	48	100	30	110	128	46	21	36	54	22	29	12	101	24	46	109	24	98	33	46
209	7	60	91	33	109	122	43	20	28	49	26	23	15	106	25	46	97	16	98	32	35
210	*10*	56	*95*	37	*107*	126	47	16	32	52	23	25	12	110	29	43	116	*26*	—	30	42
211	*9*	52	100	30	106	132	42	17	32	52	21	24	14	107	26	50	112	25	99	31	41
212	10	55	*97*	*33*	*102*	*120*	*46*	*19*	31	54	25	20	14	—	24	54	*109*	*23*	—	28	44
213	11	67	116	32	105	123	46	20	36	56	25	29	16	115	21	55	112	31	97	36	52
214	7	55	*97*	33	*105*	*123*	48	*18*	—	51	22	*25*	—	—	18	49	—	—	—	29	47
215	9	68	*94*	34	*107*	*122*	42	*18*	28	45	22	*25*	14	97	24	45	105	20	96	33	40
216	*8*	64	—	31	*105*	*125*	45	*19*	31	50	*22*	—	—	—	—	—	—	*23*	—	—	—
217	—	—	*95*	*32*	—	—	—	—	30	51	23	26	14	104	*22*	—	102	*21*	94	29	40
218	6	*63*	84	29	100	127	41	16	31	46	20	*23*	—	104	*25*	—	107	*23*	—	27	39
219	10	60	97	28	107	122	48	19	30	50	24	23	13	107	25	51	107	23	97	30	39
220	11	57	*98*	33	100	125	*44*	19	33	49	20	*25*	*14*	*104*	25	52	113	22	*98*	32	47
221	7	54	87	32	106	118	43	20	29	48	21	25	12	103	19	47	99	22	106	28	40
222	8	51	92	36	100	112	44	19	31	50	23	26	12	106	20	47	102	22	100	33	44
223	9	63	96	33	101	127	42	19	28	46	25	23	12	100	21	46	105	21	*98*	30	*42*
224	8	62	96	33	107	124	43	19	31	48	24	24	13	105	26	50	113	23	92	33	43
225	10	61	98	31	105	120	48	20	*31*	50	26	22	13	*104*	25	46	106	20	100	35	44
226	9	64	100	33	105	127	50	22	31	48	22	29	13	106	21	46	101	20	101	31	40
227	9	46	98	32	95	125	45	18	29	48	23	26	13	106	22	46	101	23	101	29	45
228	9	50	*96*	*32*	*105*	*125*	*44*	*18*	30	51	21	*25*	—	—	22	49	*107*	*23*	—	*30*	*42*
229	9	63	106	32	108	131	48	20	30	49	24	26	13	103	26	54	110	27	94	36	42
230	—	—	—	31	*110*	122	43	—	—	—	—	—	—	—	—	—	—	—	—	—	—
231	8	60	*97*	*33*	98	111	43	20	32	54	22	23	13	*104*	23	52	103	19	*98*	31	43
232	6	64	*95*	36	*105*	*120*	*47*	*19*	26	48	24	23	13	—	19	45	107	19	—	29	48
233	12	57	86	28	99	125	42	17	30	46	20	*24*	*14*	*104*	24	50	110	24	*98*	30	45
234	*9*	59	92	30	100	125	48	18	30	46	18	22	13	*104*	25	52	110	26	95	28	40
235	14	67	99	34	101	116	50	20	33	49	24	*25*	*14*	110	22	50	111	24	*98*	30	42
236	9	48	*94*	29	107	126	42	19	34	54	22	26	14	—	*23*	—	109	21	—	30	43
237	9	60	*100*	32	94	119	46	16	32	50	20	*25*	*14*	*104*	21	42	111	25	97	41	41
238	10	68	*96*	—	*103*	—	—	19	—	—	*21*	*25*	—	—	18	45	—	—	—	*30*	*42*
239	9	51	97	32	103	121	46	14	29	49	20	*25*	—	—	20	45	*105*	*22*	105	29	42
240	*10*	66	100	34	*105*	*122*	46	*19*	32	50	20	*25*	*14*	104	*23*	—	112	24	—	35	45
241	7	62	*97*	35	110	132	43	*19*	34	53	23	27	14	98	23	50	111	24	99	32	45
242	—	*56*	*93*	29	104	135	44	18	—	48	—	*24*	—	—	*23*	—	108	24	—	26	37
Klunk Late Woodland:																					
243	8	61	98	31	102	123	48	17	*29*	*48*	20	24	16	99	24	49	106	22	98	32	39
244	9	51	99	34	107	126	46	20	33	52	22	20	18	98	23	53	115	27	93	32	47
245	11	62	99	34	104	116	47	20	36	53	22	21	14	106	27	43	115	26	94	34	50
246	6	61	101	32	103	128	45	20	29	47	20	25	16	103	26	48	103	20	93	30	41

Case	Bur. no.	Mound/ knoll	Analytical status	Age	Deformation score				Measurement											
					Frontal	Bifrontal	Occipital	Lambdoid	L	MF	FC	MFB	IOB	SIOB	AIB	LOBM	LOH	NH	NB	DC
Klunk Late Woodland (cont.):																				
247	20	8	D	M	0	0	0	1	171	80	105	91	91	18	20	40	31	48	25	22
248	21	8	D	M	0	0	0	1	175	88	107	91	91	15	17	39	31	46	25	21
249	23	8	D	M	0	0	0	1	177	87	114	91	90	16	16	38	32	50	26	26
250	24	8	D	M	0	0	0	1	172	90	104	92	94	12	17	39	34	47	24	20
251	27	8	D	Y	0	1	0	1	175	88	106	99	96	19	20	44	33	52	28	23
252	28	8	D	M	0	0	0	4	172	94	104	94	90	*17*	17	40	33	48	25	20
253	29	8	D	O	0	0	0	4	172	87	108	91	92	19	19	41	34	50	26	20
254	31	8	D	Y	0	3	0	1	177	96	104	97	97	18	19	42	33	48	22	19
Ledders Late Woodland:[a]																				
255	10	1	D	Y					169	93	112	94	91	14	14	40	36	50	25	17
256	53	1	D	Y					*176*	88	112	98	99	21	21	41	39	54	28	22
257	63	1	D	M					173	94	106	*99*	95	17	20	40	34	*52*	23	22
258	79	1	D	Y					173	89	111	94	86	*17*	*18*	38	*32*	45	26	*20*
259	93	1	D	M					*173*	*91*	109	102	95	16	17	43	34	50	22	19
260	116	1	D	Y					175	88	105	94	94	19	20	40	31	47	23	21
261	121	1	D	O					*178*	*87*	109	99	90	*16*	20	41	35	50	27	21
262	138	1	D	Y					*177*	88	112	95	91	16	22	38	35	52	25	20
263	146	1	D	M					*169*	92	110	91	99	18	21	42	34	51	29	25
264	130	1	—	M					177	94	*110*	*101*	106	*18*	*22*	*45*	—	—	*27*	*21*
265	8	1	D	M					164	89	110	90	93	16	21	40	36	50	29	20
266	40	1	—	M					—	—	—	—	—	—	—	—	*35*	*52*	27	*21*
267	55	1	—	Y					—	—	—	—	—	—	—	—	—	—	—	—
268	131	1	—	M					*170*	—	—	96	—	*17*	—	—	—	—	*26*	—
269	2	2	—	Y					169	—	103	—	—	—	—	—	—	—	—	—
270	19	1	D	O					182	93	113	102	100	17	22	42	33	53	28	24
271	4	1	—	Y					—	—	—	—	—	—	—	—	—	—	—	—
272	78	1	—	Y					—	—	—	*100*	—	*17*	—	—	*34*	52	*26*	*21*
273	28	1	—	Y					—	—	—	—	—	—	—	—	—	—	—	—
274	36	2	D	Y					175	89	105	94	94	*16*	21	*41*	*34*	51	24	*22*

[a]Deformation in the Ledders cranial series is effectively absent, and crania were not scored individually. Hence, the Ledders data file does not discriminate between *lack of deformation* (0) and *unscorable due to incompleteness of cranium* (—).

											Measurement										
Case	MN	BNB	BA	RL	LM	GL	ZZ	CYL	IML	XML	WMH	LCD	BCD	ASB	FRS	FRF	PAC	PAS	OCC	MDB	MLN
Klunk Late Woodland (cont.):																					
247	10	55	87	29	99	124	46	18	32	53	24	23	12	102	19	50	104	20	*98*	31	44
248	*8*	50	99	29	104	137	43	16	26	45	21	28	13	108	25	41	103	19	100	32	41
249	9	52	96	34	121	130	45	18	*31*	*51*	22	24	14	104	23	52	112	23	96	31	37
250	12	54	96	36	106	128	48	18	32	51	24	24	15	104	22	42	103	21	96	28	45
251	10	67	104	32	99	124	46	18	32	50	23	23	16	108	20	47	110	23	100	30	51
252	5	60	100	35	96	120	42	20	32	50	22	*25*	*14*	102	22	48	105	26	88	32	40
253	10	62	87	31	102	126	42	20	35	53	21	23	14	102	25	44	108	26	90	29	40
254	9	52	102	36	106	113	48	18	33	52	23	25	15	110	22	45	106	24	105	32	48
Ledders Late Woodland:																					
255	6	54	97	30	104	126	45	16	31	49	21	23	14	106	28	49	105	22	98	29	43
256	9	64	102	30	102	124	48	20	34	52	25	*25*	15	*104*	18	46	107	24	*98*	35	49
257	12	*59*	86	33	106	119	46	19	26	46	25	*24*	14	*104*	*22*	*48*	105	20	*98*	24	38
258	*8*	62	95	29	100	132	43	16	26	46	21	22	13	97	*24*	*48*	106	22	95	25	46
259	9	53	86	33	*104*	127	46	20	33	54	22	*24*	14	*104*	*22*	*48*	*109*	*24*	*98*	30	36
260	11	52	90	34	100	125	44	16	29	50	20	24	16	104	22	45	101	21	102	33	43
261	11	60	91	34	106	115	43	*18*	27	46	22	24	12	100	*23*	*48*	109	20	94	28	37
262	12	53	95	30	107	135	45	19	32	50	23	24	13	*104*	21	53	113	25	100	26	39
263	9	62	91	33	101	120	42	18	*32*	51	24	26	12	*104*	24	51	96	*19*	*98*	36	47
264	*9*	*66*	*98*	36	—	*120*	*45*	*21*	28	47	24	*25*	—	108	*22*	—	112	24	—	*34*	*44*
265	12	53	93	28	109	133	44	17	28	48	20	24	15	104	21	48	105	26	94	33	36
266	*9*	—	*100*	33	*105*	*123*	50	—	30	49	24	27	14	*104*	—	—	—	*23*	—	33	44
267	—	—	*96*	28	—	128	—	19	26	50	25	*25*	—	—	—	—	—	*22*	—	30	44
268	—	60	*94*	34	—	122	*45*	20	—	—	24	26	13	110	—	—	103	22	—	27	37
269	—	—	*96*	29	—	134	—	—	28	48	21	*25*	—	101	18	44	103	22	99	30	43
270	11	57	*97*	*32*	*107*	*121*	*47*	*20*	33	56	20	25	14	106	22	43	115	25	105	35	50
271	—	—	*96*	39	110	115	46	20	—	—	—	*25*	15	109	—	—	—	—	—	29	50
272	11	58	98	34	107	126	46	21	—	—	26	26	13	—	—	—	—	—	—	31	40
273	—	—	101	33	110	123	—	—	—	—	—	*25*	—	—	—	—	—	—	—	—	—
274	11	60	100	30	102	129	46	*18*	29	44	18	28	14	100	21	44	94	15	107	30	37

References Cited

Acsádi, Gy., and J. Nemeskéri
1970 *History of human life span and mortality.* Akadémiai Kiadó, Budapest.

Anderson, T. W.
1958 *An introduction to multivariate statistical analysis.* John Wiley, New York.

Asch, D. L.
1976 The Middle Woodland population of the lower Illinois Valley: a study in paleodemographic methods. *Northwestern Univ. Archeol. Program, Sci. Pap.* 2.

Asch, D. L., and N. B. Asch
1978 The economic potential of *Iva annua* and its prehistoric importance in the lower Illinois Valley. *In* The nature and status of ethnobotany, R. I. Ford (ed.), pp. 300–341. *Univ. Mich. Mus. Anthropol., Anthropol. Pap.* 67.

Asch, N. B., and D. L. Asch
1980 The Dickson Camp and Pond sites: Middle Woodland archaeobotany in Illinois. *In* Dickson Camp and Pond: two Early Havana tradition sites in the central Illinois Valley, A. Cantwell, Appendix B. *Ill. State Mus., Rep. Invest.* 36.

Asch, D. L., K. B. Farnsworth, and N. B. Asch
1979 Woodland subsistence and settlement in west central Illinois. In *Hopewell archaeology: the Chillicothe Conference,* D. S. Brose and N. Greber (eds.). Kent State University Press, Kent, Ohio.

Baer, M. J.
1956 Dimensional changes in the human head and face in the third decade of life. *Am. J. Phys. Anthropol.* 14:557–575.

Baer, M. J., and J. E. Harris
1969 A commentary on the growth of the human brain and skull. *Am. J. Phys. Anthropol.* 30:39–44.

Bareis, C. J.
1976 The Knoebel site, St. Clair County, Illinois. *Ill. Archaeol. Surv. Circ. 1.*

Barnard, M. M.
1935 The secular variation of skull characters in four series of Egyptian skulls. *Ann. Eugenics* 6:352–371.

Barnett, H. C.
1955 The Coast Salish of British Columbia. *University of Oregon Monographs, Studies in Anthropology* 4.

Bass, W. M.
1971 Human osteology: a laboratory and field manual of the human skeleton. Missouri Archaeological Society, Columbia.
Basu, A., K. K. Namboodiri, L. R. Weitkamp, W. H. Brown, W. S. Pollitzer, and M. A. Spivey
1976 Morphology, serology, dermatoglyphics, and microevolution of some village populations in Haiti, West Indies. *Human Biol.* 48:245–269.
Bennett, K. A.
1969 The typological versus the evolutionary approach in skeletal population studies. *Am. J. Phys. Anthropol.* 30:407–414.
1973 The Indians of Point of Pines, Arizona: a comparative study of their physical characteristics. *Univ. of Ariz., Anthropol. Pap.* 23.
Berry, A. C., and R. J. Berry
1967 Epigenetic variation in the human cranium. *J. Anat.* 11:361–379.
Berry, R. J.
1968 The biology of non-metrical variation in mice and men. In *The skeletal biology of earlier human populations*, D. R. Brothwell (ed.), pp. 103–133. Pergamon Press, Oxford.
Biddle, N.
1814 *History of the expedition under the command of Captains Lewis and Clark to the sources of the Missouri* (2 vol.). Philadelphia.
Binford, L. R.
1964 A consideration of archaeological research design. *Am. Antiq.* 29:425–441.
Björk, A., and L. Björk
1964 Artificial deformation and cranio-facial asymmetry in ancient Peruvians. *J. Dent. Res.* 43:353–362.
Blackith, R. E., and R. A. Reyment
1971 *Multivariate morphometrics.* Academic Press, New York.
Blackwood, B., and P. M. Danby
1955 A study of artificial cranial deformation in New Britain. *J. Roy. Anthropol. Inst.* 85:173–191.
Blakely, R. L.
1973 Biological variation among and between two prehistoric Indian populations at Dickson Mounds. Unpublished Ph.D. dissertation, Indiana University.
1977 Sociocultural implications of demographic data from Etowah, Georgia. *In* Biocultural adaptation in prehistoric America, R. L. Blakely (ed.), pp. 45–66. *Southern Anthropol. Soc. Proc.* 11.
Blalock, H. M., Jr.
1972 *Social statistics* (2nd ed.). McGraw-Hill, New York.
Boas, F.
1891 Second general report on the Indians of British Columbia. *Rep. British Assoc. Advancement Sci.* 60:562–715.
Bodmer, W. F., and L. L. Cavalli-Sforza
1976 *Genetics, evolution, and man.* W. H. Freeman, San Francisco.
Bronowski, J., and W. M. Long
1951 Statistical methods in anthropology. *Nature* 168:794–795.
1952 Statistics of discrimination in anthropology. *Am. J. Phys. Anthropol.* 10:385–394.
Brooks, S. T.
1955 Skeletal age at death: the reliability of cranial and pubic age indicators. *Am. J. Phys. Anthropol.* 13:567–597.

Brothwell, D. R.

1965 *Digging up bones: the excavation, treatment, and study of human skeletal remains.* Trustees of the British Museum of Natural History, London.

1975 Possible evidence of a cultural practice affecting head growth in some Late Pleistocene East Asian and Australasian populations. *J. Archaeol. Sci.* 2:75–77.

Brown, J. A.

1971 The dimensions of status in the burials at Spiro. *In* Approaches to the social dimensions of mortuary practices, J. A. Brown (ed.), pp. 92–112. *Mem. Soc. Am. Archaeol.* 25.

1977 Current directions in midwestern archaeology. *Annu. Rev. Anthropol.* 6:161–179.

Brown, J. A., and S. Struever

1973 The organization of archaeological research: an Illinois example. In *Research and theory in current archaeology,* C. L. Redman (ed.), pp. 261–280. John Wiley, New York.

Brown, W. A. B.

1973 Forty-five Northern Irish families: a cephalometric radiographic study. *Am. J. Phys. Anthropol.* 39:57–86.

Büchi, E. C.

1950 Änderungen der Körperform beim erwachsenen Menschen; eine Untersuchung nach der Individual Methode. *Anthropologische Forschungen, Anthropologischen Gesellschaft in Wien* 1:1–44.

Buikstra, J. E.

1971 Ledders site excavation. *Ill. Assoc. Advance. of Archaeol., Newsl.* 3:4.

1974 Cultural dimensions of archaeological study: a regional perspective. Paper presented at annual meeting of the Society for American Archaeology, Washington.

1975 Cultural and biological variability: a comparison of models. Paper presented at annual meeting of the American Association of Physical Anthropologists, Denver.

1976 Hopewell in the lower Illinois Valley: a regional study of human biological variability and prehistoric mortuary behavior. *Northwestern Univ. Archeol. Program, Sci. Pap.* 2.

1977 Biocultural dimensions of archaeological study: a regional perspective. *In* Biocultural adaptation in prehistoric America, R. L. Blakely (ed.), pp. 67–84. *Southern Anthropol. Soc. Proc.* 11.

Buikstra, J. E., and L. Goldstein

1973 The Perrins Ledge crematory. *Ill. State Mus., Rep Invest.* 28, and *Ill. Valley Archaeol. Program, Res. Pap.* 8.

Butel-Dumont, G. M.

1753 *Mémoires historiques sur la Louisiane.* (2 vol.). Paris.

Caldwell, J. R.

1959 The Mississippian period. *In* Illinois archaeology, pp. 33–39. *Ill. Archaeol. Surv., Bull.* 1.

1964 Interaction spheres in prehistory. *In* Hopewellian studies, J. R. Caldwell and R. L. Hall (eds.), pp. 133–143. *Ill. State Mus., Sci. Pap.* 12.

1967 New discoveries at Dickson Mounds. *Ill. State Mus., Living Mus.* 29:139–142.

Carlsson, G. E., B. Bergman, and B. Hedegård

1967 Changes in contour of the maxillary alveolar process under immediate dentures. A longitudinal clinical and x-ray cephalometric study covering 5 years. *Acta Odontologica Scandinavica* 25:45–75.

Carlsson, G. E., and G. Persson
1967 Morphologic changes of the mandible after extraction and wearing of dentures. A longitudinal, clinical, and x-ray cephalometric study covering 5 years. *Odontologisk Revy* 18:27–54.

Chai, C. K.
1972 Biological distances between indigenous populations of Taiwan. In *The assessment of population affinities in man*, J. S. Weiner and J. Huizinga (eds.), pp. 182–221. Clarendon Press, Oxford.

Chmurny, W. W.
1973 The ecology of the Middle Mississippian occupation of the American Bottom. Unpublished Ph.D. dissertation, University of Illinois.

Clark, P. J.
1956 The heritability of certain anthropometric characters as ascertained from measurements of twins. *Am. J. Human Genetics* 8:49–54.

Cole, F., et al.
1951 *Kincaid: a prehistoric Illinois metropolis.* University of Chicago Press, Chicago.

Cook, D. C.
1972 Human growth rate as a measure of subsistence base changes in Middle and Late Woodland Indians. Paper presented at annual meeting of the Canadian Archaeological Association, St. Johns.
1974 Mortuary practice: an assessment of sources of error in paleodemography. Paper presented at annual meeting of the American Association of Physical Anthropologists, Amherst.
1975a Developmental disturbances: a measure of adaptive efficiency. Paper presented at annual meeting of the American Association of Physical Anthropologists, Denver.
1975b Pathologic states and disease process in Illinois Woodland populations: an epidemiological approach. Unpublished Ph.D. dissertation, University of Chicago.
1976 Human growth: a perspective on subsistence base change. Paper presented at annual meeting of the Society for American Archaeology, St. Louis.

Cook, D. C., and J. E. Buikstra
1973 Circular caries: postnatal correlates of prenatal stress. Unpublished manuscript based on paper presented at annual meeting of the American Association of Physical Anthropologists, Dallas.

Cook, T. G.
1976 Multidimensional models of bio-social change. Paper presented at annual meeting of the Society for American Archaeology, St. Louis.

Cooley, W. W., and P. R. Lohnes
1971 *Multivariate data analysis.* John Wiley, New York.

Corruccini, R. S.
1972 The biological relationships of some prehistoric and historic Pueblo populations. *Am. J. Phys. Anthropol.* 37:373–388.
1974 An examination of the meaning of cranial discrete traits for human skeletal biological studies. *Am. J. Phys. Anthropol.* 40:425–446.
1975 Multivariate analysis in biological anthropology: some considerations. *J. Human Evol.* 4:1–19.

Cybulski, J. S.
1975 Skeletal variability in British Columbia coastal populations: a descriptive and comparative assessment of cranial morphology. *Nat. Mus. Can., Nat. Mus. Man, Mercury Ser., Archaeol. Survy Can., Pap.* 30.

Dahlberg, G.
1926 *Twin births and twins from a hereditary point of view.* Tidens Tryckeri, Stockholm.

De Jong, G. F.
1972 Patterns of human fertility and mortality. In *The structure of human populations,* G. A. Harrison and A. J. Boyce (eds.), pp. 32–56. Clarendon Press, Oxford.

Deniker, J.
1900 *The races of man.* Charles Scribner, New York.

DeRousseau, C. J.
1973 Mortuary site survey and paleodemography in the lower Illinois River Valley. Paper presented at annual meeting of the American Anthropological Association, New Orleans.

Deuel, T.
1958 American Indian ways of life. *Ill. State Mus., Story of Ill. Ser.* 9.

Dingwall, E. J.
1931 *Artificial cranial deformation: a contribution to the study of ethnic mutilations.* John Bale, Sons, and Danielsson, London.

Dixon, R. B.
1923 *The racial history of man.* Charles Scribner, New York.

Dorsey, G. A.
1897 Wormian bones in artificially deformed Kwakiutl crania. *Am. Anthropol.* 10:169–173.

Dragoo, D. W.
1976 Some aspects of eastern North American prehistory: a review 1975. *Am. Antiq.* 41:3–27.

Eickstedt, E. von
1934 *Rassenkunde und rassengeschichte der menschheit.* Gustav Fischer Verlag, Stuttgart.

El-Najjar, M. Y.
1978 Southwestern physical anthropology: do the cultural and biological parameters correspond? *Am. J. Phys. Anthropol.* 48:151–157.

Eveleth, P. B., and J. M. Tanner
1976 *Worldwide variation in human growth.* International Biological Programme 8. Cambridge University Press, Cambridge.

Ewing, J. F.
1950 Hyperbrachycephaly as influenced by cultural conditioning. *Pap. Peabody Mus. Am. Archaeol. Ethnol.* 23(2).

Falkenburger, F.
1938 Recherches anthropologiques sur la déformation artificielle du crâne. *J. Société Américanistes Paris* 30:1–69.

Farnsworth, K. B.
1973 An archaeological survey of the Macoupin Valley. *Ill. State Mus., Rep. Invest.* 26, *Ill. Valley Archaeol. Program, Res. Pap.* 7.

Fisher, R. A.
1936 The use of multiple measurements in taxonomic problems. *Ann. Eugenics* 7:179–188.

Flower, W. H.
1881 *Fashion in deformity, as illustrated in the customs of barbarous and civilised races.* MacMillan, London.

Ford, R.
1974 Northeastern archaeology: past and future directions. *Ann. Rev. Anthropol.* 3:385–413.

Fowler, M. L. (ed)
1973 Explorations into Cahokia archaeology. *Ill. Archaeol. Surv. Bull.* 7.

1974 Cahokia: ancient capital of the Midwest. *Addison-Wesley Module in Anthropology* 48.

Fowler, M. L., and R. L. Hall

1972 Archaeological phases at Cahokia. *Ill. State Mus., Res. Ser. Pap. Anthropol.* 1.

Friedlaender, J. S.

1975 *Patterns of human variation. The demography, genetics, and phenetics of Bougainville islanders.* Harvard University Press, Cambridge.

Genovés, S. T.

1959 *Diferencias sexuales en el hueso coxal.* Instituto de Historia, Mexico City.

Gilbert, B. M., and T. W. McKern

1973 A method for aging the female os pubis. *Am. J. Phys. Anthropol.* 38:31–38.

Giles, E., and H. K. Bleibtreu

1961 Cranial evidence in archaeological reconstructions: a trial of multivariate techniques for the southwest. *Am. Anthropol.* 63:48–61.

Gill, G. W.

1977 Manifestations of a conceptual artistic ideal within a prehistoric culture. *Am. Antiq.* 42:101–110.

Goodman, M. M.

1974 Genetic distances: measuring dissimilarity among populations. *Yearbook of Phys. Anthropol.* 1973, 17:1–38.

Goldstein, L. G.

1976 Spatial structure and social organization: regional manifestations of Mississippian society. Unpublished Ph.D. dissertation, Northwestern University.

1980 Mississippian mortuary practices: A case study of two cemeteries in the lower Illinois Valley. *Northwestern Univ. Archeol. Program, Sci. Pap.* 4.

Goldstein, M. S.

1936 Changes in dimensions and form of the face and head with age. *Am. J. Phys. Anthropol.* 22:37–89.

Gosse, L. A.

1885 Essai sur les déformations artificielles du crâne. *Annales Hygiène Publique Médecine Légale,* 2 Sér., 3:317–393, 4:5–83.

Gower, J. C.

1971 Statistical methods of comparing different multivariate analyses of the same data. In *Mathematics in the archaeological and historical sciences,* F. R. Hodson, D. G. Kendall, and P. Tautu (eds.), pp. 138–149. Edinburgh University Press, Edinburgh.

Gravier, J.

1859 *Relation ou Journal du Voyage . . . en 1700.* New York.

Griffin, J. B.

1964 The northeast woodlands area. In *Prehistoric man in the New World,* J. D. Jennings and E. Norbeck (eds.), pp. 223–258. University of Chicago Press, Chicago.

1967 Eastern North American archaeology: a summary. *Science* 156:175–191.

Griffin, J. B., R. E. Flanders, and P. F. Titterington

1970 The burial complexes of the Knight and Norton Mounds in Illinois and Michigan. *Univ. Mich., Mus. Anthropol., Mem.* 2.

Gustafson, G.

1950 Age determinations on teeth. *J. Am. Dent. Assoc.* 41:45–54.

Hall, R. L.

1975 Chronology and phases at Cahokia. *In* Perspectives in Cahokia archaeology, pp. 15–31. *Ill. Archaeol. Surv., Bull.* 10.

Harn, A. D.

1971a An archaeological survey of the American Bottoms in Madison and St. Clair Counties, Illinois. *In* Archaeological surveys of the American Bottoms and adjacent bluffs, Illinois, pp. 19–39. *Ill. State Mus., Rep. Invest.* 21.

1971b The prehistory of Dickson Mounds: a preliminary report. *Ill. State Mus., Dickson Mounds Mus. Anthropol. Stud.* 1.

1975 Cahokia and the Mississippian emergence in the Spoon River area of Illinois. *Trans. Ill. State Acad. Sci.* 68:414–434.

Hellman, M.

1927 Changes in the human face brought about by development. *Internat. J. Orthodontics* 13:475–516.

Hiernaux, J.

1963 Heredity and environment: their influence on human morphology. A comparison of two independent lines of study. *Am. J. Phys. Anthropol.* 21:575–589.

1966 Human biological diversity in central Africa. *Man* 1:287–306.

1972 The analysis of multivariate biological distances between human populations: principles, and applications to sub-saharan Africa. In *The assessment of population affinities in man*, J. S. Weiner and J. Huizinga (eds.), pp. 96–114. Clarendon Press, Oxford.

Hooton, E. A.

1930 *The Indians of Pecos Pueblo: a study of their skeletal remains.* Yale University Press, New Haven.

1946 *Up from the ape.* Macmillan, New York.

Hooton, E. A., and C. W. Dupertuis

1951 Age changes and selective survival in Irish males. *Am. Assoc. Phys. Anthropol. Stud. Phys. Anthropol.* 2. Wenner-Gren Foundation, New York.

Horowitz, S. L., R. H. Osborne, and F. V. DeGeorge

1960 A cephalometric study of craniofacial variation in adult twins. *Angle Orthod.* 30:1–5.

Houart, G. L.

1971 Koster: a stratified Archaic site in the Illinois Valley. *Ill. State Mus., Rep. Invest.* 28, and *Ill. Valley Archaeol. Program, Res. Pap.* 4.

1975 Stylistic identification of social groups in the Illinois Valley Middle Woodland period. Paper presented at annual meeting of the American Association of Physical Anthropologists, Denver.

Howell, N.

1973 The feasibility of demographic studies in "anthropological" populations. In *Methods and theories of anthropological genetics*, M. H. Crawford and P. L. Workman (eds.), pp. 249–262. University of New Mexico Press, Albuquerque.

Howells, W. W.

1953 Correlations of brothers in factor scores. *Am. J. Phys. Anthropol.* 11:121–140.

1966a Craniometry and multivariate analysis: the Jomon population of Japan. A study by discriminant analysis of Japanese and Ainu crania. *Pap. Peabody Mus. Am. Archaeol. Ethnol.* 57:1–43.

1966b Variability in family lines vs. population variability. *Ann. N.Y. Acad. Sci.* 134:624–631.

1969a Criteria for selection of osteometric dimensions. *Am. J. Phys. Anthropol.* 30:451–458.

1969b The use of multivariate techniques in the study of skeletal populations. *Am. J. Phys. Anthropol.* 31:311–314.

1972 Analysis of patterns of variation in crania of recent man. In *The functional and evolutionary biology of primates*, R. Tuttle (ed.), pp. 123–151. Aldine-Atherton, Chicago.

1973 Cranial variation in man: a study by multivariate analysis of patterns of difference among recent human populations. *Pap. Peabody Mus. Am. Archaeol. Ethnol.* 67.

Howells, W. W., and H. K. Bleibtreu

1970 Hutterite age differences in body measurements. *Pap. Peabody Mus. Am. Archaeol. Ethnol.* 57 (2).

Hrdlička, A.

1908 Physiological and medical observations among the Indians of the south-western United States and northern Mexico. *Bur. Am. Ethnol., Bull.* 34.

1910 Report on skeletal material from Missouri Mounds, collected in 1906–7 by Mr. Gerald Fowke. *Bur. Am. Ethnol., Bull.* 37.

1922 The anthropology of Florida. *Publ. Florida State Hist. Soc.* 1.

1931 Catalogue of human crania in the United States National Museum collections. *U.S. Nat. Mus., Proc.* 78:1–95.

1936 Growth during adult life. *Proc. Am. Philos. Soc.* 76:847–897.

1939 *Practical anthropometry.* Wistar Institute of Anatomy and Biology, Philadelphia.

Hughes, D. R.

1968 Skeletal plasticity and its relevance in the study of earlier populations. In *The skeletal biology of earlier human populations*, D. R. Brothwell (ed.), pp. 31–55. Pergamon Press, Oxford.

Imbelloni, J.

1938 Formas, esencia y metódica de las deformaciones cefálicas intencionales. *Universidad Tucumán, Revista Instituto Antropología* 1:1–37.

1950 Cephalic deformations of the Indians in Argentina. *In* Handbook of South American Indians, Vol. 6, J. Steward (ed.), pp. 53–55. *Bur. Am. Ethnol., Bull.* 143.

Israel, H.

1968 Continuing growth in the human cranial skeleton. *Archives Oral Biol.* 13:133–138.

1971 The impact of aging upon the adult craniofacial skeleton. Unpublished Ph.D. dissertation, University of Alabama, Birmingham.

1973a Age factor and the pattern of change in craniofacial structures. *Am. J. Phys. Anthropol.* 39:111–128.

1973b The failure of aging or loss of teeth to drastically alter mandibular angle morphology. *J. Dent. Res.* 52:83–90.

1977 The dichotomous pattern of craniofacial expansion during aging. *Am. J. Phys. Anthropol.* 47:47–52.

Jantz, R. L.

1973 Microevolutionary change in Arikara crania: a multivariate analysis. *Am. J. Phys. Anthropol.* 38:15–26.

Jennings, J. D.

1968 *Prehistory of North America.* McGraw-Hill, New York.

Johnston, F. E.

1961 Sequence of epiphyseal union in a prehistoric Kentucky population from Indian Knoll. *Human Biol.* 33:66–81.

1962 Growth of the long bones of infants and young children at Indian Knoll. *Am. J. Phys. Anthropol.* 20:249–254.

Kaplan, B. A.

1954 Environment and human plasticity. *Am. Anthropol.* 56:780–800.

Kim, J., and F. J. Kohout
1975 Multiple regression analysis: subprogram REGRESSION. In *SPSS statistical package for the social sciences* (2nd ed.), by N. H. Nie, C. H. Hull, J. G. Jenkins, K. Steinbrenner, and D. H. Bent, pp. 320–367. McGraw-Hill, New York.

Klecka, W. R.
1975 Discriminant analysis. In *SPSS statistical package for the social sciences* (2nd ed.), by N. H. Nie, C. H. Hull, J. G. Jenkins, K. Steinbrenner, and D. H. Bent, pp. 434–467. McGraw-Hill, New York.

Kohler, G.
1901 *Künstliche deformation des schädels.* Erlangen.

Kowalski, C. J.
1972 A commentary on the use of multivariate statistical methods in anthropometric research. *Am. J. Phys. Anthropol.* 36:119–132.

Krogman, W. M.
1962 *The human skeleton in forensic medicine.* Charles C. Thomas, Springfield.

Lane, R. A., and A. J. Sublett
1972 Osteology of social organization: residence pattern. *Am. Antiq.* 37:186–201.

Larson, L. H., Jr.
1971 Archaeological implications of social stratification at the Etowah site, Georgia. *In* Approaches to the social dimensions of mortuary practices, J. A. Brown (ed), pp. 58–67. *Mem. Soc. Am. Archaeol.* 25.

Lasker, G. W.
1953 The age factor in bodily measurements of adult male and female Mexicans. *Human Biol.* 25:50–63.

Laughlin, W. S., and J. B. Jørgensen
1956 Isolate variation in Greenlandic Eskimo crania. *Acta Genet.* 6:3–12.

Lawson, J. A.
1709 *A New Voyage to Carolina.* London.

Lewis, M., and W. Clark
1814 *Travels to the Source of the Missouri River. . . .* London.

Lewis, T. M. N., and M. Kneberg
1946 *Hiwasee Island: an archeological account of four Tennessee Indian peoples.* University of Tennessee Press, Knoxville.

Long, J. K.
1966 A test of multiple-discriminant analysis as a means of determining evolutionary changes and intergroup relationships in physical anthropology. *Am. Anthropol.* 68:444–464.

Lunier, L.
1869 Déformations artificielles du crâne. *Nouv. Dict. Méd. Chir.* 10:182–192.

MacKay, R. H.
1961 *Skeletal maturation* (chart). Eastman Kodak, Rochester, New York.

Mackey, J.
1977 A multivariate, osteological approach to Towa culture history. *Am. J. Phys. Anthropol.* 46:477–482.

McGibbon, W.
1912 Artificially deformed skulls with special reference to the temporal bone and its tympanic portion. *Laryngoscope* 22:1165–1184.

McGregor, J. C.
1958 *The Pool and Irving villages: a study of Hopewell occupation in the Illinois River Valley.* University of Illinois Press, Urbana.

McHenry, H., and E. Giles
1971 Morphological variation and heritability in three Melanesian populations: a multivariate approach. *Am. J. Phys. Anthropol.* 35:241–253.

McKern, T. W., and T. D. Stewart
1957 Skeletal age changes in young American males, analyzed from the standpoint of identification. *Headquarters Quartermaster Research and Development Command, Natick, Mass., Technical Report* EP-45.

McNeill, R. W., and G. N. Newton
1965 Cranial base morphology in association with intentional cranial vault deformation. *Am. J. Phys. Anthropol.* 23:241–254.

Magitot, E.
1884 Essai sur les mutilations ethniques. *Comptes-Rendus Congrès Internat. Anthropol. Archéol. Préhist., 9 Sess., Lisbonne,* 549–622.

Mahalanobis, P. C.
1936 On the generalized distance in statistics. *Proc. Nat. Inst. Sci. India* 2:49–55.

Martin, R.
1928 *Lehrbuch der anthropologie in systematischer darstellung.* (2nd ed.) Gustav Fischer, Jena.

Maxwell, M. S.
1947 A summary of Illinois archeology. *Wis. Archeol.* 28:19–31.

Mayr, E.
1959 Darwin and the evolutionary theory in biology. In *Evolution and anthropology: a centennial appraisal,* pp. 1–10. Anthropological Society of Washington, Washington.
1963 *Animal species and evolution.* Harvard University Press, Cambridge.
1969 *Principles of systematic zoology.* McGraw-Hill, New York.
1970 *Populations, species, and evolution.* Harvard University Press, Belknap Press, Cambridge.

Michaelson, T.
1925 The autobiography of a Fox Indian woman. *Bur. Am. Ethnol., Annu. Rep. (1918–1919)* 40:291–349.

Miles, A. E.
1963 The dentition in the assessment of individual age in skeletal material. In *Dental anthropology,* D. R. Brothwell (ed.), pp. 191–209. Pergamon Press, Oxford.

Moore, J. A., A. C. Swedlund, and G. J. Armelagos
1975 The use of life tables in paleodemography. *In* Population studies in archaeology and biological anthropology: a Symposium, A. C. Swedlund (ed.), pp. 57–70. *Mem. Soc. Am. Archaeol.* 30.

Morant, G. M.
1936 A biometric study of the human mandible. *Biometrica* 28:84–122.

Morrison, D. G.
1974 Discriminant analysis. In *Handbook of marketing research,* R. Ferber (ed.) pp. 442–457. McGraw-Hill, New York.

Morton, S. G.
1839 *Crania Americana.* Dobson, Philadelphia.

Moss, M. L.
1958 The pathogenesis of artificial cranial deformation. *Am. J. Phys. Anthropol.* 16:269–286.

Moss, M. L., and R. W. Young
1960 A functional approach to craniology. *Am. J. Phys. Anthropol.* 18:281–292.

Munizaga, J. R.
1976 Intentional cranial deformation in the preColumbian populations of Ecuador. *Am. J. Phys. Anthropol.* 45:687–694.
Munson, P. J.
1971a An archaeological survey of the Wood River terrace and adjacent bottoms and bluffs in Madison County, Illinois. *In* Archaeological surveys of the American Bottoms and adjacent bluffs, Illinois, pp. 1–17. *Ill. State Mus., Rep. Invest.* 21.
1971b Subsistence ecology of Scovill, a terminal Middle Woodland village. *Am. Antiq.* 36:410–431.
Munson, P. J., and J. P. Anderson
1973 A preliminary report on Kane Village: a Late Woodland site in Madison County, Illinois. *In* Late Woodland site archaeology in Illinois I: investigations in south-central Illinois, pp. 34–48. *Ill. Archaeol. Surv., Bull.* 9.
Nakata, M., P. Yu, and W. E. Nance
1974 Multivariate analysis of craniofacial measurements in twin and family data. *Am. J. Phys. Anthropol.* 41:423–430.
Neumann, G. K.
n.d. Laboratory manual of bioanthropology. Unpublished manuscript on file at Department of Anthropology, Indiana University.
1942 Types of artificial cranial deformation in the eastern United States. *Am. Antiq.* 7:306–310.
1952 Archaeology and race in the American Indian. In *Archaeology of the eastern United States*, J. B. Griffin (ed.), pp. 13–34. University of Chicago Press, Chicago.
Newman, H. H., F. N. Freeman, and K. J. Holzinger
1937 *Twins: a study of heredity and environment.* University of Chicago Press, Chicago.
Newman, M. T.
1947 Indian skeletal material from the central coast of Peru. *Pap. Peabody Mus. Archaeol. Ethnol.* 27 (4).
1975 Nutritional adaptation in man. In *Physiological anthropology*, Albert Damon (ed.), pp. 210–259. Oxford Univ. Press, New York.
Newman, M. T., and C. Snow
1942 Preliminary report on the skeletal material from Pickwick Basin, Alabama. *Bur. Am. Ethnol. Bull.* 129.
Nicolucci, G.
1890 Anomalie e deformazioni artificiali del cranio. *Anomalo (L'): Gazzettino Anthropologico, Psichiatrico, Medico-Legale* 2:65–72.
Nie, N. H., C. H. Hull, J. G. Jenkins, K. Steinbrenner, and D. H. Bent
1975 *SPSS statistical package for the social sciences* (2nd ed.). McGraw-Hill, New York.
O'Brien, P. J.
1972 A formal analysis of Cahokia ceramics from the Powell Tract. *Ill. Archaeol. Surv., Mono.* 3.
1973 Some ceramic periods and their implications at Cahokia. *In* Explorations into Cahokia archaeology, M. L. Fowler (ed.), pp. 100–120, *Ill. Archaeol. Surv., Bull.* 7.
O'Connell, B. H.
1975 Fluctuating asymmetry as a measure of developmental stability in Illinois Woodland populations. Paper presented at annual meeting of the American Association of Physical Anthropologists, Denver.
1976 Adaptive efficiency in the lower Illinois Valley: fluctuating asymmetry as a measure of developmental homeostasis. Paper presented at annual meeting of the Society for American Archaeology, St. Louis.

Ortner, D. J., and R. S. Corruccini
1976 The skeletal biology of the Virginia Indians. *Am. J. Phys. Anthropol.* 45:717–722.

Osborne, R. H., and F. V. DeGeorge
1959 *Genetic basis of morphological variation. An evaluation and application of the twin study method.* Harvard University Press, Cambridge.

Otteking, B.
1930 Craniology of the North Pacific Coast. The Jesup North Pacific Expedition. *Mem. Am. Mus. Nat. Hist.* 15:1–391.

Oxnard, C.
1973 *Form and pattern in human evolution.* University of Chicago Press, Chicago.

Peebles, C. S.
1971 Moundville and surrounding sites: some structural considerations of mortuary practices II. *In* Approaches to the social dimensions of mortuary practices, (J. A. Brown (ed.), pp. 68–91. *Mem. Soc. Am. Archaeol.* 25.

Pérez-Martínez, C.
1960 Cranial deformations among the Guanes Indians of Columbia. *Am. J. Orthodontics* 46:539–543.

Perino, G. H.
n.d. The Yokem site Late Woodland mounds, Pike County, Illinois. Unpublished manuscript.
1968 The Pete Klunk mound group, Calhoun County, Illinois: the Archaic and Hopewell occupations. *In*: Hopewell and Woodland site archaeology in Illinois, pp. 9–124. *Ill. Archaeol. Surv., Bull.* 6.
1971a The Mississippian component at the Schild site, Greene County, Illinois. *In* Mississippian site archaeology in Illinois I, pp. 1–141. *Ill. Archaeol. Surv., Bull.* 8.
1971b The Yokem site, Pike County, Illinois. *In* Mississippian site archaeology in Illinois I, pp. 149–186. *Ill. Archaeol. Surv., Bull.* 8.
1973a The Koster mounds, Greene County, Illinois. *In* Late Woodland site archaeology in Illinois I: investigations in south-central Illinois, pp. 141–210. *Ill. Archaeol. Surv., Bull.* 9.
1973b The Late Woodland component at the Pete Klunk site, Calhoun County, Illinois. *In* Late Woodland site archaeology in Illinois I: investigations in south-central Illinois, pp. 58–89. *Ill. Archaeol. Surv., Bull.* 9.
1973c The Late Woodland component at the Schild sites, Greene County, Illinois. *In* Late Woodland site archaeology in Illinois I: investigations in south-central Illinois, pp. 90–140. *Ill. Archaeol. Surv., Bull.* 9.

Phenice, T. W.
1969 A newly developed visual method of sexing the os pubis. *Am. J. Phys. Anthropol.* 30:297–302.

Pollitzer, W. S.
1958 The Negroes of Charleston (S.C.): a study of hemoglobin types, serology, and morphology. *Am. J. Phys. Anthropol.* 16:241–263.

Pollitzer, W. S., D. Rucknagel, R. Tashian, D. Shreffler, W. Leyshon, K. Namboodiri, and R. C. Elston
1970 The Seminole Indians of Florida: morphology and serology. *Am. J. Phys. Anthropol.* 32:65–82.

Porter, J. W.
1973 The Mitchell site and prehistoric exchange systems at Cahokia: A.D. 1000 ± 300. *In* Explorations into Cahokia archaeology, M. L. Fowler (ed.), pp. 137–164. *Ill. Archaeol. Surv., Bull.* 7.

Rao, C. R.
1948 The utilization of multiple measurements in problems of biological classification. *J. Royal Stat. Soc. B* 10:159–203.
1952 *Advanced statistical methods in biometric research*. John Wiley, New York.
Redfield, A.
1970 A new aid to aging immature skeletons: development of the occipital bone. *Am. J. Phys. Anthropol.* 33:207–220.
Reed, E. K.
1949 The significance of skull deformation in the southwest. *El Palacio* 56:106–119.
1963 Occipital deformation in the northern southwest. *Regional Research Abstract* 310. Santa Fe.
Rightmire, G. P.
1970a Bushman, Hottentot and South African Negro crania studied by distance and discrimination. *Am. J. Phys. Anthropol.* 33:169–195.
1970b Iron age skulls from southern Africa re-assessed by multiple discriminant analysis. *Am. J. Phys. Anthropol.* 33:147–167.
1972 Cranial measurements and discrete traits compared in distance studies of African Negro skulls. *Human Biol.* 44:263–276.
Romero, J.
1970 Dental mutilation, trephination, and cranial deformation. In *Handbook of Middle American Indians, Vol. 9*. T. D. Stewart (ed.), pp. 50–67. University of Texas Press, Austin.
Sanghvi, L. D.
1953 Comparison of genetical and morphological methods for a study of biological differences. *Am. J. Phys. Anthropol.* 11:385–404.
Schour, I., and M. Massler
1941 The development of the human dentition. *J. Am. Dent. Assoc.* 28:1153–1160.
Schultz, A.
1930 The skeleton of the trunk and limbs of higher primates. *Human Biol.* 2:303–438.
Scott, J. H.
1955 Craniofacial regions. *Dent. Practitioner*, 5:208–214.
Sears, W. H.
1964 The southeastern United States. In *Prehistoric man in the New World*, J. D. Jennings and E. Norbeck (eds.), pp. 259–287. University of Chicago Press, Chicago.
Service, E. R.
1962 *Primitive social organization: an evolutionary perspective*. Random House, New York.
Shapiro, H. L.
1928 A correction for artificial deformation of skulls. *Am. Mus. Nat. Hist., Anthropol. Pap.* 30:1–38.
Shryock, H. S., J. S. Siegel, and Associates
1973 *The methods and materials of demography*. U. S. Bureau of the Census, Washington.
Smail, J. K.
1964 The use of female crania in demonstrating racial relationships as exemplified in two upper Mississippi Amerind groups. *Proc. Indiana Acad. Sci.* 74:72–80.
Sokal, R., and P. H. A. Sneath
1963 *Principles of numerical taxonomy*. W. H. Freeman, San Francisco.
Spielman, R. S.
1973 Differences among Yanomama Indian villages: do the patterns of allele fre-

quencies, anthropometrics and map locations correspond? *Am. J. Phys. Anthropol.* 39:461–480.

Spielman, R. S., F. J. da Rocha, L. R. Weitkamp, R. H. Ward, J. V. Neel, and N. A. Chagnon

1972 The genetic structure of a tribal population, the Yanomama Indians. VII. Anthropometric differences among Yanomama villages. *Am. J. Phys. Anthropol.* 37:345–356.

Steward, J.

1955 *Theory of culture change: the methodology of multilinear evolution.* University of Illinois Press, Urbana.

Stewart, T. D.

1939a A new type of artificial cranial deformation from Florida. *J. Washington Acad. Sci.* 29:460–465.

1939b Two new types of cranial deformity in the Southeast: a) fronto-parieto-occipital; b) obelionic. Abstracts No. 5 and 6. *Am. J. Phys. Anthropol.* 25:10.

1940 New evidence on the physical type of the bearers of the Hopewellian culture. Abstract No. 22. *Am. J. Phys. Anthropol.* 27:15.

1943 Skeletal remains with cultural associations from the Chicama, Moche, and Virú valleys, Perú. *U.S. Nat. Mus., Proc.* 93:153–185.

1950 Deformity, trephining, and mutilation in South American Indian skeletal remains. *In* Handbook of South American Indians, Vol. 6. J. Steward (ed.), pp. 43–48. *Bur. Am. Ethnol., Bull.* 143.

1973 *The people of America.* Charles Schribner, New York.

Stini, W. A.

1974 Adaptive strategies of human populations under nutritional stress. In *Biosocial interrelations in population adaptation,* F. E. Johnston, E. Watts, and G. Lasker (eds.) pp. 19–41. Mouton, The Hague.

1975 *Ecology and human adaptation.* Wm. C. Brown, Dubuque.

Struever, S.

1964 The Hopewell interaction sphere in Riverine-western Great Lakes culture history. *In* Hopewellian studies, J. R. Caldwell and R. L. Hall (eds.), pp. 85–106. *Ill. State Mus., Sci. Pap.* 12.

1965 Middle Woodland culture history in the Great Lakes-Riverine area. *Am. Antiq.* 31:211–223.

1968 Woodland subsistence-settlement systems in the lower Illinois Valley. In *New perspectives in archaeology,* S. R. Binford and L. R. Binford (eds.) pp. 285–312. Aldine, Chicago.

1971 Comments on archaeological data requirements and research strategy. *Am. Antiq.* 36:9–19.

Struever, S., and G. L. Houart

1972 An analysis of the Hopewell interaction sphere. *In* Social exchange and interaction, E. N. Wilmsen (ed.), pp. 47–79. *Univ. Mich. Mus. Anthropol., Anthropol. Pap.* 46.

Susanne, C.

1977 Heritability of anthropological characters. *Human biol.* 49:573–580.

Swanton, J. R.

1911 Indian tribes of the lower Mississippi Valley and adjacent coast of Mexico. *Bur. Am. Ethnol., Bull.* 43.

1946 The Indians of the southeastern United States. *Bur. Am. Ethnol., Bull.* 137.

Szpunar, C., and J. Lambert
1977 Analysis of human bone from Woodland sites. Paper presented at annual meeting of the American Anthropological Association, Houston.

Tainter, J. A.
1975 The archaeological study of social change: Woodland systems in west-central Illinois. Unpublished Ph.D. dissertation, Northwestern University.

Tallgren, A.
1974 Neurocranial morphology and ageing. A longitudinal roentgen cephalometric study of adult Finnish women. *Am. J. Phys. Anthropol.* 41:285–294.

Tanner, J. M.
1977 Human growth and constitution. In *Human biology: an introduction to human evolution, variation, growth, and ecology* (2nd ed.) by G. A. Harrison, J. S. Weiner, J. M. Tanner, and N. A. Barnicot, pp. 299–385. Oxford University Press, Oxford.

Tatsuoka, M. M.
1971 *Multivariate analysis: techniques for educational and psychological research.* John Wiley, New York.

Thoma, K., and H. Goldman
1960 *Oral pathology.* C. V. Mosby, St. Louis.

Thomas, D. H.
1976 *Figuring anthropology: first principles of probability and statistics.* Holt, Rinehart, and Winston, New York.

Todd, T. W.
1920 Age changes in the pubic bone. I: the male white pubis. *Am. J. Phys. Anthropol.* 3:285–334.
1921 Age changes in the pubic bone. III: The pubis of the white female. *Am. J. Phys. Anthropol.* 4:1–70.

Todd, T. W., and D. W. Lyon, Jr.
1924 Endocranial suture closure. I: adult males of white stock. *Am. J. Phys. Anthropol.* 7:325–384.

Topinard, P.
1879 Des déformations ethniques du crane. *Revu d'Anthropologie,* 2e Sér., 2:496–506.

Van de Geer, J. P.
1971 *Introduction to multivariate analysis for the social sciences.* W. H. Freeman, San Francisco.

Vandenberg, S. G.
1962 How "stable" are heritability estimates? A comparison of heritability estimates from six anthropometric studies. *Am. J. Phys. Anthropol.* 20:331–338.

Vandenberg, S. G., and H. H. Strandskov
1964 A comparison of identical and fraternal twins on some anthropometric measures. *Human Biol.* 36:45–52.

Vogel, J. O.
1975 Trends in Cahokia ceramics: preliminary study of the collections from Tracts 15A and 15B. *In* Perspectives in Cahokia archaeology, pp. 32–125. *Ill. Archaeol. Surv., Bull.* 10.

Ward, R. H.
1972 The genetic structure of a tribal population, the Yanomama Indians. V. Comparison of a series of genetic networks. *Ann. Human Genetics* 36:21–43.

Washburn, S. L.
1948 Sex differences in the pubic bone. *Am. J. Phys. Anthropol.* 6:199–208.

1949 Determination of sex of skeletons. *Anatomical Record* 103:516–545.

Watson, P. J., S. A. LeBlanc, and C. L. Redman

1971 *Explanation in archaeology: an explicitly scientific approach.* Columbia University Press, New York.

Webb, W. S., and C. E. Snow

1945 The Adena people. *Univ. Ky., Rep. Anthropol. Archaeol.* 6.

Weiner, J. S.

1977 Human ecology. In *Human biology: an introduction to human evolution, variation, growth, and ecology* (2nd ed.), by G. A. Harrison, J. S. Weiner, J. M. Tanner, and N. A. Barnicot, pp. 387–483. Oxford Univ. Press, Oxford.

Weiss, K. M.

1973 Demographic models for anthropology. *Mem. Soc. Am. Archaeol.* 27.

1975 Demographic disturbance and the use of life tables in anthropology. *In* Population studies in archaeology and biological anthropology: a symposium, A. C. Swedlund (ed.), pp. 46–56. *Mem. Soc. Am. Archaeol.* 30.

Whatley, B. L., and N. B. Asch

1975 Woodland subsistence: implications for demographic and nutritional studies. Paper presented at annual meeting of the American Association of Physical Anthropologists, Denver.

Wilkinson, R. G.

1971 Prehistoric biological relationships in the Great Lakes region. *Univ. Mich. Mus. Anthropol., Anthropol. Pap.* 43.

Willey, G. R.

1966 *An introduction to American archaeology: North and Middle America.* Prentice-Hall, Englewood Cliffs.

Wolánski, N., and J. Charzewska

1967 Similarity of some anthropological characteristics of parents and their offspring in different phases of ontogenetic development. *Acta Genet.* 17:365–381.

Wolf, D. J.

1976 A population model for the analysis of osteological materials. Unpublished Ph.D. dissertation, University of Arizona.

Wray, D. E.

1952 Archaeology of the Illinois Valley: 1950. In *Archaeology of the eastern United States,* J. Griffin (ed.), pp. 152–164. University of Chicago Press, Chicago.

Wray, D. E., and R. S. MacNeish

1961 The Hopewellian and Weaver occupations of the Weaver site, Fulton County, Illinois. *Ill. State Mus. Sci. Pap.* 7 (2).

Zawacki, A. A. and G. Hausfater

1969 Early vegetation of the lower Illinois Valley. *Ill. State Mus., Rep. Invest.* 17, and *Ill. Valley Archaeol. Program, Res. Pap.* 1.

Subject Index

A

Age changes in adult crania
  cross-sectional studies of, 117–119, 121, 130
  effects on biological distance, estimates of, 7, 135–138, 200–201, 203
    Late Woodland series, 148, 150–153, 156–158, 160, 166, 198
    Late Woodland and Mississippian series, 169–171, 173–174, 180–185, 192–194, 199
  effects on cranial measurements of, *see* Cranial measurements, effects of age on
  longitudinal studies of, 120–122
  nature of in study series, 122–137
Age determination of skeletons, 45–47, 118
Age structures of study series, 47–48, 50–53, 137–138
  and age effects, 148, 153, 157–158, 169, 171, 184, 193, 201, 203
Agriculture, *see* Cultivation
American Bottoms, archeological survey of, 111, 114
Angel site, 22
Annular deformation, 93–94, 112
Anthropometric traits, heritability of, 65–66, *see also* Cranial measurements, heritability of
Anthropometrics, 57–60, *see also* Cranial measurements
Apple Creek site, 12–13
Archaic components
  Klunk site, 36, 38
  Koster site, 34
Archeological methods, effects on demographic structure of skeletal series, 48–49
Artifacts, nonceramic
  Late Woodland, 11–12, 14, 17, 19
  Middle Woodland, 11
  Mississippian, 24
Artificial cranial deformation, 81
  and age effects, 131
  eastern United States, 90–91, 93, 97
  effects on biological distance estimates of, 7, 110–116, 200
    Late Woodland series, 149–151, 155–156, 161, 164–166, 198
    Late Woodland and Mississippian series, 169, 172–173, 179, 183–184, 189–194
  effects on cranial measurements of, 112–116, 200, 202
  effects on growth curves of, 131, 169
  ethnographic accounts of, 90, 92, 94–96
  incidence of in study series, 97, 99–101, 108, 109, 200
  Mexico, 90, 93, 97
  Northwest Coast, 90, 93–95, 97, 112
  procedures for scoring, 98–99, 200, 203
  reasons for, 94–97
  and selection of cases, 88, 111–112
  and selection of measurements, 110, 112–113

severity of in study series, 97–98, 101, 114, 200
sex differences in, 95–97, 101, 108–110, 131, 200
South America, 93–94, 96–97
Southeast, 91–93, 95
Southwest, 90–92, 97, 112
unintentional, 90–92
varieties of, 90–94
Artificial cranial deforming devices, 90, 94–98, 100–101, 111
Asymmetry of cranial nonmetric traits, 4, 16
Aymara deformation, *see* Annular deformation
Aztalan, 27, 205

B

Basu *et al.* biodistance study, 59
Bifrontal deformation, *see* Artificial cranial deformation
Bifrontal-occipital deformation, 92, 97, 101
Biological distance
and geographical separation of groups, 6, 57–58, 60, 64, 149–150, 152–155, 159–160, 162–165, 176, 177, 184–185, 198
among Late Woodland and Mississippian series
alternative models for, 6, 171, 172, 175–179, 184–187, 190, 193–195, 198–199
based on face measurements, 171–187
based on other measurement subsets, 187–191
univariate results, 167–171, 192–193
among Late Woodland series
alternative models for, 5, 149, 153–155, 158–161, 164, 197–198
based on face measurements, 149–161
based on other measurement subsets, 161–164
compared to Middle Woodland, 139, 154, 160, 164–165
univariate results, 139–148, 164
and temporal separation of series, 149, 153–154, 159, 162–163, 176, 186, 190, 199
Biological distance estimates
effects of age-related variation on, *see* Age changes in adult crania, effects on biological distance estimates of
effects of artificial cranial deformation on, *see* Artificial cranial deformation, effects on biological distance estimates of
Biological distance results, sex differences in, 164–166, 183, 185, 188, 192–194, 198, 199
Biological distance studies
of living populations, 56–60
of skeletal series, 27, 60–64, 165
Blakely biological distance study, 30–31, 64, 113
Blood polymorphisms, 56–57, 59–60, 62
Bluff, 38, 41, 43
Early, *see also* Late Woodland
ceramics, 11, 27, 34
dates for, 11
nonceramic artifacts, 11–12, 14
settlement patterns, 14
Late, *see also* Late Woodland
ceramics, 11, 34
dates for, 11
nonceramic artifacts, 12, 14
settlement patterns, 14
subsistence, 13, 14
Buikstra biodistance study, 4–5, 7, 139, 165, 194–195, 202, 206
Burial customs, *see* Mortuary practices

C

Cahokia, 22, 23, 177, 195, 205
ceramic complex, 23, 27–28
house forms, 14, 28
influence of, 22, 29–31, 43
Late Woodland phases at, 10, 11, 27
Mississippian phases at, 27–29
Canteen wares, 10, 19
Carbon-14 dates, *see* Radiocarbon dates
Cases, selection of, 88, 111
Ceramics
Late Woodland, 5, 10–11, 17, 19, 27–28, 34
Middle Woodland, 4, 10
Mississippian, 20, 23–24, 27, 29, 36
Chai biodistance study, 59
Chinook cranial deformation, *see* Parallelo-fronto-occipital deformation
Circular cranial deformation, *see* Annular deformation
Coefficient of divergence, 61–62
Congruence of results from different data sets, 6–8, 57–58, 164, 188–192, 194, 197, 201–202
Corruccini biodistance study, 63

Cowitchin deformation, *see* Fronto-verticoöccipital deformation
Cradleboard deformity, *see* Occipital deformation
Cradleboards, 90–92, 94–96, 98, 100, 111
Cranial base measurements
difference among Late Woodland and Mississippian groups in, 168, 170, *see also* Biological distance
differences among Late Woodland groups in, 141–142, 147, 148, *see also* Biological distance
Cranial measurement subsets
congruence of results from alternative, *see* Congruence of results from different data sets
proportion of missing data in, 149
selection and definition of, 87
Cranial measurements
correlations among, 74, 76, 86, 136–146
definition of, 67–69
effects of age on, 118–121
controlling for dental loss, 131–137
in study series, 122–130
effects of artificial cranial deformation on, 112–116, 200, 202
heritability of, 8, 56, 59, 65–67, 86
means and standard deviations of, 141–142
procedures for taking, 67, 71–72
selection of, 67, 80, 86–87, 110, 112–113, 137
use in skeletal studies, 27, 30–31, 60–64, 203
use in studies of the living, 56–60
Cranial nonmetric traits
asymmetry of, 4, 16
hereditary basis of, 8
use of for biological distance estimates, 4, 7, 27, 60–64, 165, 194–195, 202, 206
Cranial size differences among study series, 147, 148, 155, 164–165, 168–170, 192–193, 205
Cranial vault measurements, *see also* Biological distance
differences among Late Woodland and Mississippian series in, 168–169
differences among Late Woodland series in, 141–142, 147
Craniometrics, *see* Cranial measurements
Cremation, 16–18
Cultivation, 13, 20–21, 26, 28
maize, 13–14, 20–21, 28
native North American species, 12–13

D

Deformation, cranial, *see* Artificial cranial deformation
Demographic structure of study series, 47–54, 137–138
Dental loss
correlation with age, 132
effects on cranial morphology of, 118–121, 128–129, 131–136, 192, 194, 201
sex differences in, 132–133, 192
Dermatoglyphics, 58–59
Developmental disturbances, 4
Dickson cranial series,
age structure of, 53
artificial cranial deformation in, 97, 108, 110, 113
biological distance among, 30–31
Dickson site, 29, 205
Discrete traits, *see* Cranial nonmetric discrete traits
Discriminant analysis, 61, 63–64, 74–76
advantages and disadvantages of, 76–78
assumptions of statistical model, 77
classification procedure, 76, 80
results of for Late Woodland and Mississippian series, 174–175, 182–183
results of for Late Woodland series, 152, 154–155, 158, 166
Discriminant analysis results, *see* Biological distance
Discriminant function coefficients
derivation of, 75, 78
as measures of discriminatory power, 79, 138, 150–152, 156–157, 160, 173–174, 180–183, 201
Discriminant function, general form of, 75
Disease patterns, 4, 205

E

Early Bluff, *see* Bluff, Early
East St. Louis site, 23
Ecology
differences between groups in, 6, 130, 139, 155, 179
of west-central Illinois, 12
Environmental stress, biological effects of, 4, 15–16, 50, 66, 205
Etowah site, 22, 53

F

Face measurements
differences among Late Woodland and

Mississippian series, 167–171, *see also* Biological distance
differences among Late Woodland series, 140–142, 147, *see also* Biological distance
variability of, 149
Fairmount phase, Cahokia, 27, 28
Fort Ancient, 26
Fox Creek, 10
Friedlaender biodistance study, 58
Frontal deformation, *see* Artificial cranial deformation
Fronto-occipital deformation, *see* Fronto-verticoöccipital deformation
Fronto-parieto-occipital deformation, 93
Fronto-verticoöccipital deformation, 92–93, 97–98, 101

G

Gene flow, 6, 60, 63–64, 154
Genetic distance, 56, 58–59
Gibson series, 53
Gower's R^2 statistic, 59
Growth curves, 205
Growth of cranium
effects of artificial cranial deformation on, 131, 169
in adulthood, *see* Age changes in adult crania
Growth patterns of subadults, 130

H

Havana wares, 10
Helton site, 17
Heritability of cranial measurements, 8, 56, 59, 65–67, 86
Hiwasee Island site, 27
Homer Adams site, 19, 53
Hopewell, *see* Middle Woodland
House forms
Late Woodland, 14–15, 28, 29
Mississippian, 28, 29
Howells biodistance studies, 61
Hunting and gathering, 12–14, 21
Hypothesis of nonspecificity, *see* Nonspecificity hypothesis

I

Irving site, 10
Ischio-pubic index, 44
distribution of in Schild Mississippian series, 45

J

Jantz biodistance study, 63
Jersey Bluff, *see* Bluff
Joe Gay site, 17, 53

K

Kane Village site, 15
Kincaid site, 205
Klunk (Ben) site, 36
Klunk (Pete) site
excavation of, 36
location of, 3, 33, 36–37
radiocarbon dates for, 34, 36
Knight mound group, 10
Knoebel site, 29
Koskimo deformation, *see* Annular deformation
Koster habitation site, 13, 34
Koster mortuary site
excavation of, 33–34
location of, 3, 33–35
radiocarbon dates for, 34

L

Lambdoid deformation, 91–92, 97, 101, *see also*, Artificial cranial deformation
Lambdoid flattening, natural, 92, 98, 101, 111
Late Bluff, *see* Bluff, Late
Late Woodland
biological distances, *see* Biological distance, among Late Woodland series
ceramics, 5, 10–11, 17, 19, 27–28, 34, 206
dates for, 9
environmental stress in, 15–16
house forms, 14–15, 28, 29
mortuary practices, 16–19
nonceramic artifacts, 11–12, 14, 17, 19
phases of, 10–11, 27
population density, 15
residence patterns, 165, 198
settlement patterns, 5, 13–15
subsistence, 4, 5, 12–15, 26
trade, 5, 12
Late-Woodland–Mississippian biological distances, *see* Biological distance, among Late Woodland and Mississippian series
Late-Woodland–Mississippian relationships,
archeological evidence, 25–26, 28–31, 40, 43
biological evidence, *see* Biological distance, among Late Woodland and Mississippian series

Laughlin and Jørgensen biodistance study, 60–61
Ledders site
excavation of, 38
location of, 3, 33, 38–39
radiocarbon dates for, 34, 38

M

Macon Plateau site, 27
Macoupin Valley, archeological survey of, 14
Mahalanobis D^2 estimates, 62, 64, 110
associations with cranial deformation scores, 114–116, 200, 203
derivation of, 74, 79
among Late Woodland and Mississippian series, 175–179, 183–186, 187–191
among Late Woodland series, 152–155, 158–165
Maize, cultivation of, 13–14, 20–21, 28
Mandible measurements
differences among Late Woodland and Mississippian groups in, 168, 170, *see also* Biological distance
differences among Late Woodland groups in, 141–142, 147, 161–164, *see also* Biological distance
effects of age on, 125, 127–129, *see also* Cranial measurements, effects of age on
controlling for dental loss, 132, 135–136
variability of, 149
Marriage patterns, 5, 56, 112, 165, 185, 187, 194, 198–199
Measurement error, intraobserver, *see* Replicability
Measurements, cranial, *see* Cranial measurements
Measuring points, definition of, 67, 69–71
Mesoamerica, influence of, 20, 25–26, 28, 90
Middle Woodland, 5, 6, 9–10, 36, 38, 53
artificial cranial deformation in, 92, 100–101, 155
ceramics, 4, 10
environmental stress in, 15–16
mortuary practices, 16–19
nonceramic artifacts, 11
population density, 15
settlement patterns, 14
skeletal material, 161, 166
subsistence, 4, 12–13
trade, 12, 15
Middle Woodland groups, biological distance among, 139, 149–150, 154, 160, 164–165, 198
Migration
Mesoamerican, 26
Mississippian, 6, 25–27, 29–31, 167, 171–172, 175–179, 184–187, 190, 193, 195, 198, 199
Migration rates and biological distance, 56, 59, 60
Missing data, 71, 74
and case selection, 88
comparison of methods for estimating, 82–83
estimation of, 80–85
multiple regression procedure for estimation of, 84–85
proportion of in measurement subsets, 149
and variable selection, 86
Mississippian
beginning date, 20
ceramics, 20, 23–24, 27, 29, 36
general characteristics, 20
house forms, 28–29
mesoamerican influences on, 20, 25–26, 28
migration, *see* Migration, Mississippian
mortuary practices, 19–20, 22, 24
nonceramic artifacts, 24
origin of, 20, 25–26
population density, 20, 22, 28
settlement patterns, 20–23
association with biological distance, 167, 179, 187, 194, 199
social structure, 24–25
spread of, 20–21, 25–27, 29–31
subsistence patterns, 6, 20–21, 26, 28
association with biological distance, 167
temple mounds, 20, 22, 40
trade, 12, 20–22, 28
Mitchell site, 23
Moorehead phase, 29
Moss site, 29
Mortality
general human pattern of, 47–48, 54
in Late Woodland, 15, 50–53
in Middle Woodland, 15
in Mississippian, 50–53
Mortuary practices
effects on demography, 48
Late Woodland, 16–19
Middle Woodland, 16–19
Mississippian, 19–20, 22, 24
Moundville site, 22

Multidisciplinary research program, 2, 204

N
Natchez Indians, 21, 95
Nonmetric discrete traits, *see* Cranial nonmetric traits
Nonspecificity hypothesis, 7, 194, 202

O
Obelionic deformation, 91–92
Occipital deformation, 92, 97, *see also* Artificial cranial deformation
Odontometrics, 58–60
Oneota, 26
Orbicular deformation, *see* Annular deformation
Ortner and Corruccini biodistance study, 64

P
Parallelo-fronto-occipital deformation, 93
Pathology, skeletal, 15
Patrick phase, 27–29
Penrose coefficients, 64
Perrins Ledge crematory site, 17
Pike phase, 10
Point of Pines series, 53
Pollitzer *et al.* biodistance studies, 59
Pool site, 10
Population density, 50
  in Late Woodland, 5, 15
  in Middle Woodland, 15
  in Mississippian, 20, 22, 28, 179
Pottery, *see* Ceramics
Process school of archeology, 1
Projectile points, *see* Artifacts, nonceramic
Pulcher site, 23

R
Radiocarbon dates, 30, 31
  Bluff, 11
  Klunk site, 34, 36
  Koster site, 34
  Ledders site, 34, 38
  Schild site, 29, 34, 40
  Yokem site, 29, 34, 41, 43
Raymond pottery, 27
Regional approach, 2, 204
Replicability
  of cranial measurements, 72–74, 76
  of deformation scores, 99
Research problems, 5–6, 139, 197
Residence patterns, Late Woodland, 165, 198
Rightmire biodistance studies, 61–62

S
Sample size, 80, 88
  cranial series, 33–34, 36, 38, 41, 43
  Klunk, 140, 166, 175
  Schild knolls, 177, 179
Sampling error, 161, 166, 194
Sanghvi biodistance study, 57
Schild site
  excavation of, 38, 40
  location of, 3, 33–35, 38, 40
  radiocarbon dates for, 29, 34, 40
Scovill site, 12–13
Secular change, 119, 120
Selective survival, 119, 120
Seneca cemeteries, 165
Sepo Late Woodland, 31
Settlement patterns
  Late Woodland, 5, 13–15
  Middle Woodland, 14
  Mississippian, 20–23
    association with biological distance, 167, 179, 187, 194, 199
Sex determination of skeletons, 44–45
Sex ratios of study series, 53–54
Sexual dimorphism, 44, 45
Size differences, cranial, *see* Cranial size differences
Social structure, Mississippian, 24–25
Spielman *et al.* biodistance studies, 57–58
Spoon River Mississippian, 30
St. Louis, 22, 23
Stirling phase, 27, 29
Subsistence
  Late Woodland, 4, 5, 12–15, 26
  Middle Woodland, 4, 12–13
  Mississippian, 6, 20, 21, 26, 28
Subsistence patterns, Mississippian, association with biological distance, 167
Systems theory, 1

T
Tabular erect deformation, *see* Fronto-verticoöccipital deformation
Tabular oblique deformation, *see* Parallelo-fronto-occipital deformation
Teeth, loss of, *see* Dental loss
Temple mounds, 20, 22, 40
Trade
  Late Woodland, 5, 12
  Middle Woodland, 12, 15
  Mississippian, 12, 20–22, 28
Twin studies, 65–66

U
Unnamed phases, Cahokia, 27–28
Upper Mississippian cultures, 26

V
Variability, within-group,
 contribution of sexual dimorphism, 44
 in Schild series, 178–179, 186–187, 194, 199
Variables, selection of, *see* Cranial measurements, selection of
Vertico-occipital deformation, *see* Occipital deformation

W
Warfare, 15
Weaver focus, 10–12
Weeden Island site, 27
West–central Illinois,
 ecology of, 12
 research program, 2, 204
White Hall, 10–12, 14, 16, 34
Wolf biodistance study, 27, 64
Wood River Terrace, 11

Y
Yokem site
 excavation of, 41
 location of, 3, 33, 39, 41, 42
 radiocarbon dates for, 29, 34, 41, 43